Exercise Immunology

T0174158

Exercise immunology is an important, emerging subdiscipline within exercise physiology, concerned with the relationship between exercise, immune function and infection risk. This book offers a comprehensive, up-to-date and evidence-based introduction to exercise immunology, including the physiological and molecular mechanisms that determine immune function and the implications for health and performance in sport and everyday life.

Written by a team of leading exercise physiologists, the book describes the characteristics of the immune system and how its components are organised to form an immune response. It explains the physiological basis of the relationship between stress, physical activity, immune function and infection risk, and identifies the ways in which exercise and nutrition interact with immune function in athletes and non-athletes. The book shows students how to evaluate the strengths and limitations of the evidence linking physical activity, immune system integrity and health, and explains why exercise is associated with anti-inflammatory effects that are potentially beneficial to long-term health.

Every chapter includes useful features, such as clear summaries, definitions of key terms, discussions of seminal research studies and practical guidelines for athletes on ways to minimise infection risk, with additional learning resources available on a companion website. This is an essential textbook for any course on exercise immunology or advanced exercise physiology.

Visit the companion website for this book at www.routledge.com/cw/gleeson

Michael Gleeson is Professor of Exercise Biochemistry at Loughborough University, UK. Over the past 20 years he has published over 150 papers on exercise physiology, biochemistry and immunology and sports nutrition. He is a member of several sports science societies in the UK and worldwide, as well as being a past president of the International Society of Exercise and Immunology. He is also an elected Fellow of the European College of Sport Science, a past editor of the *Journal of Sports Sciences* and is currently associate editor of *Exercise Immunology Review*.

Nicolette Bishop is Senior Lecturer in Exercise Physiology at Loughborough University, UK where she leads the Performance Health Research Theme within the Peter Harrison Centre for Disability Sport. She is widely published in the area of exercise immunology, is a member of the International Society of Exercise and Immunology, a physiology advisory board member for the *Journal of Sports Sciences* and acts as a consultant for the English Institute of Sport.

Neil Walsh is Professor, and Director of the Extremes Research Group, in the School of Sport, Health and Exercise Science at Bangor University, UK. He is physiology section editor for the *Journal of Sports Sciences*, and a full member of BASES, the Physiology Society, the International Society of Exercise and Immunology and the American College of Sports Medicine.

Exercise Immunology

Edited by Michael Gleeson, Nicolette Bishop
and Neil Walsh

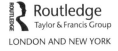
Routledge
Taylor & Francis Group

LONDON AND NEW YORK

First published 2013
by Routledge
2 Park Square, Milton Park, Abingdon, Oxon OX14 4RN

Simultaneously published in the USA and Canada
by Routledge
711 Third Avenue, New York, NY 10017

Routledge is an imprint of the Taylor & Francis Group, an informa business

British Library Cataloguing in Publication Data
A catalogue record for this book is available from the British Library

Library of Congress Cataloging in Publication Data
Exercise immunology / edited by Michael Gleeson, Nicolette Bishop, and Neil Walsh.
page cm
Includes bibliographical references.
1. Exercise–Immunological aspects. I. Gleeson, Michael, 1956– II. Bishop, Nicolette. III. Walsh, Neil.
QP301.E954 2013
612.7'6–dc23
2012050416

ISBN: 978-0-415-50725-7 (hbk)
ISBN: 978-0-415-50726-4 (pbk)
ISBN: 978-0-203-12641-7 (ebk)

Typeset in Garamond
by FiSH Books, London

Contents

Figures

Tables

Technique boxes and group activities

TECHNIQUE BOXES

GROUP ACTIVITIES

Contributors

Stéphane Bermon, MD, PhD
Stéphane Bermon is a sports physician and exercise physiologist at the Monaco Institute of Sports Medicine and Surgery since 2006. He is a member of the Medical and Antidoping Commission of the International Association of Athletics Federations (IAAF). Stéphane is the author and co-author of more than 30 books or peer-reviewed scientific papers. He graduated (MD) from Nice University Medical School and also holds a PhD in Exercise Physiology from the University of Aix-Marseille II. He also holds a Specialised Master's degree (École Centrale de Paris) in Health Engineering. He was team physician for a professional soccer team (four years) and for professional road cycling teams (three years). Dr Bermon was a professional snowboarder in his earlier years. He still practices endurance sports such as the long-distance triathlon.

Nicolette C. Bishop, PhD
Nicolette (Lettie) Bishop is a Senior Lecturer in Exercise Physiology in the School of Sport, Exercise and Health Sciences at Loughborough University. Her research interests lie in the effect that exercise has on immune function and inflammation in healthy individuals and in those with chronic conditions. Her recent research has focused on the effects of acute exercise and training on immune function and respiratory infection incidence in elite and recreational athletes with spinal cord injuries. She has published over 50 papers on exercise immunology and is co-author of the International Society of Exercise and Immunology Position Statement on Immune function and Exercise (Walsh *et al.* 2011a). She is also a member of the Peter Harrison Centre for Disability Sport at Loughborough University, a role that she really enjoys for both the research and the team camaraderie. She leads a module in exercise immunology for Masters students at Loughborough. For the past six years, Lettie has somehow juggled working 'part-time' with looking after her two young boys – how she manages this remains a mystery to her and she knows which one leaves her the most exhausted!

Jos A. Bosch, PhD

Jos Bosch is an associate professor in the Department of Psychology of the University of Amsterdam. He is a biopsychologist with an expertise in health psychology, psychophysiology and psychoneuroimmunology; a field that studies the interactions between psychological, neuroendocrine and immunological processes. His work involves both experimental research and epidemiological studies in healthy and clinical populations. A main focus is on the role of the immune system and immune-regulating neuroendocrine factors, such as glucocorticoids and catecholamines, in depression and anxiety. He has also carried out several studies on the effects of exercise and psychological stress on immune function. In addition to his work in Amsterdam, Jos has adjunct appointments at the University of Houston (Department of Health and Human Performance, TX, USA) and the University of Heidelberg (Mannheim Institute of Public Health and Preventive Medicine, Germany). He is an associate editor of *Health Psychology* and ad-hoc associate editor of *Psychological Bulletin*.

Michael Gleeson, PhD

Michael (Mike) Gleeson is Professor of Exercise Biochemistry in the School of Sport, Exercise and Health Sciences at Loughborough University. He has published over 150 papers on exercise biochemistry, physiology, immunology and nutrition. He is co-author of textbooks on exercise biochemistry, exercise immunology and sport nutrition and has taught these subjects to undergraduate and postgraduate students for the past 20 years. His recent research has focused on the effects of acute exercise, repeated exercise and intensified training on the immune system and the modifying effects of nutritional interventions such as carbohydrate, antioxidants and probiotics. He is also interested in the hormonal responses to stress and overtraining and the factors that make some individuals more susceptible to infection than others. He is on the Editorial Board of several international journals. He is a member of the Physiological Society and is a past president of the International Society of Exercise and Immunology (www.isei.dk). He is also a Fellow of the British Association of Sport and Exercise Sciences and the European College of Sport Science. He has provided advice on minimising risks of infection and nutritional strategies to maintain immune function to numerous sports clubs and organisations and has been involved in immunoendocrine monitoring studies of several professional athlete groups including swimmers, rugby union and football players in recent years. In his spare time, Mike enjoys playing tennis, watching football and drinking beer.

Samuel J. Oliver, PhD

Samuel (Sam) Oliver is a lecturer in human physiology in the School of Sport, Health, and Exercise Science at Bangor University. He gained his PhD in 2007, studying the influence of nutritional deficiencies on human health and performance. Funded by the Ministry of Defence, the findings had implications for soldier training and performance. He is a member of the Extremes Research Group (http://extremes. bangor.ac.uk) and his research focuses on the effect of extreme environments (e.g. altitude, heat, cold, dehydration, nutrient restriction and sleep loss) on human performance and health. Current research themes include understanding the mechanisms responsible for illness and decreased performance at high altitude, which involves both field research expeditions and laboratory studies. A second research theme examines the effects of thermal stress and dehydration on thermal tolerance and performance. In his spare time, Sam enjoys climbing mountains and surfing waves.

Paula Robson-Ansley, PhD

Paula Robson-Ansley is a reader in the Department of Sport and Exercise Sciences at Northumbria University, where she leads the exercise-immunology research group. She has a wide range of research interests, including the impact of exercise on immune function and the role of nutrition in maintenance of immune function in athletes. Paula spent four years as a research fellow in South Africa at the South African Sport Science Institute, Cape Town University and Stellenbosch University. Aside from research, she was fortunate enough to work with elite South African and visiting British athletes as a fatigue-management consultant. During her time in South Africa, Paula also investigated the effect of 80-km races on endurance Arab horse's immune system function as well as red blood cell tyrosine metabolism in rhinos! More recently, she has developed a novel theory to explain the unexplained underperformance syndrome and extends this to individuals with chronic fatigue syndrome. Paula's current research interest is the role of cytokines, namely interleukin-6, in fatigue during exercise, chronic fatigue syndrome and inflammatory disorders, as well as the impact of exercise in allergic thresholds. Paula is a co-director of Sport Asthma, which provides gold-standard testing for exercise-induced asthma and air-borne allergy.

Richard J. Simpson, PhD

Richard (Rickie) Simpson is a lecturer in human physiology in the Department of Health and Human Performance at the University of Houston, USA. His main research interests are concerned with the effects that exercise, age and disease has on immune function. Immune-cell senescence is a state of immunological dysfunction that is acquired with age and exposure to various stressors, leaving the host at an increased risk of infection and development of autoimmune disorders. Progressive erosion of chromosome telomeres owing to excessive rounds of cell division and/or exposure to oxidative stress are the most accepted mechanisms underpinning T-lymphocyte senescence. Senescent T-cells are known to have short telomeres, which, in turn, has been shown to be a reliable predictor of human lifespan and morbidity.

Neil P. Walsh, PhD

Neil Walsh is a professor in the School of Sport, Health and Exercise Science at Bangor University. He graduated in Sports Science from Manchester Metropolitan University in 1994 and studied for his Masters degree in Sports Science at Loughborough University in 1995. He became a Lecturer in Exercise Physiology at Trinity and All Saints College, University of Leeds, in 1995 and completed his PhD in Exercise Immunology and Nutrition at the University of Birmingham in 2000. In the summer of 2000, Neil became a Lecturer in Physiology at Bangor University, where he is currently a professor and Director of the Extremes Research Group. Neil has published many papers and a number of book chapters on topics including the immune response to exercise and markers of hydration status. Much of Neil's recent work has been funded by the Ministry of Defence (UK) and has included studies looking at the effects of infantry training on immune function and infection incidence and the effects of fluid and energy restriction on immune function, hydration status and exercise performance. Neil is currently the Physiology Editor of the *Journal of Sports Sciences* and also contributes as a guest writer for *Runners World*. He has edited the two landmark position statements on exercise immunology (Walsh *et al.* 2011a, 2011b) that were commissioned by the International Society of Exercise and Immunology. In his spare time, Neil is a keen road cyclist.

Preface

Exercise immunology is a subdiscipline of exercise physiology that is concerned with the effects of acute and chronic physical activity on immune function. It is a relatively new area of research. Before 1970, there were only a handful of papers describing the effects of exercise on the numbers of circulating white blood cells. Since the mid-1970s there has been an increasing number of papers published on this subject and in recent years at least 400 new papers have appeared in the scientific literature each year.

Interest in exercise immunology was prompted by mostly anecdotal reports by athletes, coaches and team doctors in the 1970s and 1980s that athletes seemed to suffer from a high incidence of infections (predominantly colds and flu). This was about the time that many sports were changing from amateur to professional status and athletes were increasingly able to devote more time to hard training. A few epidemiological studies in the 1980s and early 1990s appeared to confirm this higher incidence of upper respiratory tract infection during heavy training in endurance athletes and following competitive prolonged exercise events, such as marathon and ultramarathon races. Since then, over a thousand studies have reported that prolonged exercise results in a temporary depression of various immune cell functions. A substantially smaller number of studies indicate that a chronic impairment of immune function can occur during periods of intensified training. Even fewer studies suggest that moderate regular exercise is associated with improved immune function and a reduced incidence of infection compared with a completely sedentary lifestyle. Thus, exercise is not universally bad for the immune system; rather, it is excessive amounts of exercise (possibly in combination with other stressors, e.g. psychological) that result in immune system depression and increased susceptibility to infection. In recent years, studies have focused on the possible mechanisms by which exercise improves or impairs immune function. Intervention studies have investigated the effects of diet and nutritional supplements on immune responses to exercise. Other studies have looked at exercise in environmental extremes (heat, cold, altitude and microgravity) and in particular subpopulations (elderly, obese, HIV and cancer patients).

Exercise immunology is now established as an important field of research in the discipline of exercise physiology and is therefore being introduced as an area of study in sport and exercise science degree programmes in many countries around the world.

At present, this probably takes the form of a few lectures within a module devoted to exercise physiology, physiology of training, health of the athlete or exercise and health. In some universities, however, a full module is devoted to the study of this fascinating subject at undergraduate or master's level. More institutions would probably introduce the subject if a suitable undergraduate text was available. This book is intended to provide such a text. The subject of exercise immunology is still generally ignored in standard exercise physiology texts and only a couple of books aimed more at researchers and postgraduates have been written on the subject and these are now somewhat out of date.

In this book, we examine the evidence for the relationship between exercise load and infection risk. This is followed by a description of the components of the human immune system and how they function to protect the body from invasion by potentially disease-causing micro-organisms. The subject is not covered to the same depth as in a clinical immunology text but this book does cover the essential details of the structure and function of different immune system cells, soluble factors, the immune response to infection and how the immune system is organised and regulated. The main factors that influence immune function including age, sex, stress and diet are also mentioned. Subsequent chapters describe the known effects of acute exercise and heavy training on the numbers of circulating white blood cells, innate (nonspecific) and acquired (specific) immunity, the effect of exercise in environmental extremes on immune function and the impact of nutrition on immunity and immune responses to exercise. Other chapters consider the anti-inflammatory effects of exercise (one of the main reasons why regular exercise can reduce the risk of chronic metabolic and cardiovascular diseases), allergies in athletes and the impact of exercise on immune function in special populations such as the elderly, people who are obese, or have diabetes or HIV. One chapter provides evidence-based guidelines on how athletes can minimise their risk of immunodepression and infection.

This book has been written with the needs of both students and course instructors in mind. The aim of the book is to enable the student to understand and evaluate the relationship between exercise, immune function and infection risk. After reading this book students should be able to:

- appreciate the influence of habitual physical activity on infection risk;
- describe the characteristics of the components of the immune system and explain how these components are organised to form an immune response;
- appreciate the ways in which immune function can be assessed;
- understand the physiological basis of the relationship between stress, physical activity, immune function and infection risk;
- identify the ways in which exercise and nutrition interact with immune function in athletes and non-athletes;
- evaluate the strengths and limitations of the evidence linking physical activity, immune system integrity and health;
- provide guidelines to athletes on ways of minimising infection risk.

To reinforce learning, each chapter begins with a list of learning objectives and ends with a list of key points and suggestions for further reading. Several chapters contain technique boxes that explain the different ways in which immune function can be measured; the emphasis here is on the principles of the tests used and their limitations rather than on the minute detail of the assay methods. There are also text boxes which focus on specific issues of general interest, key concepts, student group activities and biographies of some of the eminent scientists whose research efforts have greatly contributed to the field of exercise immunology. At the end of the book, there is an extensive bibliography listing all the cited references and a glossary provides definitions of all key terms and abbreviations.

The book is designed to provide the basis of a module in exercise immunology that could run over one or two semesters. Each chapter is structured in a logical sequence, as it would be presented in a lecture, and the tables and figures used are ones that we and the other contributors currently use in our lectures. This should reduce the time that course instructors have to spend preparing lectures and tutorials.

The editors and other contributors are all active researchers in exercise and/or stress immunology. They also teach the subject of exercise immunology to undergraduate and masters students and supervise postgraduate research students, so they are well versed in communicating information about this subject, which is being continually updated by new research. All the contributors are members of the International Society of Exercise and Immunology.

This book is primarily written for students of sport science, exercise science and human physiology. It is also relevant to students of medicine, biomedical sciences, physiotherapy and health sciences. The more practical aspects may also be of interest to athletes, coaches and team doctors. We hope that this book inspires instructors as well as students to delve more deeply into the subject of exercise immunology. Most of all, we hope that you enjoy reading our book on this fascinating subject.

Michael Gleeson
Nicolette C. Bishop
Neil P. Walsh

1 The influence of exercise on infection risk

Nicolette C. Bishop

LEARNING OBJECTIVES

After studying this chapter, you should be able to:

- appreciate the different agents that cause common infections;
- appraise the J-shaped model of upper respiratory tract infection risk and exercise volume;
- appreciate the strengths and limitations of the methods used to measure the incidence of infection;
- evaluate the evidence concerning the effect of single bouts of prolonged exercise and intensive endurance training on infection risk;
- appreciate the influence of airway inflammation on symptoms of respiratory infection;
- evaluate the evidence concerning the effect of regular moderate exercise on infection risk compared with a sedentary lifestyle;
- appreciate other factors that influence symptoms of infection.

INTRODUCTION

Acute upper respiratory tract infections (URTI, such as coughs and colds, influenza, sinusitis, tonsillitis, other throat infections and middle ear infections) are among the most common illnesses experienced at all ages. These infections lead to absence from school and work, visits to general practitioners (GPs) and heavy use of 'over the counter' medicines. In the UK, respiratory infections account for approximately 5.5 million GP visits annually and an estimated cost of £170 million (Health Protection Agency, 2005). These infections are also one of the main reported causes of illness in athletes. For example, analysis of the 126 reported illnesses in athletes competing at the World Athletics Championships in Daegu, South Korea, in 2011 revealed that 40% of illnesses affected the upper respiratory tract, with confirmed infection in around 20% of cases (Alonso *et al.* 2012). Other than sickness associated with exercise-induced dehydration (12%), gastroenteritis/diarrhoea was the next most common illness reported (10%).

CAUSES OF INFECTIONS

Pathogens are disease-causing microorganisms and these can include viruses, bacteria, fungi and parasites. The causes of upper respiratory infections can be viral or bacterial and they are most commonly transmitted by airborne droplets or nasal secretions. Pathogens involved as causal agents in respiratory infections can lead to a wide variety of illnesses (Table 1.1) and many are seasonal in their activity, tending to have higher levels during the winter months.

Table 1.1 Examples of common causes of upper respiratory tract infections	
INFECTION	ORGANISM
Common cold/cough	Rhinovirus, coronavirus, adenovirus, influenza A and B, human parainfluenza virus, enterovirus
Middle ear infection (otitis media)	Rhinovirus and other common-cold viruses, *Streptococcus pneumoniae*, *Haemophilus influenza*, *Moraxella catarrhalis*
Sinusitis	Rhinovirus, coronavirus, enterovirus, adenovirus, influenza A and B, *S. pneumoniae*, *H. influenza*, *M. catarrhalis*
Sore Throat	Adenovirus, influenza virus, rhinovirus, Epstein-Barr virus, cytomegalovirus, *S. pyogenes*, *Mycoplasma pneumoniae*

Note. Viral causes are in plain text; bacterial causes are in italics.

A virus is a microscopic organism that cannot replicate or express its genes without a host living cell. Viruses invade living cells and use the nucleic acid material that they contain to replicate themselves. A single virus particle (virion) is in and of itself essentially inert. It lacks the necessary components that cells need to reproduce. When a virus infects a cell, it marshals the cell's enzymes and much of the cellular machinery to replicate; viral replication produces many progeny that, when complete, leave the host cell to infect other cells in the organism.

Viruses may contain double-stranded DNA, double-stranded RNA, single-stranded DNA or single-stranded RNA. The type of genetic material found in a particular virus and the exact nature of what happens after a host is infected varies depending on the nature of the virus. Double-stranded DNA viruses typically must enter the host cell's nucleus before they can replicate. Single-stranded RNA viruses, however, replicate mainly in the host cell's cytoplasm. Once a virus infects its host and the viral progeny components are produced by the host's cellular machinery, the assembly of the viral capsid (the protein coat that envelopes viral genetic material) is usually a non-enzymatic, spontaneous process.

The virus may mutate during the process of its replication; this ability to change slightly in each infected person is the reason why treating viruses can be difficult. Viruses are responsible for several common diseases in humans, not least upper respiratory infections (Table 1.1). For example, there are more than 200 different viruses that can cause the common cold, most of which are rhinoviruses but other viruses such as coronaviruses and adenoviruses can also be responsible.

Bacteria are single-celled microscopic organisms that are larger than viruses and lack nuclei and other organised cell structures. As you can see in Table 1.1, several bacterial species are capable of causing respiratory infections (pathogenic bacteria), yet most are non-infectious and many play critical roles; for example, bacteria in the gut aid digestion. Bacteria come in a variety of shapes (e.g. rod-like, spheres and spirals) and sizes. Bacteria are usually classified as Gram-positive or Gram-negative, based on a basic microbiological staining procedure called the Gram stain, which reveals the presence (Gram-negative) or absence (Gram-positive) of an outer membrane. For example, the streptococcal species of bacteria are rod-like gram positive bacteria and, as outlined in Table 1.1, pathogenic species of streptococci (*Streptococcus pyogenes, S. pneumoniae*) are causes of sore throats, ear infections and sinusitis.

Gastroenteritis/diarrhoea is worthy of mention here, not least because it was the second most common infectious illness reported in athletes attending both the 2009 and 2011 World Championships (Alonso *et al.* 2010, 2012). The major cause of viral gastroenteritis in adults is norovirus (although other viruses such as adenoviruses can also be responsible). Close contact with infected individuals and poor personal hygiene, in particular not washing hands after using the toilet, is the major route of transmission. Bacterial causes (mainly through poor food hygiene practices or competing in polluted water) include bacteria of the *Campylobacter* species, *Escherichia coli* and *Salmonella*. Travellers' diarrhoea is a term used to refer to gastroenteritis that is acquired when travelling abroad and this can affect athletes travelling to competition. Travellers' diarrhoea is usually the result of drinking infected water or eating infected foods. It is caused by a range of different bacteria or, less commonly, parasites such as cryptosporidium and *Giardia intestinalis*. These parasites are microorganisms that live in the gut and derive nutrients from the host, causing symptoms such as abdominal pain, vomiting and diarrhoea.

IS THERE A J-SHAPED RELATIONSHIP BETWEEN EXERCISE TRAINING LOAD AND INFECTION RISK?

The amount of exercise that a person does has an effect on respiratory infection incidence. It has been suggested that the relationship between exercise intensity/volume and susceptibility to URTI is J-shaped (Nieman 1994a, 1994b; Figure 1.1). According to this model, taking part in some regular moderate physical activity decreases the relative risk of infection below that of a sedentary individual. However, performing prolonged, high-intensity exercise or periods of strenuous exercise training is associated with an above average risk of infection. When first proposed, the J-shaped model was based on the findings of a relatively small number of studies and the majority of these explored the relationship between single bouts of endurance exercise and URTI risk in the following one to two weeks. Recent evidence (Matthews *et al.* 2002; Nieman *et al.* 2011a) from several large-scale longitudinal studies provides us with additional evidence to evaluate the validity of the J-shaped relationship.

Figure 1.1 The J-shaped model of the relationship between risk of upper respiratory tract infection (URTI) and exercise volume (Adapted from Nieman, 1994)

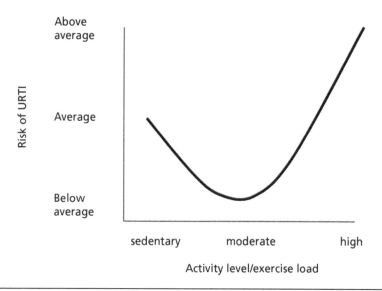

Box 1.1 The amount of exercise a person does can influence their susceptibility to infection

We all suffer from colds at some time but recent research indicates that a person's level of physical activity influences their risk of respiratory tract infections such as a cold, most probably by affecting immune function. Moderate levels of regular exercise seem to reduce our susceptibility to illness compared with an inactive lifestyle but long, hard bouts of exercise and periods of intensified training put athletes at increased risk of colds and flu.

Effects of single bouts of prolonged strenuous exercise on infection incidence

Most studies that have explored the effect of a single (acute) exercise session on subsequent risk of URTI have looked at responses from athletes involved in endurance-type events. That is not to say that athletes involved in resistance or sprint events are not at risk of infections; those training heavily with insufficient recovery periods between sessions appear to be at as much risk of symptoms of URTI as those who perform endurance sports.

A description of the methods commonly used to measure infection risk is detailed in Technique box 1.1. Many of the studies of infection in athletes, particularly the earlier studies, have been survey-based epidemiological studies, with self-reporting of symptoms of URTI, rather than a confirmed clinical diagnosis. As mentioned in Technique box 1.1, these studies have the advantage of allowing large numbers of athletes to be studied. On the other hand, it should be recognised that the self-reporting of URTI by athletes may be influenced by a degree of positive response bias in the data: those who have symptoms of URTI may be more likely to return these questionnaires (a positive response). It could also be argued that highly trained athletes are more self-aware and may report symptoms that less active individuals would not take any notice of.

Technique box 1.1

Measurement of incidence of infection

Studies that have looked at the relationship between both moderate and more intense exercise and infection risk have largely relied on data collected by means of self-report survey. In the majority of these studies, the presence of an infectious pathogen has not been confirmed; rather subjects have completed a questionnaire or a daily logbook in which they noted their symptoms of illness (including URTI) either during the study or retrospectively. For example, in one randomised exercise training study, subjects recorded health problems each day by means of codes including: cold (runny nose, cough, sore throat); allergy (itchy eyes, stuffy nose); headache; fever; nausea/vomiting/diarrhoea; fatigue/tiredness; muscle/joint/bone problem or injury; menstrual cramps; other (describe); or none (Nieman et al. 1990b). An episode of URTI was defined as coding for a cold with or without supporting symptoms of headache, fever, fatigue/tiredness or nausea/vomiting/diarrhoea for 48 hours and separated from a previous episode by at least one week. Jackson et al. (1958) validated a cold symptom questionnaire (see questionnaire below) after administering by nasal instillation a dilute, cell-free, nasal secretion from donors with a common cold to over 1000 human volunteers and recording symptoms in those who became infected.

More recent studies (e.g. Spence et al. 2007; Nieman et al. 2011a) have chosen to administer the Wisconsin Upper Respiratory Symptom Survey (WURSS) or a modified version of this (http://www.fammed.wisc.edu/research/external-funded/wurss), which were developed from the original Jackson score questionnaire. This is a reliable and multi-validated questionnaire that provides data on symptom duration and severity as well as absolute episodes.

The move towards email administration of self-report questionnaires (as used by Fondell et al. (2011)) appears to have a positive effect on response rates and also allows investigators to monitor participants more regularly. In most studies, physical activity patterns are also assessed by questionnaire, such as the International Physical Activity

Questionnaire (IPAQ; http://www.ipaq.ki.se/downloads.htm). These studies have the advantage in that they allow large cohorts to be studied, although the reliability of the data gained from these studies will depend upon the reproducibility and validity of the questionnaires administered and the period of recall; memory recall over long periods of time has obvious potential for error.

Clinical confirmation of infection requires the collection of a throat swab and/or saliva sample for later culture and identification of potential bacterial pathogens. Viral pathogens can be identified from viral nuclear material present in saliva samples. From a practical standpoint, laboratory-based identification of respiratory pathogens is neither practical nor cost effective and results are rarely available before the symptoms are resolved. On the other hand, physician diagnosis, long considered the 'gold standard' method of confirming the presence of true URTI is perhaps not as robust as once thought; large discrepancies between physician and laboratory diagnosed infection were apparent in elite athletes presenting at an Australian Sports Medicine Clinic (Cox *et al.* 2008).

Jackson score upper respiratory tract illness questionnaire

Do you think that you are suffering from a common cold or flu today?

Fill in the circle if your answer is YES ○

If yes please complete all the questions below:

Are any of the following symptoms of the common cold or flu present today? Please indicate your response by filling in one circle for each of the following symptoms:

Symptom	Degree of discomfort			
	None at all	Mild	Moderate	Severe
Sneezing	○	○	○	○
Headache	○	○	○	○
Malaise (feeling generally unwell)	○	○	○	○
Nasal discharge (runny nose)	○	○	○	○
Nasal obstruction (blocked nose)	○	○	○	○
Sore throat	○	○	○	○
Cough	○	○	○	○
Earache	○	○	○	○
Hoarseness	○	○	○	○
Chilliness	○	○	○	○

Note: Participants should complete the questionnaire at the end of each day to document the severity of their ten cold-related symptoms on a four-point scale (0 = no symptom, 1 = mild symptom, 2 = moderate symptom, 3 = severe symptom). The total symptom score is calculated by summing the daily scores for all ten symptoms. Any consecutive two-day total symptom score greater than 14 can be considered as the first criterion to indicate a Jackson-verified cold; these are used in the analysis of number of cold (URTI) episodes. A second criterion is the subjective self-report that the participant had the impression that they were suffering from a cold (the first circle is filled in) on three or more consecutive days.

The findings of two early studies looking at incidence of self-reported URTI following marathon-type events suggest that participating in competitive endurance events is associated with an increased risk of URTI during the 7–14 days following the event (Peters and Bateman 1982; Nieman *et al.* 1990a). In a randomly selected sample of 140 runners in the 1982 Two Oceans Marathon (a distance of 56 km) in Cape Town, 33% of the runners reported symptoms of URTI in the two-week period following the race, compared with 15% of a group of age-matched non-running controls, each of whom lived in the same household as one of the runners (Peters and Bateman 1982). Further examination of the data revealed a significant negative relationship between race time and post-race illness (symptoms of URTI were far more prevalent in those runners who completed the race in less than four hours, suggesting a relationship between acute exercise stress, or previous training load, and susceptibility to URTI). Similar findings were reported from a cohort of over 2000 runners who took part in the 1987 Los Angeles Marathon (Nieman *et al.* 1990a). During the week after the marathon, 12.9% of the runners reported symptoms of URTI compared with only 2.2% in a control group of experienced runners who had entered the race but did not compete for reasons other than illness (Figure 1.2).

Figure 1.2 Percentage of runners reporting episodes of upper respiratory tract infection (URTI) during the week after the 1987 Los Angeles Marathon (Nieman *et al.* 1990). Controls were runners who had entered the race but did not compete for reasons other than illness

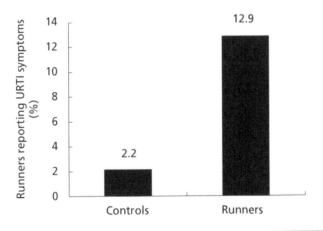

It is important to keep this relationship in perspective; the findings of these studies suggest that the relative risk of an episode of URTI is increased following heavy exercise but the majority of athletes do not experience an episode of URTI after prolonged strenuous activity. For example, in the cohort of over 2000 marathon runners who completed the 1987 Los Angeles marathon, only one in every seven marathon runners reported symptoms of URTI in the week following the event (Nieman *et al.* 1990a). Exercise duration may be an additional critical factor in

---

Box 1.2 Does excessive exercise increase infection risk?

- Studies of single bouts of prolonged endurance exercise (e.g. marathon and ultra-marathon events) have been typically associated with an increase in reported upper respiratory symptoms, which have been assumed to be representative of URTI (e.g. Peters and Bateman 1983; Nieman *et al*. 1990a).
- Intensive endurance training is often associated with an increase in episodes of clinically confirmed URTI or self-reported upper respiratory symptoms. This relationship has also been reported in athletes involved in intermittent sports, including football, rugby and tennis.
- In the absence of clinical confirmation, caution needs to be taken when interpreting reported upper respiratory symptoms as actual infections. In many cases, self-reported symptoms of respiratory illness may reflect airway inflammation or allergic reaction rather than an illness with an identifiable infectious cause.

---

determining post-race susceptibility for respiratory illness because performing 5-km, 10-km and 21.1-km events do not appear to increase the reporting of symptoms of URTI in the week after the race above that reported in the week before (Nieman *et al*. 1989a).

Recurrence of recent infection may also account for a significant proportion of infections reported after endurance events. One-third of runners who reported upper respiratory tract symptoms (URTS) in the three weeks before the 2000 Stockholm Marathon also reported post-race episodes (Ekblom *et al*. 2006). This suggests a recurrence of recent infection, perhaps caused by performing strenuous exercise before recovering fully.

Effects of intensive endurance training on infection incidence

In addition to the higher incidence of respiratory symptoms reported by the runners who completed the 1987 Los Angeles Marathon, 40% of the runners also reported experiencing at least one episode of URTS during the two months prior to the marathon itself (Nieman *et al*. 1990a). After controlling for confounding factors such as age, perceived stress levels and illness in the home, it was found that those who ran more than 96 km (60 miles) per week in training were twice as likely to suffer illness compared with those who trained less than 32 km (20 miles) per week (Figure 1.3).

Although many of the investigations of the relationship between exercise training and URTI incidence (with or without concurrent measures of immune function) have concentrated on runners, there are now several published reports detailing a relationship between heavy volumes of training and competition and URTS in athletes involved in other sports including swimming (Gleeson *et al*. 1999a), football (Bury *et al*. 1998), tennis (Novas *et al*. 2003), American Football (Fahlman and Engels 2005) and rugby union (Cunniffe *et al*. 2011) For example, in elite Australian swimmers, URTI incidence was higher in swimmers than in moderately exercising

Figure 1.3 Training load (running distance per week) and relative risk of upper respiratory tract infection (URTI) in the two months prior to the 1987 Los Angeles Marathon (Nieman *et al.* 1990a); 40% of the runners reported experiencing at least one episode of upper respiratory symptoms during the two months before the marathon; after controlling for confounding factors, it was found that those who ran more than 96 km (60 miles) per week in training were twice as likely to suffer illness compared with those who trained less than 32 km (20 miles) per week

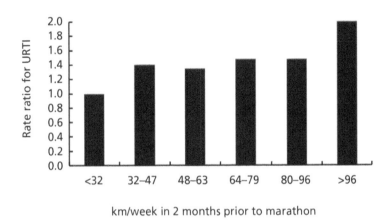

support staff (Gleeson *et al.* 1999a). Furthermore, an 11-month observation of elite Welsh Rugby Union players found peaks in URTI occurred after periods of increased training intensity and reduced game activity (Cunniffe *et al.* 2011). However, a relationship between training volume and occurrence of URTS is not always found. Analysis of the training volume of around 1,500 runners in the six months prior to the 2000 Stockholm Marathon found no relationship with reported URTS either in the three weeks before or in the three weeks after the race (Ekblom *et al.* 2006). Furthermore, clinically confirmed URTI was not related to the weekly combined sailing and training load of elite America's Cup yachtsmen over a 50-week monitoring period (Neville *et al.* 2008).

The need to distinguish between 'elite' and 'highly trained' has been suggested to be an important influencing factor in the relationship between exercise training load and infection risk. It has been argued by some exercise immunologists that much of the literature has focused on the sub-elite athletic population but infection incidence in truly elite athletes is actually lower than in highly-trained athletes, resulting in an S-shaped, rather than J-shaped curve (Malm 2006; Figure 1.4). Although this view has sparked some debate, there is perhaps some logic to the argument that an increased susceptibility for infection is simply incompatible with the training required to perform to the levels achieved by elite athletes. Moreover, the ability to withstand infections during periods of heighted physiological and psychological strain could actually be a prerequisite for elite performance.

Figure 1.4 The proposed S-shaped relationship between physical activity/exercise load and risk of upper respiratory tract infection (URTI) (adapted from Malm 2006); this model proposes that true elite athletes suffer fewer infections than their highly trained counterparts; it is suggested that the ability to withstand infections during periods of heighted physiological and psychological strain could actually be a prerequisite for elite performance

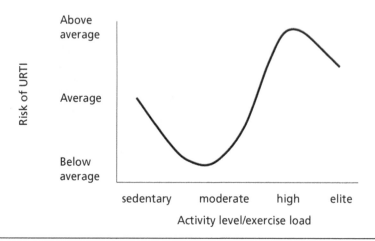

Infection or airway inflammation?

Current guidance to help athletes to avoid illness, particularly of the upper respiratory tract, is focused on minimising transmission of infectious pathogens and maintaining immune competence (Bishop 2012). This seems sensible if we assume that these symptoms all have an infectious cause. However, several reports suggest that a substantial proportion of URTI symptoms experienced by athletes are not caused by identifiable infectious pathogens. A study examining the causes of URTS in both elite and recreational triathletes and sedentary control subjects of similar age over a five-month period found that only 11 of 37 illness episodes had an identifiable infectious cause (Spence *et al.* 2007; Figure 1.5). Rhinovirus was the most commonly identified pathogen, with a small number of bacterial pathogens, including *S. pyogenes*, *Haemophilus influenza* and *Mycoplasma pneumoniae* also responsible. This aside, almost 75% of reported cases of URTS tested negative for detectable infectious agents. This study demonstrates the difficulties that researchers face when attempting to identify true infectious episodes from observation or self-reporting of symptoms alone. Even sports physicians can overestimate the occurrence of actual infections. In an evaluation study of URTS in elite Australian athletes, physicians characterised 89% of cases as viral or bacterial URTI, yet only 57% of cases were actually associated with an identified pathogen or laboratory measure consistent with infection (Cox *et al.* 2008). These findings strongly suggest that not all URTI are in fact associated with the commonly identifiable infectious agents and, for this reason, the term URTI should be used with due caution. Given this uncertainty about the aetiology of URTS in athletes, scientists are encouraged to use the term upper respiratory illness (URI) instead.

Figure 1.5 Breakdown of episodes of upper respiratory illness into those with and without identified pathogenic cause during the five-month monitoring period in sedentary (*n* = 20), recreational athletes (*n* = 30) and elite athletes (*n* = 20); although a J-shaped relationship is apparent when all episodes are considered, the relationship is less clear when only infectious illnesses are considered (adapted from Spence *et al.* 2007); URTI = upper respiratory tract infection

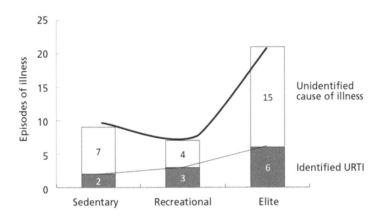

These findings lead us to the question of the cause of the unidentifiable illnesses because, infectious or not, these illnesses still lead to loss of training and competition days. The fact that the causes were unidentified does not necessarily mean that these illnesses were not infectious; there are many reasons why a pathogen may not be identified, including the limitations of current diagnostic techniques and the existence of as yet unknown pathogens. Having said that, there is now a convincing line of thought that airway inflammation may be at least partly responsible for those illnesses without identifiable pathogenic cause. Lung ventilation rates at rest are typically about 5–10 L/minute but during strenuous exercise (such as running at marathon pace) can increase to 100–200 L/minute. This increased ventilatory load with exercise can damage the airways, causing an increase in airway osmolarity and stimulating bronchial epithelial cells to release chemical signals (chemoattractants) to promote the movement of immune cells into the airways (Bermon 2007). The resulting non-infectious inflammation leads to many of the same symptoms as infectious respiratory illnesses.

In addition to exercise hyperventilation, allergy and exposure to environmental factors such as cold dry air, pollutants and chlorine-related products can all trigger an inflammatory response and subsequent URTS. In the evaluation study of URTS in elite Australian athletes discussed previously, laboratory investigation identified allergy in almost 40% of the athletes presenting with URI, yet the sports physicians did not consider allergy as a possible cause of these symptoms for any of the episodes (Cox *et al.* 2008). The prevalence of an allergic (rather than an infectious) cause of symptoms is highlighted in a study that found a strong correlation between the prevalence of allergy and post-race reporting of symptoms of URI in over 200 runners who had taken part in the 2010 London Marathon (Robson-Ansley *et al.* 2012). Furthermore, it is possible that some of the self-reported episodes of apparent URTI following the marathon events in large cities such as Cape Town and Los Angeles were actually related to pollutant-related airway inflammation and/or inflammation caused by sustained high ventilatory loads. With this in mind, strategies to prevent respiratory illness in athletes also need to look beyond avoidance of bacterial or viral pathogen transmission. Clarification of the causes of symptoms of respiratory illness in athletes alongside identification of those athletes who are most vulnerable to these symptoms is necessary to help in identifying the most appropriate treatment and management strategies (Bishop 2012).

Other factors influencing infection risk in athletes

Despite the limitations in the identification of infectious URTS, it is clear that infections of the upper respiratory tract do exist and do appear to be more prevalent in the athletic population. While subsequent chapters will look at the effects of exercise on different aspects of immune function, there are several other factors that can also influence the risk of infection in athletes. As described in Chapters 9 and 10, heightened psychological stress, poor sleep quality and poor dietary practices all impact on immune function and subsequent risk of infection. Furthermore, practices such as sharing drinking bottles, a lack of hand washing, drinking tap water or melted ice cubes when travelling and living in close proximity to others, for example on training camps, can all increase the transmission of infectious pathogens. Practical guidelines on minimising infection risk are discussed in detail in Chapter 10.

Summary of effects of heavy exercise on infection risk

The J-shaped model suggests that participating in acute bouts of intense exercise and involvement in heavy schedules of training and competition increases the relative risk of URTS to above that of a sedentary individual. Research in this area has generally concentrated on survey-based studies of large cohorts of competitive endurance-trained athletes and, while the findings do provide support for a negative relationship between heavy exercise and risk of URTS, it is important to acknowledge the existence of both infectious and non-infectious episodes of upper respiratory illness. A number of other factors may contribute to the higher number of illness episodes experienced by athletes, including impaired immune function, airway inflammation caused by exercise hyperventilation, allergy or environmental pollutants, increased exposure to pathogens, poor nutritional practices and increased psychological stress.

Moderate exercise and risk of URTI

The J-shaped relationship between exercise training load and infection risk suggests that regular participation in moderate recreational physical activity is associated with a lower risk of infection than that of sedentary individuals. Certainly, many fitness enthusiasts would agree wholeheartedly that regular exercise helps to keep illness at bay and there are now some quite convincing epidemiological data to support this notion. There have been two main experimental designs employed by researchers to look at this area: (1) longitudinal intervention studies, where small cohorts of sedentary individuals undertake a short period (typically 6–12 weeks) of prescribed, supervised regular exercise. Illness rates are compared with a control group who either continued with their sedentary lifestyle or who undertook some passive or very low intensity activity; and (2) longitudinal observational studies, where the activity patterns and illness rates are recorded over much longer periods of time, sometimes up to one year. These studies rely on greater recall of activity and illness but do allow considerably larger cohorts to be observed over a longer period of time. However, as highlighted in the above section, issues concerning the classification of true URTI must be taken into consideration.

Box 1.3 Does regular moderate exercise reduce infection risk compared with a sedentary lifestyle?

- It is a widely held belief that doing regular moderate exercise is good for health and may also lower the incidence of URTI.
- A small number of studies show that regular moderate exercise can decrease the incidence of the common cold (Matthews *et al.* 2002; Nieman *et al.* 2011a).
- It is not clear whether this is because regular exercise improves one or more aspects of immune function, although a few studies have reported modest increases in saliva immunoglobulins and natural killer cell activity with moderate exercise training in previously sedentary subjects.
- Regular exercise could also reduce the incidence of common colds by indirect effects in improving psychological mood state, improving sleep quantity and quality, improving nutritional status (by increasing appetite and nutrient intake in undernourished individuals) and encouraging other aspects of a healthy lifestyle (e.g. improved quality of diet, good personal hygiene).
- Summary: regular exercise may be immuno-stimulatory in those with compromised immune function (such as the elderly or people who are obese) and there is some evidence that it can reduce the incidence of respiratory tract infection. However, it remains contentious whether doing regular moderate exercise improves immune function in otherwise healthy individuals.

Interventional studies

One of the earliest interventional studies involved a group of 36 previously sedentary young women who were mildly obese (body mass index of around 28 $kg.m^{-2}$) randomly assigned to either 15 weeks of supervised exercise training (five 45-minute sessions of brisk walking at 60% heart rate reserve each week) or to a control group who did not participate in any exercise outside of normal daily activity (Nieman *et al.* 1990b). Symptoms of illness were recorded daily in a logbook using a coding system, whereby different numbers coded for different symptoms (e.g. 1 for a runny nose, 2 for a cough, and so on). Importantly, all of the women were unaware of the aims of the study in attempt to reduce the over-reporting of symptoms. Over the 15-week study period, the actual number of URTI episodes did not differ between the two groups. However, the women in the exercising group reported significantly fewer days with URTI symptoms compared with the sedentary controls (5.1 ± 1.2 days versus 10.8 ± 2.3 days in the exercising and control groups, respectively), which suggests that the exercising women were able to 'get over' their colds more quickly.

In a similar study, 14 previously sedentary elderly women (aged 67–85 years) completed 12 weeks of supervised brisk walking with another group of 16 of their sedentary peers participating in supervised sessions of callisthenics (light exercise involving muscular strength and flexibility work) over the same period (Nieman *et al.* 1993a). Only three of the walkers experienced an episode of URTI during the study period, compared with eight of the individuals in the callisthenics group. Both groups were also compared with a group of 12 highly conditioned elderly women who were still actively involved in 'masters' level endurance competitions; only one of these women experienced an episode of URTI during the same period.

Both of these studies had relatively small numbers of participants and the exercise programmes lasted three to four months. In a year-long intervention study, 115 postmenopausal women who were overweight or obese were randomly assigned to either an exercise group (45 minutes of moderate exercise on five days per week) or a control group who attended weekly 45-minute stretching sessions (Chubak *et al.* 2006). At the start of the study and at three-month intervals thereafter, the women completed self-administered questionnaires. The women had been educated in how to fill in the questionnaires and they had received instructions on how to discriminate between allergic and infectious illness symptoms. To assess the reproducibility of the questionnaire responses, a subgroup of women filled in the questionnaire again within five weeks of the initial response and it was found that there was a high level of agreement in reporting of URTI episodes. Over 12 months, the risk of self-reported colds (but not all URTI) decreased in exercisers relative to stretchers and, in the final three months of the study, the risk of colds in the stretchers was more than threefold that of the exercisers (Figure 1.6). Interestingly, exercise appeared to particularly reduce the number of cold episodes in participants who did not already take multivitamins.

Observational studies

Interventional observational studies have investigated the relationship between exercise and self-reported URTI episodes in women who were either older, overweight/obese or both. This is important to acknowledge because, as we will see in Chapter 13, there are differences between males and females in both immunity and immune responses to exercise and immune function generally decline with age. One study that focused on the association between activity levels and URTI in younger adults (aged 20–23 years) failed to find any relationship (Schouten *et al.* 1988). The

Figure 1.6 Exercisers and stretchers reporting either 0, 1, 2 or 3 episodes of cold infection over the 12-month observation period (data from Chubak *et al.* 2006)

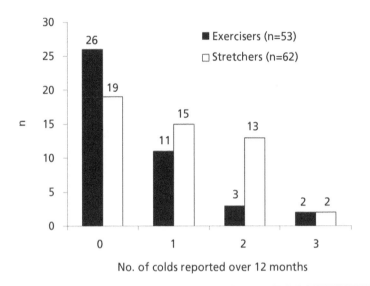

92 men and 107 women in that study had been asked to recall habitual physical activity over the previous three months and symptoms of URTI over the previous six months. While these findings may suggest that any benefits of regular activity on symptoms of respiratory illness are confined to older adults, the long period of recall used in these studies, particularly the six-month period of recall of URTI, does question the reliability of the reported findings.

A more robust study design was employed by Matthews *et al.* (2002). The relationship between exercise and infection risk was explored across a broad range of age (20–70 years) and habitual physical activity level. Over 500 adults were asked to recall episodes of colds, flu or allergic episodes at three-month intervals over a period of one year. Physical activity levels were assessed by 24-hour recall occurring on three occasions within seven weeks of each URTI recall and took into consideration physical activity at home, at work and during leisure time. The data were also adjusted for many of the known risk factors for infection, such as age, smoking, anxiety, depression and dietary factors such as macronutrient and vitamin supplement intake. The findings suggested that regular moderate physical activity was associated with a 20–30% reduction in annual risk of URTI, compared with low levels of habitual activity (Figure 1.7). Although this study was based on three-month recall of 'colds' and 'allergies' rather than any specific symptoms of URTI, the patterns of seasonal variation in episodes of colds were in agreement with the accepted annual distribution of URTI. As can be seen in Figure 1.8, colds were four times more prevalent in the winter months (November to March) than in the summer (June to August), whereas allergies were more common in the summer.

Figure 1.7 Relative risk of upper respiratory tract infection (URTI) across habitual physical activity quartiles; units of physical activity are expressed as MET-h/day 1; MET = resting metabolic rate (i.e. 3.5 ml O_2/kg body mass/minute) so, for example, a value of 6 MET-h/day is equivalent to 1 hour of moderate exercise (where metabolic rate is six times the resting value) per day

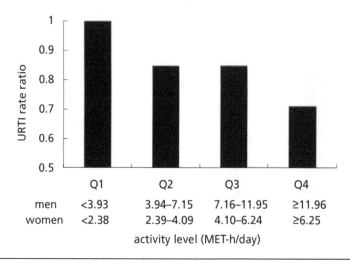

	Q1	Q2	Q3	Q4
men	<3.93	3.94–7.15	7.16–11.95	≥11.96
women	<2.38	2.39–4.09	4.10–6.24	≥6.25

activity level (MET-h/day)

Figure 1.8 Seasonal variation (percentage within 95% confidence interval) in reported colds (upper respiratory tract infections), influenza (flu) and allergies in a USA general population sample (data from Matthews *et al.* 2002)

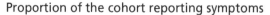

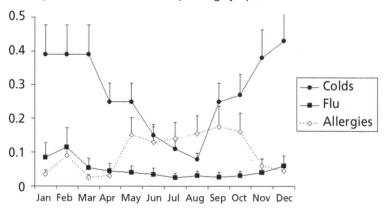

In a robust study that addresses many of the study design issues we have highlighted in this chapter Nieman *et al.* (2011a) provide strong support for a protective effect of regular physical activity on episodes of respiratory illness. Over 1000 males and females of a wide age range (18–85 years) completed a validated questionnaire of symptoms, the Wisconsin Upper Respiratory Symptom Survey, on a daily basis over a 12-week winter period (the season when URTS are most prevalent). Leisure time activity levels were assessed, as was self-perceived level of fitness and confounders, such as age, gender, body mass index, stress, fruit intake, marital status and education level, were taken into account. The key findings from the study were a reduction in days with URTS during the 12-week period with increasing levels of activity. Those who exercised on at least five days each week had a 43% fewer number of days with URTS compared with those who were largely sedentary (reporting activity on less than one day each week) (Figure 1.9). Furthermore, compared with the sedentary group, a significantly lower incidence of symptom days was also found in those reporting activity on one to four days per week. Similar findings have been reported in a four-month prospective study of over 1500 Swedish adults aged 20–60 years (Fondell *et al.*, 2011). Here URTS (classified as colds *and* influenza) were assessed via self-report questionnaires that were emailed to participants at three-week intervals and physical activity was assessed by questionnaire at baseline. There was an 18% reduction in URTS risk between high and low physical activity quartiles that improved to a 42% reduction in URTS risk in those with high levels of perceived stress. This relationship was stronger in men who reported higher stress levels compared with women.

It is important to emphasise that, in these studies, someone in the most active group is unlikely to be performing the large quantities of vigorous training that form the focus of the studies of athletes described in the earlier parts of this chapter. They are more likely to engage in regular moderate-vigorous but non-fatiguing exercise, such as going to the gym or jogging on most days of the week and being moderately active in the rest of their free time (such as performing household chores, walking, gardening, and actively playing with young children).

Figure 1.9 Total number of days with upper respiratory symptoms over the 12-week observation period across physical fitness and exercise frequency tertiles; * $P < 0.05$ compared with the low fitness or exercise frequency tertile (data from Nieman *et al.* 2011a)

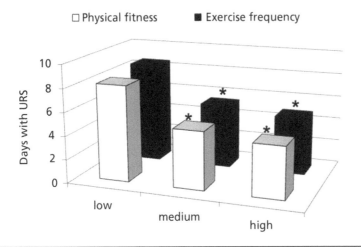

Group activity 1.1

Discuss the strengths and weaknesses of the epidemiological studies that investigate the effects of habitual physical activity level on infection incidence

The problem

There are only a limited number of studies that have investigated relatively large populations (e.g. Matthews *et al.* 2002; Nieman *et al.* 2011a) and even these have not included individuals engaged in large volumes of training. There is the problem of possible confounding factors (such as age, gender, psychological stress, diet) that need to be controlled for, and the history of infection episodes is often limited to self-reporting and recall rather than the use of validated infection symptom questionnaires or physician diagnosis. The studies of athletes have mostly been limited to examining URTS by self-report in the weeks following long-distance running events (e.g. Peters and Bateman 1983; Nieman *et al.* 1990a).

Questions for group discussion

- What are the strengths and weaknesses of the epidemiological studies that investigate the effects of habitual physical activity level on infection incidence?
- What confounding factors need to be considered in such studies?
- What would be the best ways of monitoring infection incidence in large scale population studies?

Moderate exercise and URTS duration and severity

On balance, the evidence from the available randomised controlled studies and larger survey-based studies does suggest some association between moderate exercise and reduced risk of URTS. In addition, for each episode of URTS, symptom severity and duration may also be lower in physically active individuals. Nieman *et al.* (2011a) reported that daily URTS severity was 32% and 41% lower between the high and low perceived fitness and aerobic activity tertiles. Number of daily symptoms reported (symptomology) were also 34% and 41% lower between the high and low perceived fitness and aerobic activity tertiles. This is not to say that exercising during an upper respiratory illness will hasten recovery. Weidner *et al.* (1998) vaccinated 50 moderately trained college students with human rhinovirus on two consecutive days. Thirty-four of the students then went on to exercise at 70% heart rate reserve for 40 minutes every other day for ten days, with the remaining 16 students assigned to a no exercise condition. Over the ten days, symptom severity and duration were assessed using a checklist and by weighing collected facial tissues. Throughout the ten days post-vaccination, mean scores on the symptom questionnaire did not differ between the two groups, neither were there any differences in mass of the collected tissues. While these findings suggest that continuing to exercise during an URTI episode in moderately fit individuals does not affect symptom severity or duration, any extrapolation of these findings should be taken with caution. There was no sedentary control group to act as comparison and, as we saw at the beginning of this chapter, human rhinovirus is just one of many respiratory pathogens and symptom profiles may differ between different causative microorganisms. Since this study only investigated rhinovirus-caused URTI, this may account for the discrepancies between the findings of this study and those of Nieman *et al.* (1990b, 2011a) where the episodes of URTS experienced were naturally occurring.

Summary of effects of moderate exercise on infection risk

The J-shaped relationship between exercise and infection risk suggests that regularly taking part in moderate levels of physical activity decreases the relative risk of URTI to below that of a sedentary individual. The findings of several interventional and observational studies certainly lend support to this relationship. Previously, it has been argued that the selection criteria used may well present some degree of bias towards those with a 'healthy lifestyle' and, hence, the findings are not valid for the general population. However, this argument is not as strong as perhaps it once was; the large cohort studies have adjusted their data to take into account confounders such as age, gender, body mass index, dietary factors such as vitamin intake, smoking habits, education and perceived stress among many other demographical and lifestyle influences, yet the protective effect of regular exercise on risk of URTS remains.

KEY POINTS

- Acute upper respiratory tract infections (URTI; e.g. coughs and colds, influenza, sinusitis, tonsillitis, other throat infections and middle ear infections) are among the most common illnesses experienced at all ages and lead to absence from school and work, visits to GPs, and heavy use of 'over the counter' medicines.
- The causes of upper respiratory infections can be viral or bacterial and are most commonly transmitted by airborne droplets or nasal secretions. Many are seasonal in their activity, tending to circulate in higher levels during the winter months.
- The J-shaped relationship between exercise and infection risk suggests that participating in regular moderate exercise is associated with a lower risk of URTI compared with that of a sedentary individual. Performing acute bouts of prolonged, intense exercise or heavy volumes of training is associated with an above average risk of URTI.
- Studies of single bouts of endurance exercise have been typically associated with an increase in reported upper respiratory tract symptoms (URTS).
- Intensive endurance training is often associated with an increase in episodes of clinically confirmed URTI or self-reported URTS. This relationship has also been reported in athletes involved in intermittent sports including football, rugby and tennis.

- In the absence of clinical confirmation, caution needs to be exercised when interpreting reported URTS as actual infections. In many cases, self-reported symptoms of respiratory illness may reflect airway inflammation or allergic reaction rather than an illness with an identifiable infectious cause.
- Regular participation in moderate amounts of physical activity is associated with fewer episodes of URTS compared with sedentary individuals.
- For each episode of URTS, symptom severity and duration may also be lower in physically active individuals compared with sedentary individuals.
- This positive effect of regular activity on infection risk persists even when confounders such as age, gender, dietary factors, body mass index and stress are taken into account.

FURTHER READING

Bermon, S. (2007) Airway inflammation and upper respiratory tract infection in athletes: is there a link? *Exercise Immunology Review* 13: 6–14.

Moreira, A., Delgado, L., Moreira, P. and Haahtela T. (2009) Does exercise increase the risk of upper respiratory tract infections? *British Medical Bulletin* 90: 111–31.

Nieman, D.C. (1994) Exercise, upper respiratory tract infection, and the immune system. *Medicine and Science in Sports and Exercise* 26: 128–39.

Nieman, D.C., Henson, D.A., Austin, M.D. and Sha, W. (2011) Upper respiratory tract infection is reduced in physically fit and active adults. *British Journal of Sports Medicine* 45: 987–992.

Spence, L., Brown, W.J., Pyne, D.B., Nissen, M.D., Sloots, T.P., McCormack, J.G., Locke, A.S. and Fricker, P.A. (2007) Incidence, etiology, and symptomatology of upper respiratory illness in elite athletes. *Medicine and Science in Sports and Exercise* 39: 577–86.

Walsh, N.P., Gleeson, M., Shephard, R.J., Gleeson, M., Woods, J.A., Bishop, N.C., Fleshner, M., Green, C., Pedersen, B.K., Hoffman-Goetz, L., Rogers, C.J., Northoff, H., Abbasi, A. and Simon, P. (2011) Position statement. Part one: Immune function and exercise. *Exercise Immunology Review* 17: 6–63. [Note: Information on pages 11–16 relates specifically to respiratory infections in athletes.]

2 The human immune system

Michael Gleeson and Jos Bosch

LEARNING OBJECTIVES

After studying this chapter, you should be able to:

- describe the main components of the immune system and their functions;
- distinguish between innate and acquired (adaptive) immunity;
- explain the basis of how the body recognises and responds to non-self material;
- describe the components and actions of humoral and cell-mediated immune mechanisms;
- appreciate some of the factors that affect immune function;
- describe the principle of enzyme-linked immunosorbent assay (ELISA) methods to measure the concentration of specific soluble proteins in body fluids.

INTRODUCTION AND OVERVIEW OF THE IMMUNE SYSTEM

The body is constantly under attack by viruses, bacteria and parasites. The immune system provides us with numerous complex and potent layers of defence that can resist these attacks. When successful, this system of defence establishes a state of immunity against infection (Latin: *immunitas*, freedom from). The immune system protects against, recognises, attacks and destroys elements that are foreign to the body. This function is essential to body homeostasis. It involves the precise coordination of many different cell types and molecular messengers, yet, like any other homeostatic system, the immune system is composed of redundant mechanisms to ensure that essential processes are carried out. The immune system is particularly important in defending the body against pathogenic (disease-causing) micro-organisms including bacteria, protozoa, viruses and fungi.

Micro-organisms have inhabited Earth for at least 2.5 billion years and the power of immunity is a result of coevolution in which indigenous bacteria particularly have shaped the body's defence functions. In humans, the critical role of the immune system becomes clinically apparent when it is defective. Thus, inherited and acquired immunodeficiency states are characterised by increased susceptibility to infections, sometimes caused by commensal micro-organisms not normally considered to be pathogenic. The immune system also plays an important role in defending us against cancer by identifying and destroying tumour cells. However, excessive activity of the immune system can also be damaging rather than protective. This is seen in the case of autoimmune diseases, where the immune system inappropriately attacks tissues or organs, and in hypersensitivity reactions, where an excessive allergic response causes a high level of inflammation that can be fatal.

Box 2.1 Components of the immune system

The components of the immune system comprise both cellular and soluble elements.

- All blood cells originate in the bone marrow from common stem cells. The latter are capable of differentiating into erythrocytes (red blood cells, important in oxygen transport), megakaryocytes (precursors of platelets, important in blood clotting) and leukocytes or white blood cells, which have diverse functions in immune defence.
- Leukocytes consist of the granulocytes (60–70% of circulating leukocytes), monocytes (5–15%) and lymphocytes (20–25%). Various subsets of the latter, including B cells, T cells and natural killer (NK) cells can be identified by the use of fluorescent-labelled monoclonal antibodies to identify cell surface markers (known as clusters of differentiation or cluster designators, CD).
- All T cells express CD3 on the cell surface and so are designated as CD3+ cells. B cells do not express CD3 but do express CD19 on the cell surface so are designated as CD3–CD19+; B cells also express CD20 and CD22. NK cells are designated as CD3–CD16+CD56+.

THE CELLULAR COMPONENTS OF THE IMMUNE SYSTEM

The characteristics of the various leukocytes are described below and summarised in Table 2.1.

Granulocytes: neutrophils, basophils and eosinophils

Granulocytes are a type of leukocyte that includes neutrophils, eosinophils and basophils. The name neutrophil derives from staining characteristics on haematoxylin and eosin-stained histology preparations. Whereas the cytoplasmic granules of basophils stain dark blue and eosinophils stain bright red, neutrophils stain a neutral pink. They are called granulocytes because their cytoplasm contains small granules, that contain proteins with potent protein-digesting and bactericidal properties. Granulocytes are very important in helping the body to fight bacterial infections. People who have abnormally lower numbers of granulocytes are more likely to get frequent and severe bacterial and fungal infections. Granulocytes are also called

Table 2.1 Characteristics of leukocytes

LEUKOCYTE	MAIN CHARACTERISTICS
Granulocytes:	60–70% of leukocytes
Neutrophils	> 90% of granulocytes
	Phagocytosis of foreign substances
	Have a receptor for antibody: phagocytose antigen-antibody complexes
	Display little or no capacity to recharge their killing mechanisms once activated
Eosinophils	2–5% of granulocytes
	Phagocytose parasites
	Triggered by immunoglobulin G to release toxic lysosomal products
Basophils	0–2% of granulocytes
	Produce chemotactic factors
	Tissue equivalent = the mast cell, which releases a eosinophil chemotactic factor
Monocytes/macrophages	5–15% of leukocytes
	Egress into tissues (e.g. liver, spleen) and differentiate into the mature form: the macrophage
	Phagocytose enabling antigen presentation
	Secrete immunomodulatory cytokines
	Retain their capacity to divide after leaving the bone marrow
Lymphocytes	15–25% of leukocytes
	Activate other lymphocyte subsets
	Produce lymphokines
	Recognise antigens
	Produce immunoglobulins (antibody)
	Exhibit memory
	Exhibit cytoxicity

polymorphonuclear leukocytes (PMN) because of the varying shapes of the nucleus, which is usually lobed into two to five segments connected by chromatin filaments. Granulocytes or PMN are produced and released from the bone marrow.

Neutrophils

Normally, neutrophils contain a nucleus divided into two to five lobes. Neutrophils are the most abundant leukocyte in the blood, constituting 50–70% of the total circulating leukocytes. One litre of human blood contains about five billion neutrophils (5×10^9 cells) which are about 12–15 micrometres (μm or 10^{-6} m) in diameter. Once neutrophils have received the appropriate signals, within minutes they can leave the blood and reach the site of an infection. Neutrophils do not return to the blood; they turn into pus cells and die. Neutrophils do not normally exit the bone marrow until maturity but, during an infection, neutrophil precursors called myelocytes and promyelocytes are released. These are often referred to as non-segmented 'band cells' and are thought to be not as functionally effective as mature neutrophils.

Neutrophils have three strategies for directly attacking micro-organisms: phagocytosis (ingestion) followed by intracellular killing; release of soluble antimicrobial compounds (including granule proteins); and generation of neutrophil extracellular traps (NETs). Neutrophils are phagocytes, capable of ingesting micro-organisms or other particles coated with antibody and complement proteins and damaged cells or cellular debris. This process is known as endocytosis and involves amoeboid-type movement surrounding and engulfing the target (e.g. a bacterium). Neutrophils can internalise and kill many microbes, with each phagocytic event resulting in the formation of a phagosome (a type of vacuole or membranous sack) into which reactive oxygen species and hydrolytic enzymes are secreted. The consumption of oxygen during the generation of reactive oxygen species has been termed the oxidative or respiratory burst, although unrelated to respiration or energy production. The respiratory burst involves the activation of the enzyme NADPH oxidase, which produces large quantities of superoxide, a highly reactive oxygen species (ROS). Superoxide dismutates spontaneously or through catalysis via enzymes known as superoxide dismutases (Cu/Zn-SOD and Mn-SOD), to hydrogen peroxide, which is then converted to hypochlorous acid (HClO) by the enzyme myeloperoxidase. It is thought that the bactericidal properties of HClO are enough to kill bacteria phagocytosed by the neutrophil but this may instead be a step necessary for the activation of proteases (enzymes such as elastase that break down proteins).

Neutrophils can release products that stimulate other phagocytes, including monocytes and macrophages; these secretions increase phagocytosis and the formation of reactive oxygen compounds involved in intracellular killing. The release of an assortment of proteins from the cytoplasmic granules is called degranulation. Neutrophils have two types of granules: primary (azurophilic) granules (found in young cells) and specific granules (which are found in more mature cells). Primary granules contain cationic proteins and defensins that are used to kill bacteria, proteases and cathepsin G to break down (bacterial) proteins, lysozyme to break down bacterial cell walls and myeloperoxidase (used to generate hydrochlorous acid). In addition, secretions from the azurophilic granules of neutrophils stimulate the phagocytosis of antibody-coated bacteria. The secondary granules contain compounds that are involved in the formation of reactive oxygen species, lysozyme and lactoferrin (used to chelate iron, which is essential for bacteria to multiply).

NETs are a web of fibres composed of chromatin and serine proteases that trap and kill microbes extracellularly. NETs provide a high local concentration of antimicrobial components and bind, disarm and kill microbes independent of phagocytic uptake. In addition to their possible antimicrobial properties, NETs may serve as a physical barrier that prevents further spread of pathogens. Trapping of bacteria may be a particularly important role for NETs in sepsis, where NETs are formed within blood vessels.

When circulating in the bloodstream and inactivated, neutrophils are spherical. Once activated, they change shape and become more amorphous or amoeba-like and can extend pseudopods as they hunt for microbes. The average lifespan of (non-activated) neutrophils in the circulation is about five to six days. Upon activation, they marginate (position themselves adjacent to the blood vessel endothelium), and undergo selectin-dependent capture followed by integrin-dependent adhesion in most cases, after which they migrate into tissues, where they survive for only one to two days. Because neutrophil antimicrobial products can also damage body tissues, their short lifespan limits damage to the host during inflammation.

During the beginning or acute phase of inflammation, particularly as a result of infection, neutrophils are usually one of the first cells to migrate towards the site of inflammation. They migrate through the blood vessel walls, then through interstitial tissue fluid, following chemical signals such as interleukin-8 (IL-8), complement fragment C5a and leukotriene B4 in a process called chemotaxis. They are the predominant cells in pus, accounting for its whitish/yellowish appearance.

Basophils

Basophils are one of the least abundant cells in bone marrow and blood (fewer than two percent of all leukocytes). Like neutrophils and eosinophils, they have a lobed cell nucleus; however, they have only two lobes and the chromatin filaments that connect them are barely visible. Basophils have receptors that can bind to antibodies, complement proteins and histamine. The cytoplasm of basophils contains numerous granules that contain histamine, heparin, chondroitin sulphate, peroxidase, platelet activating factor and other substances.

When an infection occurs, mature basophils will be released from the bone marrow and travel to the site of infection. When basophils are activated or damaged, they release histamine, which contributes to the inflammatory response that helps to fight invading organisms. Histamine causes dilation and increased permeability of nearby blood capillaries. Activated basophils and other leukocytes (e.g. monocytes) also release prostaglandins that stimulate increased blood flow to the site of infection. Both of these mechanisms allow blood-clotting elements to be delivered to the infected area. This begins the recovery process and blocks the travel of microbes to other parts of the body. Increased permeability of the inflamed tissue also allows more phagocytes to migrate to the site of infection so that they can ingest and kill microbes.

Eosinophils

Eosinophils also have a segmented nucleus (two to four lobes). Eosinophils play a crucial part in the killing of parasites (e.g. enteric nematodes) but these cells have a limited ability to participate in phagocytosis. They also function as antigen-presenting cells, regulate other immune cell functions (e.g. CD4+ T cell, dendritic cell, B cell, mast cell, neutrophil and basophil functions), are involved in the destruction of tumour cells and promote the repair of damaged tissue. Elevated numbers of circulating eosinophils are commonly found in persons suffering from allergies.

Monocytes

Monocytes are the largest type of leukocyte in the blood, produced by the bone marrow from haematopoietic stem cell precursors called monoblasts. They are cells that possess a large smooth nucleus, a large area of cytoplasm and many internal vesicles for processing foreign material. Monocytes circulate in the bloodstream for about one to three days and then typically move into tissues throughout the body. They normally constitute 5–15% of the leukocytes in the blood. Monocytes are also stored as a reserve in the spleen. Monocytes which migrate from the bloodstream to other tissues differentiate into tissue resident macrophages or dendritic cells.

Monocytes and their macrophage and dendritic-cell progeny serve three main functions in the immune system. These are phagocytosis and intracellular killing, antigen presentation to lymphocytes and cytokine production. Phagocytosis is the process of uptake of microbes and particles followed by digestion and destruction of this material. Monocytes can perform phagocytosis (in a similar way to neutrophils) using intermediary opsonisation proteins, such as antibody or complement that coat the pathogen, as well as by binding to the microbe directly via pattern-recognition receptors that recognise pathogens. These receptors are referred to as Toll-like receptors (TLRs). Monocytes are also capable of killing infected host cells via antibodies, termed antibody-mediated cellular cytotoxicity.

Microbial fragments that remain after such digestion can serve as antigen. The fragments can be incorporated into major histocompatibility (MHC) class II molecules and then traffic to the cell surface of monocytes (and macrophages and dendritic cells). This process is called antigen presentation and it leads to activation of T lymphocytes, which then mount a specific immune response against the antigen. Dendritic cells are often referred to as professional antigen-presenting cells as this is their main function.

Other microbial products can directly activate monocytes and this leads to production of pro-inflammatory cytokines followed somewhat later by anti-inflammatory cytokines. Typical cytokines produced by monocytes are tumour necrosis factor alpha (TNF-α), interleukin (IL)-1, IL-6 and IL-12.

Macrophages express CD14; they are widely distributed among the body tissues and can be phenotypically polarised by the microenvironment to mount specific functional actions. Polarised macrophages can be broadly classified in two main groups: classically activated macrophages (or M1), whose typical activating stimuli are interferon-gamma (IFN-γ, a cytokine secreted by activated T lymphocytes) and bacterial lipopolysaccharide (LPS, a component of the cell wall in Gram-negative bacteria) and alternatively activated macrophages (or M2). M1 macrophages exhibit potent microbicidal properties and promote strong IL-12-mediated proinflammatory T helper (Th) lymphocyte-1 responses, while M2 macrophages support Th2-associated effector functions (Martinez *et al.* 2008). Beyond infection, M2 polarised macrophages play a role in resolution of inflammation through high endocytic clearance capacities and trophic factor synthesis, accompanied by reduced proinflammatory and increased anti-inflammatory cytokine secretion.

Dendritic cells are present in tissues in contact with the external environment, such as the skin (where there is a specialised dendritic cell type called the Langerhans cell) and the inner lining of the nose, lungs, stomach and intestine. They can also be found in an immature state in the blood. Once activated, they migrate to the lymph nodes, where they interact with lymphocytes (both T and B cells) to initiate and shape the acquired (or adaptive) immune response. At certain stages of their development, they grow branched projections, the dendrites, that give the cell its name (*déndron* being Greek for tree). Immature dendritic cells are also called veiled cells, as they possess large cytoplasmic 'veils' rather than dendrites.

Lymphocytes

Lymphocytes account for 15–25% of blood leukocytes. Under the optical microscope, lymphocytes can be divided into large lymphocytes and small lymphocytes. Large granular lymphocytes include natural killer (NK) cells. The small lymphocytes are mostly T cells and B cells. Under the microscope, in a Wright's stain blood smear, a normal lymphocyte has a large, dark-staining nucleus with little to no cytoplasm. In normal situations, the coarse, dense nucleus of a lymphocyte is approximately the size of a red blood cell (about 7 μm in diameter). Polyribosomes are a prominent feature in the lymphocytes that can be seen with an electron microscope. The ribosomes are involved in protein synthesis allowing the generation of large quantities of cytokines and immunoglobulins (antibodies) by these cells.

It is impossible to distinguish between T cells and B cells in a peripheral blood smear. Normally, flow cytometry testing is used for specific lymphocyte population counts. This can be used to specifically determine the percentage of lymphocytes that contain a particular combination of specific cell surface proteins, such as the cluster of differentiation (CD) markers, or that produce particular proteins (for example, cytokines using intracellular cytokine staining).

T cells (processed in the thymus glands) and B cells (bursa of Fabricius-derived cells) are the major cellular components of the acquired immune response. T cells are involved in cell-mediated immunity, whereas B cells are primarily responsible for humoral immunity (relating to antibody whose actions are mostly restricted to the extracellular fluids). T cells are more numerous than B cells in blood; T cells account for 60–80% of blood lymphocytes and B cells 5–15%. The function of T cells and B cells is to recognise and respond to specific 'non-self' antigens, during a process known as antigen presentation. Once they have identified an invader, the cells generate specific responses that are tailored to effectively eliminate specific pathogens or pathogen-infected cells. B cells respond to pathogens by producing large quantities of antibody which then neutralise foreign molecules (e.g. toxins) or microbes like bacteria and viruses. In response to pathogens some T cells, called Th cells, produce cytokines that direct the immune response while other T cells, called T-cytotoxic (Tc) cells, produce toxic granules that contain powerful enzymes which induce the death of pathogen-infected cells. Following activation, B cells and T cells leave a lasting legacy of the antigens they have encountered, in the form of memory cells. These long-lived cells enable the body to develop a more rapid and effective immune response to a micro-organism that is encountered for a second time, even years later. Essentially, these memory cells 'remember' each specific pathogen encountered and are able to mount a strong and rapid response if the same pathogen is detected again.

NK cells are lymphocytes that are part of the innate immune system. They play a major role in defending the host from both tumours and virus infected cells. NK cells account for 5–20% of blood lymphocytes. NK cells distinguish infected cells and tumours from normal and uninfected cells by recognising changes of a surface molecule called MHC class I. NK cells are activated in response to a family of cytokines called interferons. Activated NK cells release cytotoxic (cell-killing) enzymes (e.g. perforin) from their intracellular granules, which then destroy the altered cells. They were named 'natural killer cells' because of the initial notion that they do not require prior activation to kill cells that are missing MHC class I molecules.

Group activity 2.1

Examination of a stained human blood smear

The problem

You have been given a light microscope and a slide (blood smear stained with Wright's stain). The slide is of human blood and you are going to identify the three main types of leukocytes in that slide.

What are you looking out for?

Using the information that you have from this chapter on immune cell characteristics, you should be able to identify:

• red blood cells (numerous small circular cells with no nucleus)

and the following immune cells:

• neutrophils (60% of all leukocytes)
• lymphocytes (20–25% of all leukocytes)
• monocytes (10–15% of all leukocytes)
• eosinophils and basophils (less than 2% of all leukocytes).

Tasks

1. Identify each of the main cell types outlined above.
2. When you have identified a type of leukocyte (not the red blood cells), each student should draw it and label it with its name and the characteristics that you used to help you to identify it.
3. A little extra for the neutrophils: in the sample, there should be neutrophils of different maturity (age). Identify an older and a younger neutrophil – again, draw these and label the characteristic that you used to help you differentiate between an older and younger neutrophil.
4. What is the main difference in the physical appearance of the granules in eosinophils and basophils?

Soluble components of the immune system

Soluble factors of the immune system act in several ways: (a) to activate leukocytes; (b) as neutralisers (killers) of foreign agents; and (c) as regulators of the immune system. Such factors include the cytokines and some examples of these, together with their sources and actions, are shown in Table 2.2. These polypeptide messenger substances stimulate the growth, differentiation and functional development of leukocytes via specific receptor sites on either secretory cells (autocrine function) or immediately adjacent leukocytes (paracrine function). There are various subclasses of

Table 2.2 Producers and immune actions of soluble factors	
SOLUBLE FACTOR	PRODUCER(S) AND IMMUNE ACTIONS
Cytokines:	
IL-1	Produced mainly from activated macrophages
	IL-1α tends to remain cell associated
	IL-1β acts as a soluble mediator
	Stimulates IL-2 production from CD3+ and CD4+ cells
	Increases IL-1 and IL-2 receptor expression
	Increases B-cell proliferation
	Increases TNF-α, IL-6 and CSF levels
	Stimulates secretion of prostaglandins
	Appears to be an endogenous pyrogen
IL-2	Produced mainly by CD4+ cells
	Stimulates T-cell and B-cell proliferation and expression of IL-2 receptors on their surfaces
	Stimulates release of IFN-γ by T-cells
	Stimulates NK cell proliferation and killing
IL-6	Produced by activated Th-cells, fibroblasts and macrophages
	Stimulates the differentiation of B-cells, inflammation and the acute phase response
TNF-α	Produced from monocytes, T-cells, B-cells and NK cells
	Enhances tumour cell killing and antiviral activity
IFN-γ	Produced from activated T-cells
	Enhances cell-mediated immunity
	Activates NK cells and antiviral activity
Acute-phase proteins	Made in the liver, secreted into the blood
	Encourage cell migration to sites of injury and infection
	Activate complement
	Stimulate phagocytosis
Complement proteins	Found in the serum
	Consist of 20 or more proteins
	Stimulate phagocytosis, antigen presentation, and neutralisation of infected cells
	The 'amplifier' of the immune response

Notes: CD = clusters of differentiation; IL = interleukin; IFN = interferon; CSF = colony-stimulating factor; TNF = tumour necrosis factor; Th = T helper; NK = natural killer

cytokines, including interleukins, interferons, tumour necrosis factors, lymphokines and colony stimulating factors. The actions of cytokines are not confined to the immune system; they also influence the endocrine and nervous systems including the brain. Other soluble factors include complement and acute-phase proteins that are secreted from the liver, lysozyme in mucosal secretions and the specific antibodies secreted from B lymphocytes. The actions of these other various non-specific soluble factors are summarised in Table 2.2.

Box 2.2 Innate and acquired immunity

The immune system can be divided into two general arms: innate (natural or non-specific) and acquired (adaptive or specific) immunity, which work together synergistically.

The acquired immune system developed late in the phylogeny and most animal species survive without it. However, this is not true for mammals – including humans – which have an extremely sophisticated acquired immune system that is both systemic and mucosal (local) in type. There appears to be great redundancy of mechanisms in both systems providing robustness to ensure that essential defence functions are preserved.

The attempt of an infectious agent to enter the body immediately activates the innate system. This first line of defence comprises three general mechanisms, with the common goal of restricting micro-organism entry into the body: (1) physical/structural barriers; (2) chemical barriers; and (3) phagocytic cells that can ingest and kill micro-organisms and other non-specific killer cells which can eliminate host cells that become infected.

Failure of the innate system and the resulting infection activates the acquired system, which responds with a proliferation of cells that either attack the invader directly or produce specific defensive proteins, antibodies (also known as immunoglobulins, Ig) which help to counter the pathogen in various ways. This is helped greatly by receptors on the cell surface of lymphocytes that recognise the antigen (foreign substance – usually the proteins and lipopolysaccharides located on the surface of the bacteria or virus), engendering specificity and 'memory' that enable the immune system to mount an augmented response when the host is reinfected by the same pathogen.

INNATE IMMUNITY

A pathogen that attempts to infect the body will immediately be counteracted by the innate immune system (Table 2.3), the body's first line of defence (Figure 2.1), which comprises surface barriers (Figure 2.2), soluble factors, professional phagocytes (cells that can engulf, ingest and digest foreign material) and NK cells (Figure 2.1). Together, these functions constitute a primary layer of natural defence against invading micro-organisms, with the common goal of restricting their entry into the body by providing: (1) physical/structural hindrance and clearance mechanisms via epithelial linings of skin and mucosal barriers, mucus, ciliary function and peristalsis; (2) chemical factors such as the low pH of stomach fluids, numerous antimicrobial peptides and proteins; (3) phagocytic cells including neutrophils, eosinophils, blood

COMPONENTS	CELLULAR	SOLUBLE
	Table 2.3 Main elements of the immune system	
Innate	Natural killer cells (CD16+, CD56+)	Acute phase proteins
	Phagocytes (neutrophils, eosinophils, basophils, monocytes, macrophages)	Complement proteins
		Lysozymes
		Cytokines (interleukins, interferons, colony-stimulating factors, tumour necrosis factors)
Adaptive	T-cells (CD3+, CD4+, CD8+)	Immunoglobulins: IgA, IgD, IgE, IgG, IgM
	B-cells (CD19+, CD20+, CD22+)	

CD = clusters of differentiation or cluster designators

Figure 2.1 Major components of innate immunity

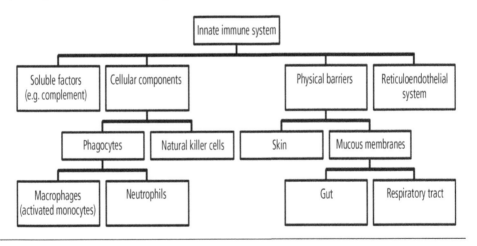

monocytes, tissue macrophages and dendritic cells capable of ingesting and killing micro-organisms; and (4) NK cells which are non-specific killer cells that can destroy host cells that become infected with viruses, thus preventing further viral replication. Challenges of the innate system often lead to activation of the acquired immune system, which aids substantially in recovery from infection, as discussed below.

Figure 2.2 Protective function of the body's surface barriers

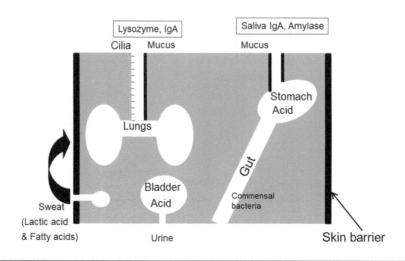

The role of antimicrobial soluble factors in innate immunity

The production and secretion of acute phase proteins by the liver is induced by cytokines, especially IL-6, which is released from activated monocytes and macrophages when they encounter pathogens. These proteins have a variety of functions, including activation of complement, binding of iron and stimulation of phagocytes. Haptoglobin removes any free haemoglobin in the plasma and transferrin (together with lactoferrin released from neutrophils) chelate-free iron; these effects are designed to reduce the availability of free iron in the body fluids, which is especially important because iron is needed by bacteria for their replication. Another acute phase protein called C-reactive protein has a similar structure to that of antibody molecules. It coats foreign material and damaged host tissue and stimulates the activity of phagocytes that can kill bacteria and remove cell debris.

The complement system consists of over 20 different proteins that normally circulate in the blood plasma in inactive forms. The presence of certain yeasts, fungi or bacteria and antibody-antigen complexes activates the complement cascade (Figure 2.3) that results in the break-up of several of the complement proteins into smaller biologically active fragments. The fragments formed from the breakup of complement proteins C3 and C5 are particularly important: C3b promotes phagocytosis, C3e promotes increased release of leukocytes from the bone marrow, C5a attracts and activates phagocytes and C5b combines with C6, C7, C8 and C9 to form a membrane attack complex. The latter attaches to bacterial cell membranes, forming pores which allow osmotic influx of water into the bacterium, causing it to swell until it bursts.

Figure 2.3 The complement cascade

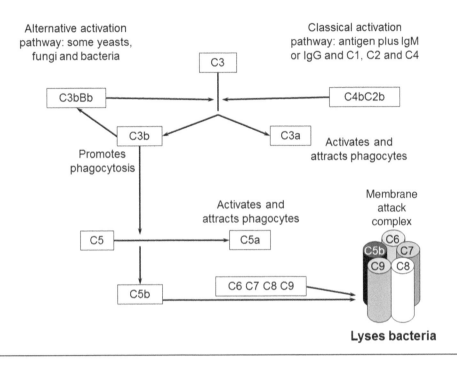

The role of phagocytic cells in innate immunity

The major phagocytic cells of the immune system are neutrophils, monocytes, macrophages and dendritic cells. Neutrophils and monocytes are found in blood and can move out of the circulation (extravasate) into the tissues when infection or tissue damage is present. Neutrophils are the most abundant type of white blood cell. Macrophages and dendritic cells are found in most tissues of the body, with large numbers present in the lymphoid tissues such as the lymph nodes, spleen and tonsils. Phagocytic cells are capable of amoeboid-type movement and can engulf and ingest foreign material, including whole bacteria. Ingested material is held within a vacuole in the cytoplasm of the cell. Granules containing digestive enzymes fuse with the vacuole releasing their contents on to the foreign material. At the same time, a respiratory or oxidative burst is initiated which generates highly reactive oxygen species such as the superoxide radical ($O_2^{-\bullet}$), hydrogen peroxide (H_2O_2) and hydrochlorous acid (HClO), which aid the killing and breakdown of bacteria, as illustrated schematically in Figure 2.4.

Engagement of other types of receptor on phagocytic cells such as immunoglobulin Fc receptors and complement receptors, triggers phagocytosis and elimination of invading micro-organisms. Although some pathogens have evolved

Figure 2.4 The killing process in phagocytes

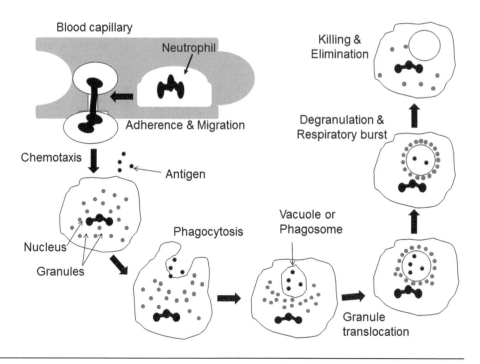

mechanisms to evade innate immunity (e.g. bacterial capsules), they cannot usually persist within the body when an acquired immune response reinforces innate immunity by providing specific antibodies directed against the invading pathogen and its toxins. Thus, the innate and acquired immune systems are not independent; innate immunity influences the character of the acquired response and the effector arm of the acquired response supports several innate defence mechanisms.

The role of natural killer cells in innate immunity

Approximately 10–15% of peripheral blood lymphocytes are neither T nor B cells (Table 2.4). Despite the fact that these previously so-called 'null cells' employ recognition mechanisms somewhat similar to T cells, they are considered to belong to the innate immune system and are therefore currently referred to as NK cells. The NK cell receptors are pattern recognition receptors (PRRs) encoded in the germ line and they recognise structures of high-molecular-weight glycoproteins expressed on virus-infected cells. After activation, NK cells release their granule contents, which include cytolysin and perforin (pore-forming proteins which cause break up of the cell membrane so that the infected host cell breaks up or lyses) and kill virally infected host cells and a variety of tumour cells without prior sensitisation (Cerwenka and

Table 2.4 Lymphocyte functions and characteristics	
LYMPHOCYTE SUBSET	MAIN FUNCTION AND CHARACTERISTIC
T-cells (CD3+):	60–80% of lymphocytes
Th (CD3+CD4+)	60–70% of T cells
	'Helper' cells
	Recognise antigen to co-ordinate the acquired response
	Secrete cytokines that stimulate T and B cell proliferation and differentiation
Tc/Ts (CD3+CD8+)	30–40% of T cells
	Ts ('suppressor') involved in the regulation of B cells and other T cells by suppressing proliferation and certain functions
	Ts may be important in 'switching off' the immune response
	Tc ('cytotoxic') kill a variety of targets, including some tumour cells
CD3+CD45RO+	T memory cells (or recently activated T cells)
CD3+CD45RA+	Naïve and inactivated T cells
B cells (CD19+ CD20+ CD22+)	5–15% of lymphocytes
	Produce and secrete Ig, specific to the activating antigen
	Exhibit memory
NK cells (CD3–CD16+ CD56+)	5–20% of lymphocytes
	Large, granular lymphocytes
	Express spontaneous cytolytic activity against a variety of tumour-and virus-infected cells
	MHC-independent
	Do not express the CD3 cell-surface antigen
	Triggered by IgG
	Control foreign materials until the antigen-specific immune system responds

CD = clusters of differentiation; Ig = immunoglobulin; MHC = major histocompatibility complex; NK = natural killer; Th = T helper; Tc/Ts= T cytotoxic/suppressor

Lanier 2001). Thus, NK cells are important both in defence against viral infection and in preventing the development of cancers.

THE RECOGNITION OF FOREIGN MATERIAL

The recognition molecules involved in innate immunity are encoded in the germ line. This system is therefore quite similar among healthy individuals and shows no apparent memory effect – that is, re-exposure to the same pathogen will normally elicit more or less the same type of response. These receptors sense conserved molecular structures that are essential for microbial survival and are present in many types of bacteria, including endotoxin or lipopolysaccharides (LPS), teichoic acids and bacterial DNA (Beutler and Rietschel 2003). Although such structures are generally called pathogen-associated molecular patterns (PAMPs), they also occur in the bacteria that live in our gut (Medzhitov 2001). However, the intestinal microflora may induce distinct molecular programming of the innate immune system, which may explain why the indigenous micro-organisms located in the large intestine are normally tolerated by the host (Nagler-Anderson 2001).

The cellular receptors of the innate immune system that recognise PAMPs as 'danger signals' are called PRRs, with many of them belonging to the so-called TLRs. They are expressed mainly by monocytes, macrophages and dendritic cells but also by a variety of other cell types such as neutrophils, B cells and epithelial cells (Medzhitov 2001). A family of ten mammalian TLRs (TLR1–10) have been identified to date and they recognise conserved pathogen-associated molecular patterns (PAMPs) including LPS, lipoproteins, peptidoglycan, lipoteichoic acid and zymosan (components of bacterial cell walls), flagellin (a protein component of the flagellum or 'tail' of motile bacteria, bacterial DNA and double-stranded RNA (found in many viruses). Most TLRs are expressed on the cell surface but some (e.g. TLR9) are located in the cytoplasm. There are also some other intracellular surveillance proteins called nucleotide-binding oligomerisation domain (NOD) receptors that can detect bacterial peptidoglycan, The peptidoglycan product sensed by NOD1 is a motif characteristic of Gram-negative bacteria plus some Gram-positive bacteria, such as *Bacillus* and *Listeria* species. In contrast, NOD2 has been implicated as a general sensor for both Gram-positive and Gram-negative bacteria, since muramyl dipeptide, which is the minimal motif in all peptidoglycans, is the structure recognised by NOD2.

As PAMPs are not expressed by host cells, TLR and NOD recognition of PAMPs permits self–non-self discrimination (Kaisho and Akira 2006). The binding of these foreign molecules to TLRs and NODs causes activation of immune cells. TLRs, in particular, control both the activation of innate immunity through the induction of antimicrobial activity (e.g. phagocytosis) and the production of inflammatory cytokines and the generation of acquired immunity through the induction of several signalling molecules on the cell surface of macrophages and dendritic cells (collectively known as antigen-presenting cells), as shown in Figure 2.5 and described in further detail below. Therefore, TLRs, through pathogen recognition and the control of innate and adaptive immune responses, play a pivotal role in the host defence response against infection. Thus, the initial activation of the innate immune system prepares the ground for a targeted and powerful protective function of the acquired immune system (Table 2.3).

ACQUIRED OR ADAPTIVE IMMUNITY

The purpose of acquired or adaptive immunity is primarily to combat infections by preventing colonisation of pathogens and keep them out of the body (immune exclusion) and to seek out specifically and destroy invading micro-organisms (immune elimination). In addition, specific immune responses are, through regulatory mechanisms, involved in avoidance of overreaction against harmless antigens (hypersensitivity or allergy) as well as discrimination between components

Figure 2.5 Binding of pathogen associated molecular patterns (PAMP) and endogenous danger signal molecules such as heat shock proteins to Toll-like receptors leads to activation of the antigen-presenting cell (APC) and subsequent activation of T-helper (Th) cells with which it interacts. APCs take up antigen via endocytic pattern recognition receptors and process (degrade) it to immunogenic peptides, which are displayed to T cell receptors (TCR) in the polymorphic grove of major histocompatibility complex molecules after their appearance at the cell surface. An interaction occurs between the APC and the T cell, as indicated, usually resulting in cellular activation. When naive CD4+ Th cells are activated by APCs that provide appropriate co-stimulatory signals (cytokines and/or accessory binding molecules), they differentiate into Th1 or Th2 cells with polarised cytokine secretion. Cytokines produced by APCs and Th cells result in proliferation and activation of other immune components

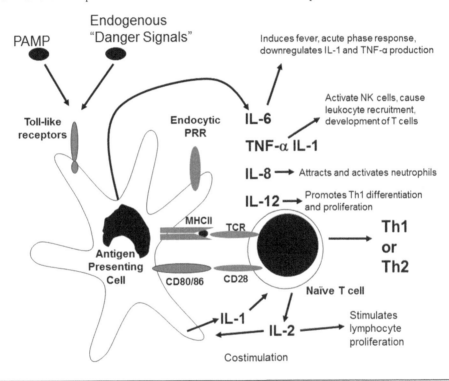

of 'self' and 'non-self'. Autoimmune diseases occur when this control mechanism breaks down. The major components of acquired immunity are shown in Table 2.3 and Figure 2.6.

The role of antigen-presenting cells in acquired immunity

The antigen-presenting cells (APCs) include monocytes, macrophages and dendritic cells. The latter are sometimes called 'professional APCs', as this is their primary function and they are able to stimulate mature yet unprimed (naïve) T cells and thus initiate primary immune responses (Moll 2003). Most other APCs re-stimulate memory T cells and thus initiate secondary responses. The TLRs on the surface of APCs are activated by binding to PAMPs, which then leads to increased expression

Figure 2.6 Major components of acquired (adaptive, specific) immunity

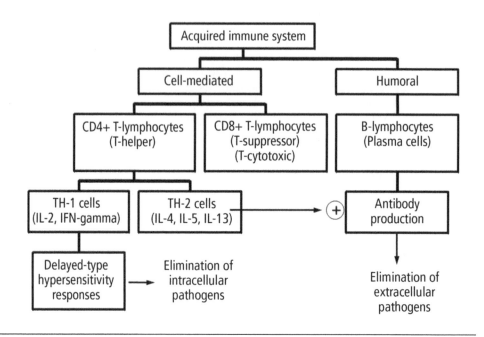

of MHC class-II proteins on the cell surface of the APC. The MHC class-II proteins contain a region called the polymorphic groove, into which parts of digested foreign proteins can be inserted. These can then be presented to T lymphocytes. In this manner, the T cell receptors specifically recognise short immunogenic peptide sequences of the antigen (Figure 2.5).

Only APCs express MHC class-II proteins; other cells in the body normally express MHC class-I proteins. The ability of the acquired immune system to distinguish self from non-self likewise depends largely on the structure of the MHC molecules, which are slightly different in each individual except for homozygous (identical) twins.

The phagocytosis (ingestion) of the invading micro-organism by an APC is the first step in a chain of events leading to the eventual elimination of the pathogen. Lysosomal digestive enzymes and oxidising substances are released into the intracellular vacuole containing the foreign material within the APC. The foreign proteins (antigens) normally found on the micro-organism's surface are processed (degraded) to immunogenic peptides which are then incorporated within the polymorphic groove of MHC class-II proteins which are then translocated to the cell surface. The antigens can now be presented to the other cellular immune components, in particular the T-cell receptors (TCRs) on T-helper (Th) cells. (Figure 2.5). The Th lymphocytes (CD4+ expressing cells) coordinate the response via cytokine release to activate other immune cells. Stimulation of mature B lymphocytes results in their proliferation and differentiation into immunoglobulin-secreting plasma cells. Immunoglobulins or antibodies are important to antigen recognition and memory of earlier exposure to specific antigens. They also help to eliminate pathogens in the extracellular fluids but they cannot enter cells and so are not effective against pathogens that have infected host cells.

The role of lymphocytes in acquired immunity

In peripheral blood, the lymphocytes comprise 20–25% of the leukocytes. Initially, all lymphocytes are alike: they are round in shape with a prominent circular nucleus surrounded by a thin layer of cytoplasm which does not contain granules. After circulating in the blood as immature lymphocytes, they continue their maturation either in the thymus, a gland in the upper chest, where they become T lymphocytes or in the bone marrow where they become B lymphocytes. The thymus and bone marrow are called the primary lymphoid organs (Figure 2.7). Naïve T and B cells enter the bloodstream and become disseminated to secondary lymphoid organs such as the spleen, lymph nodes and mucosa-associated lymphoid tissue (Figure 2.7).

Figure 2.7 The thymus and bone marrow are called the primary lymphoid tissues, as these are the tissues where maturation of lymphocytes takes place (T cells in thymus, B cells in bone marrow). Through the blood circulation, lymphocytes migrate to other (secondary) lymphoid tissues such as spleen, lymph nodes and the gut-associated lymphoid tissue (e.g. Peyer's patches in the small intestine)

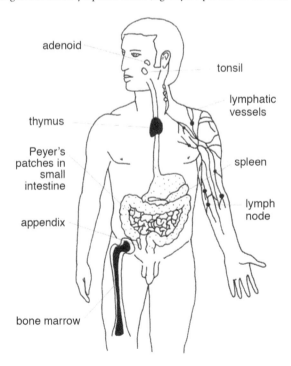

Certain adhesion molecules and receptors for chemokines (chemo-attractant cytokines) enable adherence of immune cells to specialised vascular endothelium and their migration into the lymphoid organs, which are anatomically and functionally organised to facilitate interactions between lymphocytes and various types of APCs. Lymph nodes contain large numbers of macrophages, which ingest pathogens swept into the lymph nodes by the flow of lymph fluid. As indicated above, macrophages play a key role in activating lymphocytes.

Antigens are carried into these immune-inductive structures from peripheral tissues via draining lymph, passively as soluble molecules and dead or live particles and actively by migrating dendritic cells, as well as directly from mucosal surfaces by 'membrane' or 'microfold' cells in mucosa-associated lymphoid tissue. Lymphocytes located in the lymph nodes are thus strategically located to remove antigens before they reach the blood. As macrophages and lymphocytes resist invasion, lymph nodes may swell, a common sign of infection. Lymphocytes that do not encounter antigens re-enter the bloodstream by way of efferent lymphatics and then the thoracic duct. The functional consequence of this recirculation of T and B cells is that all parts of the body are under continuous antigen-specific immunological surveillance.

The role of T and B lymphocytes in acquired immunity

Various lymphocyte subsets can be identified by the use of monoclonal antibodies (usually of mouse origin), which recognise specific proteins – that is, cellular markers known as cluster of differentiation or cluster designator (CD) molecules (see Table 2.4). Thus, all T lymphocytes (or T cells) express selectively CD3 and all B lymphocytes (or B cells) express selectively CD19 and CD20. Th cells express CD4, whereas most cytotoxic T cells express CD8. Acquired or adaptive immunity depends on the functional properties of both T and B cells and is directed by their antigen-specific surface receptors, which show a random and highly diverse repertoire.

As they mature, the lymphocytes develop immunocompetence: each cell becomes competent at recognising one particular antigen, and mounting an immune response against that antigen alone. Each T and B cell bears antigen receptors with a certain specificity; these differ between individual clones of lymphocytes. A clone consists of daughter cells derived by proliferation from a single ancestor cell, so-called clonal expansion. The total population of T and B cells in a human may be able to recognise some 10^{11} different antigens. This remarkably diverse antigen receptor repertoire is generated during lymphocyte development by random rearrangement of a limited number of receptor genes. Thus, the acquired immune system is prepared for an almost unlimited variety of potential infections. It is important to realise that the versatility of the immune system is not due to flexible cells that change their antigenic targets on demand; rather it depends on the presence of an enormous diversity of lymphocytes with different receptor specificities. Most T cells recognise protein or peptide antigens; however, there is a subset of T cells called $\gamma\delta$ T cells that recognise lipid and other non-peptide antigens. They are potent cytotoxic cells that aid the host in bacterial elimination, wound repair and delayed-type hypersensitivity reactions. γδ T cells have a high tissue-migrating phenotype and are found to infiltrate epithelial-rich tissue such as skin, intestines and the reproductive tract. They make up 2–15% of the total CD3+ blood T cell population and are mostly negative for both CD4+ and CD8+ surface antigens.

Even without priming, the acquired immune system is able to respond to an enormous number of antigens but the detection of any single antigen could be limited to relatively few lymphocytes, perhaps only one in one million. Consequently, in a primary immune response, there is generally an insufficient number of specific lymphocytes to eliminate the invading pathogen. However, when an antigen receptor is engaged by its corresponding antigen, the lymphocyte usually becomes activated (primed), ceases temporarily to migrate, enlarges and proliferates rapidly so that, within three to five days, there are numerous daughter cells – each specific for the antigen that initiated the primary immune response. Such antigen-driven clonal expansion accounts for the characteristic delay of several days before acquired immunity becomes effective in defending the body.

In addition to the effector cells generated by clonal expansion and differentiation, so-called memory cells are also generated; these may be very long-lived and are the basis of immunological memory characteristic of acquired immunity (Faabri *et al.* 2003). Functionally, immunological memory enables a more rapid and effective secondary immune response upon re-exposure to the same antigen. In contrast to innate immunity, the antigen specificities of acquired immunity reflect the individual's lifetime exposure to stimuli from infectious agents and other antigens and will consequently differ among individuals.

GENERAL MECHANISM OF THE ACQUIRED OR ADAPTIVE IMMUNE RESPONSE

As outlined above, acquired immunity is based on antigen-specific responses but it is effected by an array of humoral (fluid borne) and cell-mediated immune reactions.

Humoral immunity

The effector cells of the B-cell system are the terminally differentiated antibody-producing plasma cells. These constitute the basis for so-called humoral (fluid-borne) immunity, which is mediated by circulating antibody proteins or immunoglobulins comprising five subclasses: IgA, IgD, IgE, IgG and IgM (Table 2.5). The antigen-specific receptor on the surface of the B lymphocyte is a membrane-bound form of Ig produced by the same cell. Engagement of surface Ig by corresponding antigen will, in co-operation with 'help' provided by cognate Th cells, initiate B cell differentiation and clonal expansion (Figure 2.8). The resulting effector B cells can then transform into plasma cells that secrete large amounts of antibody with the same specificity as that of the antigen receptor expressed by the progenitor B lymphocyte.

Table 2.5 Properties of the five classes of immunoglobulin (Ig) found in extracellular fluid

Ig CLASS	MEAN ADULT SERUM LEVEL (g/L)	SERUM HALF LIFE (days)	PHYSIOLOGICAL FUNCTION
M	1.0	5	Complement fixation
			Early immune response
			Stimulation of ingestion by macrophages
G	12.0	25	Complement fixation
			Placental transfer
			Stimulation of ingestion by macrophages
A	1.8	6	Localised protection in external secretions, e.g. saliva
D	0.03	2.8	Function unknown
E	0.0003	2	Stimulation of mast cells
			Parasite expulsion

Figure 2.8 Humoral immunity: stimulation of mature B-lymphocytes by the actions of activated Th2 cells results in the proliferation and differentiation into B cell clones of immunoglobulin-secreting plasma cells

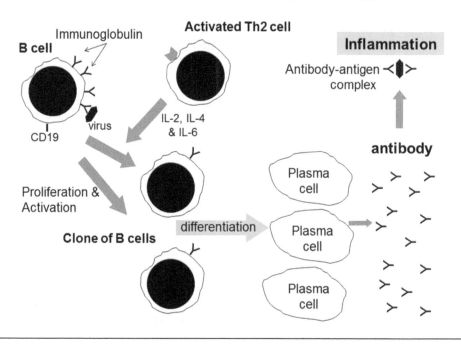

Most antigens activate B cells only when the B cells are stimulated by cytokines from Th cells: these are called T-cell-dependent antigens. Some antigens are T-cell independent; they usually have a repetitive structure and bind with several receptors on the B cell surface at once, a process called capping. The antigen is taken into the cell and activates it causing appropriate clones of B cells to proliferate and differentiate into memory cells and plasma cells which are capable of secreting large amounts of antibody during their brief life of four to five days. The antibodies circulate in the blood and lymph, binding to antigen and contributing to the destruction of the organism bearing it. Until recently, it was thought that antibodies did not cross cell membranes and so their actions were limited to within the extracellular fluids (blood plasma, lymph, interstitial fluid). However, it is now recognised that some antibodies can enter cells when they are bound to viruses and can initiate virus elimination mechanisms within the cell cytoplasm.

Each antibody molecule has the ability to: (a) bind to a specific antigen; and (b) assist with the antigen's destruction. Every antibody has separate regions for each of these two functions (Figure 2.9). The regions that bind the antigen differ from molecule to molecule and are called variable regions. Only a few humoral effector mechanisms exist to destroy antigens, so only a few kinds of regions are involved; these are called constant regions. An antibody molecule consists of two pairs of polypeptide chains – two short identical light chains and two longer identical heavy chains. The chains are joined together to form a Y-shaped molecule. The variable regions of heavy and light chains are located at the ends of the arms of the Y, where they form the antigen-binding sites. Thus, on each antibody molecule there are two antigen-binding sites, one at each tip of the antibody's two arms. The rest of the antibody molecule, consisting of the constant regions of the H and L chains, determines the antibody's effector function. There are five types of constant region and, hence, five major classes of antibody, called IgA, IgD, IgE, IgG and IgM. Their

Figure 2.9 Basic structure of an immunoglobulin molecule; the molecule consists of four polypeptide chains; two light chains (shown in red) and two heavy chains (shown in blue). Each heavy chain is linked to a light chain and the heavy chains are linked to each other by disulphide bounds. The fragment antigen-binding (Fab) unit contains two antigen-binding sites and the molecule binds to effector cells and molecules via the fragment crystallisable (Fc) unit

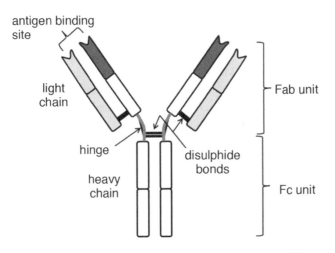

different roles in the immune response are described in Table 2.5. Within each class, there will be a multitude of subpopulations of antibodies, each specific for a particular antigen. Whereas IgM and IgG dominate systemic humoral immunity, IgA is normally the dominating antibody class of mucosal immunity (Table 2.5).

Antibodies do not have the power to destroy antigen-bearing invaders directly. Instead, they effectively tag foreign molecules and cells for destruction by various effector mechanisms. Each mechanism is triggered by the selective binding of antigens to antibodies to form antigen-antibody complexes. The antibodies may simply block the potential toxic actions of some antigens (a process called neutralisation) or they may cause clumping together of antigens or foreign cells (agglutination) which can then be ingested by phagocytes. Precipitation is a similar mechanism, in which soluble antigen molecules are cross-linked to form inactive and immobile precipitates that are captured by phagocytes. Antibody-antigen complexes on the surfaces of invading micro-organisms usually cause complement activation. As mentioned earlier, once they become activated, complement proteins attack the membrane of the invader and, by coating the surface of foreign material, make it even more attractive to phagocytes (a process known as opsonisation).

Cell-mediated immunity

When acquired immunity is mainly mediated by activated effector T cells and macrophages, the reaction is referred to as cell-mediated immunity or delayed-type hypersensitivity (DTH). Many pathogens, including all viruses, can only reproduce within host body cells. The cellular immune response fights pathogens that have already entered cells. Activated T lymphocytes, including memory cells and Tc cells, attack and kill infected host cells or foreign cells. There are also Th cells, suppressor T cells and regulatory T (Treg) cells, very important in mobilising and regulating the whole immune response. When Th cells bind to specific antigenic determinants displayed with MHC proteins on the cell surface of macrophages, the macrophage is stimulated to release a cytokine called IL-1 which stimulates the T cells to grow and divide (Figure 2.10). The activated T cells release another cytokine, IL-2, which further stimulates proliferation and growth of Th and Tc cells. T-cytotoxic cells recognise and attach to cells which have on their surface appropriate antigenic determinants coupled with MHC complex proteins. T-cytotoxic cells then release perforin (just like NK cells) which causes death of the infected host cell by lysis. The fragments of cell debris are ingested and digested by phagocytes.

Immunological memory

An antigen entering the body selectively activates only a tiny fraction of the quiescent lymphocytes, which then grow and divide to form a clone of identical effector cells. Each antigen may carry several antigenic determinants, each activating a different clone, and an invading bacterium will carry a number of different antigens. So a particular species of bacterium invading the body will activate several clones of lymphocytes.

Figure 2.10 Cell-mediated immunity: activated Th1 cells stimulate clonal proliferation of T cytotoxic cells which are capable of killing host cells that have become infected with pathogens

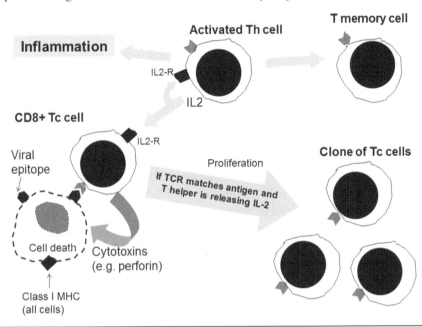

The first encounter with any antigen causes the primary immune response to that antigen. There is a lag period of several days before clones of lymphocytes selected by the antigen can multiply and differentiate to become effector B and T cells. From B cells, it takes several days for specific antibodies to appear in the blood and it is several weeks before peak antibody levels (referred to as antibody titres) are attained. Antibodies of the IgM class are predominantly produced in the primary response to antigen exposure. During the lag period, while specific antibody levels are slowly increasing, pathogenic micro-organisms may gain entry to the body and multiply in sufficient numbers to cause damage to host tissues and symptoms of illness.

A second exposure to the same antigen (even years later) produces a much more rapid, stronger and longer-lasting secondary response. This depends on memory cells, which are produced at the same time as effector cells during the primary response. Effector cells usually only last for a few days but memory cells may last for decades. When there is a second exposure to the same antigen, they rapidly multiply and differentiate to give large numbers of effector cells and large quantities of antibodies (mainly of the IgG class in the secondary response) dedicated to attacking the antigen. Thus, following a first exposure to a specific pathogen, immunity is effectively acquired, such that on a subsequent exposure to the same pathogen – even if this occurs years later – symptoms of illness do not arise. This is the basis of vaccination in which an attenuated pathogen (or specific molecules from it) are injected into a person to 'immunise' them against a particular disease (e.g. polio, rubella, diphtheria, tetanus).

Regulation and the Th1/Th2 balance

Whether humoral or cell-mediated immunity will dominate, depends largely on the type of cytokines that are released by the activated Th cells. Cell-mediated immunity depends on a so-called Th1 profile of cytokines, including particularly IFN-γ and TNF-α. These cytokines activate macrophages and induce killer mechanisms, including Tc cells. A Th2 profile includes mainly IL-4, IL-5 and IL-13, which are necessary for promotion of humoral immunity, IgE-mediated allergic reactions and activation of potentially tissue-damaging eosinophils. IL-4 and IL-13 primarily drive B cell differentiation to antibody production, while IL-5 mainly stimulates and primes eosinophils.

In recent years, great efforts have been made to elucidate the mechanisms involved in the induction and regulation of a polarised cytokine profile characterising activated Th-cell subsets. There is particularly great interest in the role of APCs in shaping the phenotypes of naïve T cells during their initial priming, partly because the differential expression level of various co-stimulatory molecules on activated and matured dendritic cells may exert a decisive impact (Liew 2002). Thus, interaction of the T cell CD28 receptor with CD80 on APCs appears to favour Th1 differentiation, whereas interaction with CD86 appears to favour the Th2 phenotype. Certain cytokines secreted by the developed Th1 and Th2 cells act in an autocrine and reciprocally inhibitory fashion: IL-4 promotes Th2 cell expansion and limits proliferation of Th1 cells, whereas IFN-γ enhances growth of Th1 cells but decreases Th2 cell development. In fact, the cytokine microenvironment clearly represents a potent determinant of Th1/Th2 polarisation, with IL-4 and IL-12 as the initiating key factors – being derived principally from innate immune responses during T-cell priming. Activated macrophages and dendritic cells are the main source of IL-12, whereas an early burst of IL-4 may come from NK cells, mast cells, basophils or already matured bystander Th2 cells (Liew 2002).

Altogether, exogenous stimuli such as pathogen-derived products, the maturational stage of APCs, as well as genetic factors will influence Th1/Th2 differentiation, in addition to complex interactions between antigen dose, TCR engagement and MHC antigen affinities. High antigen doses appear to favour Th1 development, while low doses favour the Th2 subset (Boonstra *et al.* 2003). Influential antigenic properties include the nature of the antigen, with bacteria and viruses promoting Th1-cell differentiation and flatworms (helminths) the Th2 subset. Th2 differentiation also appears to be promoted by small soluble proteins characteristic of allergens. Some important allergens (e.g. from house dust mite) are proteases and it has been suggested that this favours Th2 development because helminths secrete proteases to aid tissue penetration (Liew 2002).

Although it is somewhat of an oversimplification, the Th1 response can be seen as the major promoter of cell-mediated reactions that provide an effective defence against intracellular pathogens (i.e. viruses and some bacteria that can enter host cells). In contrast, the Th2 response primarily activates humoral immunity and the antibodies produced are usually only effective against pathogens in the extracellular fluids (Figure 2.11). As mentioned previously, Th1- and Th2-cell responses are

Figure 2.11 Th1/Th2 cytokine balance

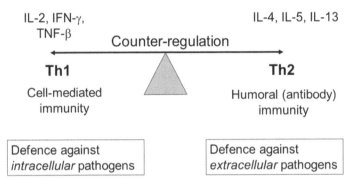

cross-regulatory and the Th1/Th2 cytokine balance is also influenced by Treg cells (Maloy and Powrie 2001), which may secrete the suppressive cytokines IL-10 and transforming growth factor-β (TGF-β). Treg cells are important in preventing excessive activity of the immune system and help to bring a stop to immune activation after a pathogen has been eliminated.

In summary, therefore, the nature of the APC (usually a dendritic cell) that stimulates the naive T cells in a primary immune response will to a large extent influence the development of Th1, Th2 and Treg cells via its co-stimulatory molecules and cytokine secretion. In this manner, the signature of the microbial environment imprinted through PRRs, is important for maintenance of homeostasis in the acquired immune system. Interestingly, the Treg cells may also exert a dampening effect directly on innate immune mechanisms (Maloy *et al.* 2003). The anti-inflammatory regulatory network may furthermore include IL-10 and TGF-β derived from other activated immune cells such as macrophages and dendritic cells (McGuirk and Mills 2002).

Activation of the immune response by endogenous danger signals

The activation of macrophages and dendritic cells, necessary for the initiation of primary and secondary immune responses, can be induced by endogenous danger signals – released by host tissues undergoing stress, damage or abnormal death – as well as by PAMPs expressed by pathogens. Some of the endogenous danger signals that have recently been discovered are heat-shock proteins, nucleotides, reactive oxygen intermediates, extracellular matrix breakdown products and interferons. Some of these are primary activators of APCs and work through activation of TLRs and others give positive feedback signals to enhance or modify an ongoing response (Galluci and Matzinger 2001).

MUCOSAL IMMUNITY

The mucosal immune system is arguably the largest immune component in the body. It not only defends the intestine from invasion by infections but also plays a similar role in the respiratory system, mouth, eyes and reproductive tract. Mucosal immunity can be viewed as a first line of protection that reduces the need for systemic immunity, which is principally proinflammatory and potentially tissue damaging and therefore a 'two-edged sword', as explained above. Numerous genes are involved in the regulation of innate and acquired immunity, with a variety of modifications introduced over millions of years. During such evolutionary modulation, the mucosal immune system has generated two non-inflammatory layers of defence: (a) immune exclusion performed by secretory antibodies to inhibit surface colonisation of micro-organisms and dampen penetration of potentially dangerous soluble substances; and (b) immunosuppressive mechanisms to avoid local and peripheral hypersensitivity to innocuous antigens. The latter mechanism is referred to as 'oral tolerance' when induced via the gut (Brandtzaeg 1996) and probably explains why overt and persistent allergy to food proteins is relatively rare. A similar downregulatory tone of the immune system normally develops against antigenic components of the commensal microbial flora in the large intestine (Duchmann *et al.* 1997). Mucosally induced tolerance is a robust adaptive immune function, since more than a ton of food may pass through the gut of a human adult every year! This results in a substantial uptake of intact antigens, usually without causing any harm.

The immune system of the gut divides into the physical barrier of the intestine and active immune components, which include both innate and adaptive immune responses. The physical barrier is central to the protection of the body to infections. Acid in the stomach, active peristalsis, mucus secretion and the tightly connected monolayer of the epithelium each play a major role in preventing micro-organisms from entering the body. The cells of the immune system in the gut are found in the lamina propria. Specialised lymphoid aggregates, called Peyer's patches, reside below specialised epithelial cells whose structure enables sampling of small particles.

Antibody-mediated mucosal defence

The intestinal mucosa contains at least 80% of the body's activated B cells, which are terminally differentiated to Ig-producing plasma cells. IgA is the predominant immunoglobulin secreted at mucosal surfaces. Secretory IgA (SIgA) is a dimer of 350 kD (whereas circulating IgA is mostly monomeric). The two monomers in SIgA are joined by a J chain and protected from proteolysis by another peptide, the secretory component, made by epithelial cells. It is acquired by IgA molecules as they pass through the epithelium on their journey from the plasma cell to the mucosal surface (further details on IgA structure and transport can be found in Chapter 6). Immune exclusion is then mediated by these antibodies in cooperation with innate nonspecific defence mechanisms. In addition, there may be some contribution to external defence by serum-derived or locally produced IgG antibodies transferred passively into the gut lumen. IgA can immobilise micro-organisms or prevent their attachment to mucosal surfaces. It is generally believed that most IgA in the blood is later available for transport to mucosal surfaces.

SIgA is also secreted in saliva in the mouth. This IgA also comes from B cells in the surrounding mucosal tissue. Saliva IgA is thought to be important in defence against infections of the upper respiratory tract. Saliva also contains other proteins with antimicrobial actions, including amylase (which can help prevent bacterial attachment to epithelial surfaces), lysozyme (which aids in the destruction of bacterial cell walls), defensins and lactoferrin (an iron-chelating protein whose actions help to limit bacterial multiplication). The concentration of IgA, lysozyme and defensins, as well as other soluble protein components of the immune system, can be measured by a technique called enzyme-linked immunosorbent assay (ELISA, described in Technique box 2.1). ELISA methods can also be used to measure the concentrations of cytokines and hormones in blood plasma and other body fluids.

REGULATION OF IMMUNE FUNCTION VIA NERVES AND HORMONES

The lymphoid tissues are innervated by nerves. Nerve cells (neurons), glia cells and immune cells share intercellular signals like hormones, neurotransmitters and modulators, cytokines and chemokines, and they express respective receptors for these signals. Some of these shared signals can cross the blood–brain barrier in both directions (Capuron and Miller 2011). Immune cells traffic to all sites throughout the body, come in close contact to nerve endings and to the brain at the meningeal borders and in the cerebrospinal fluid and can even reach the brain parenchyma. Both immune cells that circulate in the blood and those resident in lymph nodes and tissues can be influenced by the action of several hormones released from endocrine glands. Thus, immune function can be regulated to some degree by the actions of both neurotransmitters and hormones. Furthermore, cytokines secreted from immune cells can have effects on the brain including the induction of fever by resetting the hypothalamic thermostat a few degrees above normal body temperature of 37 degrees Celsius (this is caused by IL-6) and the induction of 'sickness behaviours' such as feeling tired and unwell. The important actions of stress hormones (e.g. adrenaline and cortisol) are described in more detail a little later in this chapter.

Primary lymphatic tissues (thymus and bone marrow) and secondary lymphatic tissues (spleen, lymph nodes, mucosa-associated lymphatic tissue) are innervated by sympathetic, peptidergic and partly also by sensory nerve fibres (Nance and Sanders 2007). The endocrine and autonomous nervous systems regulate immune functions not only directly via hormones and neural innervation but also indirectly via influences on blood flow, blood pressure, lymph flow, the supply of substrates (e.g. glucose, fatty acids) and oxygen and on non-immune cells in the vicinity of lymphatic tissues like adipocytes surrounding the spleen and lymph nodes. Note that some messenger molecules can serve multiple functions. For example, noradrenaline is a

Technique box 2.1

ELISA methods to measure immunoglobulins, other antimicrobial proteins, cytokines and hormones

The enzyme-linked immunosorbant assay (ELISA) is one of the simplest and most reliable tools that the exercise immunologist has at their disposal. Indeed, the development of a wide range of commercially available ELISAs was an important stimulus for research into the influence of exercise on the immune system. The use of the ELISA allows researchers to measures an enormous range of molecules but, before discussing some specific examples of the use of the ELISA as applied to exercise immunology research, let us outline of the principles behind the ELISA.

Principles of ELISA

The ELISA technique is based on a sandwich principle which is illustrated in the figure:

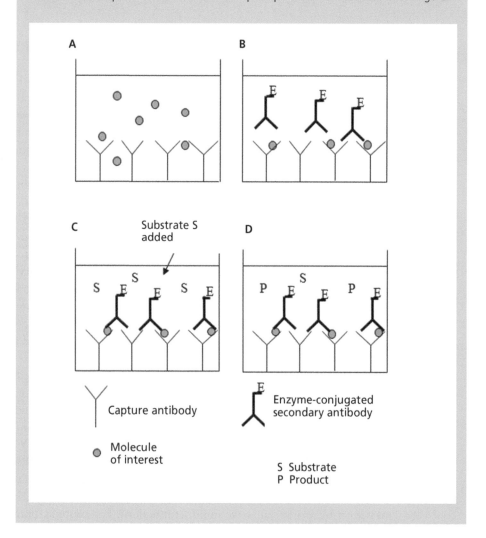

First, a 96-well plate is coated with a specific capture antibody against the molecule of interest (all commercially available ELISA plates come with the individual wells pre-coated with the specific capture antibody). Next, samples of interest, standards and control samples are added to individual wells and the plate is incubated for a fixed period of time during which the molecule of interest is captured by the specific capture antibody (Figure A). Following the incubation period, the plate is washed several times to remove any unbound molecules from the wells of the plate. Next, a secondary antibody that is conjugated to an enzyme (e.g. peroxidase) is added to each well. Importantly, this secondary antibody recognises a different epitope (an epitope is a site on a large molecule against which antibodies will be produced and to which the antibody will bind) on the molecule of interest to that recognised by the capture antibody. During a second incubation period, the enzyme-conjugated secondary antibody binds to the molecule of interest that has bound to the capture antibody, thus completing the 'sandwich' (Figure B). Following another series of washes to remove any unbound secondary antibody, a chromogenic substrate of the enzyme is added to each well (Figure C). The reaction of the enzyme with its substrate (S in Figure C) converts the substrate to a product (P in Figure D) that produces a colour change. Thus, the greater the amount of enzyme present (i.e. the greater the amount of molecule of interest bound to the capture antibody), the greater the colour development. To quantify the amount of molecule of interest present within in each well, the absorbance (also known as the optical density or extinction) is determined at a specific wavelength on a microplate reader. Next, a standard curve is generated via a set of standards of known concentration and the concentration of the molecule of interest present in each well is interpolated from the calibration curve. While all ELISAs follow a similar set of procedures and are based on the same principles as described above, variations on this theme are common.

Use of ELISA

The ELISA is an extremely sensitive, specific and versatile tool and can be used for the measurement of many biological molecules, such as cytokines, hormones, adhesion molecules, soluble receptors, intracellular signalling proteins and mRNA. However, with regard to exercise immunology research, the main use of the ELISA has been in the measurement of cytokines. In addition, ELISAs can also be used to assess cell function; this is particularly advantageous since many functional techniques (e.g. flow cytometery), require expensive equipment and a considerable degree of expertise. For example, to assess the influence of exercise on monocyte cell function, one could assess LPS-stimulated production of IL-1β, TNF-α and IL-6, to assess neutrophil function; one could assess the LPS-stimulated release of enzymes (e.g. elastase or myeloperoxidase) from intracellular granules. The concentration of secretory IgA (SIgA) in saliva can also be measured by ELISA. This can be a useful measure of mucosal immune responses to exercise or training.

hormone released from the adrenal glands and also a neurotransmitter in the central nervous system; leptin is released from adipocytes and acts as a circulating hormone but also as a paracrine cytokine signal.

Gut-associated lymphoid tissue and bronchus-associated lymphoid tissue receive both sympathetic and peptidergic innervation. The nerve network within mucosal tissues is very extensive. It has been calculated that the number of nerve-cell bodies present in the gastrointestinal tract is equivalent to that found in the spinal cord. Neuropeptides are found in very large amounts in these tissues, particularly vasoactive intestinal peptide and somatostatin. The salivary glands are also innervated and this influences saliva flow rate and IgA secretion. Evidence suggests that sympathetic nerve stimulation may upregulate IgA secretion in the submandibular glands but, otherwise, there is a lack of information of how the sympathetic innervation may affect mucosal immunity.

AUTOIMMUNE DISEASES

Failure of immune system regulation can lead to the development of autoimmune diseases. Examples of such diseases include asthma, atherosclerosis, cancer, Crohn's disease, myasthenia gravis, multiple sclerosis, rheumatoid arthritis, systemic lupus erythematosus and food allergies. For some of these diseases, symptoms may be caused or aggravated by an inappropriately activated immune system. Although the immune system is designed to destroy threatening micro-organisms, it can also damage body tissues. Usually, the inflammation and tissue destruction that are associated with the mechanisms used to eradicate a pathogen are acceptable and functionally insignificant. However, in several diseases (e.g. rheumatoid arthritis), the tissue destruction by the activated immune system is substantial, long lasting and harmful. It is because of the potentially damaging effects of the immune cells on body tissues that the system is very tightly regulated. Failure of these regulatory mechanisms can result in the full might of the immune system being inappropriately directed against the body's own tissues and the development of chronic inflammatory or autoimmune diseases.

FACTORS AFFECTING IMMUNE FUNCTION

Resistance to infection is strongly influenced by the effectiveness of the immune system in protecting the host against pathogenic micro-organisms. Immune function is influenced by genetic as well as environmental factors (Figure 2.12) and thus there is some degree of variability in resistance to infection within the normal healthy adult population. Resistance to specific infections is also affected by previous exposure to the disease-causing pathogen or inoculation with vaccines used for immunisation. Vaccines contain dead or attenuated pathogens that trigger immune responses including the development of specific memory without eliciting symptoms of disease that are associated with inoculation by live pathogens.

Figure 2.12 Factors affecting immune function

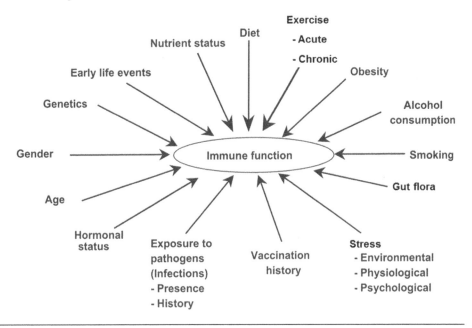

Age

Age is a critical factor in resistance to infection. Antigen-specific cellular and humoral immunity is central to the acquired immune responses generated in the adult human. In contrast, the very young rely primarily on innate immunity, although this component of the immune system is not as fully functionally developed in young children as it is in adults. Although many previous studies have demonstrated a marked decline in several aspects of immune function in the elderly, it is now recognised that some immune responses do not decline and can even increase with advancing age (Lesourd *et al.* 2002). Nowadays, the influence of ageing on the immune system is generally described as a progressive occurrence of dysregulation, rather than as a general decline in function. Indeed, it has also been shown that many decreased immune responses that were previously attributed to the ageing process are actually linked to other factors such as poor nutritional status or an ongoing disease which is not clinically apparent (Lesourd *et al.* 2002).

The activity of the thymus, an essential organ for the production of T cells, has long been recognised to decline with age, initially in terms of its structure and morphology and later in terms of its function (Gress and Deeks 2009). Although the factors underlying this decline, which normally begins in the third decade of life, are not fully understood, a link with sex steroids has been suggested. Measurements of the production of new T cells by the human thymus show a stable plateau through the second decade of life and do not normally begin to decline until the latter part of the third decade. Consequent upon this decline is a change in the distribution of cells in the peripheral circulation, with naïve T cells declining with age, while memory and effector cells increase. Essentially, these effects progressively decrease the capacity to respond to novel pathogens which requires differentiation and proliferation of the existing naïve T cell pool.

Sex

Sex also affects immune function. In females, estrogens and progesterone modulate immune function and, thus, immunity is influenced by the menstrual cycle and pregnancy (Haus and Smolensky 1999). Consequently, sex-based differences in responses to infection, trauma and sepsis are evident. Women are generally more resistant to viral infections and tend to have more autoimmune diseases than men do (Beery 2003). Estrogens are generally immune enhancing, whereas androgens including testosterone – exert suppressive effects on both humoral and cellular immune responses. In females, there is increased expression of some cytokines in peripheral blood and vaginal fluids during the follicular phase of the menstrual cycle and with use of hormonal contraceptives. In the luteal phase of the menstrual cycle, blood leukocyte counts are higher than in the follicular phase and the immune response is shifted towards a Th2-type response (Faas *et al.* 2000). In pregnancy, elevated levels of progesterone appear to suppress cell-mediated immune function and Th1 cytokine production and enhance humoral immunity and Th2 cytokine production (Wilder 1998). The inhibition of cell-mediated immunity probably reduces the risk of the mother's immune system attacking the developing embryo.

Stress

Stress, both physical and psychological, results in neuroendocrine signals being released from the brain that can affect immune function. Stress increases neuroendocrine hormones, particularly glucocorticoids (e.g. cortisol) and catecholamines (e.g. adrenaline) but, to some extent, also prolactin, growth hormone and nerve growth factor (Glaser and Kiecolt-Glaser 2005). Stress, through the action of these stress hormones, can have both salubrious and detrimental effects on immune function, such as changes in NK-cell activity, changes in the composition of lymphocyte populations in the blood, lymphocyte proliferation and antibody production and can be responsible for reactivation of latent viral infections (Glaser and Kiecolt-Glaser 2005). Stress can occur in a variety of forms, physical or psychological, acute or chronic. It is possible and probable that different forms of stress will have different effects on the stress hormones released and on immune function. For example, the effects of acute psychological stress (minutes to hours) on the immune system are sometimes the opposite of chronic forms of stress (days to years). Whereas acute stress increases the secretion of SIgA in saliva, chronic stress is typically associated with a decrease (Bosch *et al.* 2002). Likewise, NK-cell activity increases during acute stress but is decreased during chronic forms of stress (Segerstrom and

Miller 2004). The negative effects of prolonged stressors on the immune system have received most attention, as they can have significant consequences on health which include, but are not limited to, increased infection risk (Cohen 2005), delayed wound healing (Walburn *et al.* 2009), impaired responses to vaccination (Burns 2012) and possibly even the progression of some cancers (Antoni *et al.* 2006).

The main two neuroendocrine pathways activated in response to stress that control the immune system are the hypothalamic–pituitary–adrenal (HPA) axis, which results in release of glucocorticoids, and the sympathetic nervous system, which results in release of catecholamines, adrenaline (which is the same as epinephrine) and noradrenaline (also called norepinephrine). However, there are other neuroendocrine factors that are released following stress that also regulate the immune system, including prolactin, growth hormone and nerve growth factor (NGF).

One of the main mechanisms by which the brain controls the immune system is through activation of the HPA axis. Upon stimulation, corticotrophin-releasing hormone is secreted from the paraventricular nucleus of the hypothalamus. This then stimulates the anterior pituitary gland to secrete adrenocorticotrophic hormone (ACTH) into the systemic circulation. This, in turn, induces the adrenal glands to synthesise and secrete glucocorticoids. In humans, the natural glucocorticoid is cortisol, whereas in rodents it is corticosterone. Physiological levels of glucocorticoids are thought to be immunomodulatory whereas high stress-induced levels are immunosuppressive (Dhabhar 2009). In humans, a variety of stressors cause increases in plasma ACTH and cortisol levels. These stressors include intense or prolonged exercise and various forms of psychological stress such as fear, worry and anxiety.

Cortisol elicits its many actions through a cytosolic receptor, the glucocorticoid receptor. Upon ligand binding, the glucocorticoid receptor dissociates from a protein complex and translocates to the nucleus, where it binds to specific DNA sequences to modulate gene transcription. In addition, glucocorticoid receptors can also interfere with the signalling pathways of other transcription factors, such as nuclear factor-κB to repress transcription of many inflammatory molecules.

The activation of the sympathetic nervous system induces secretion of adrenaline into the systemic blood supply. Noradrenaline is released from the nerve terminals in the vicinity of immune cells. These catecholamines bind to the β2-adrenergic receptor and stimulate activation of a G-coupled protein, which results in increased intracellular cyclic adenosine monophosphate (cAMP) production. This results in an inhibition of the intracellular signalling pathways that normally activate the immune response to pathogens.

Prolactin and glucocorticoid receptors are also released during stress. Like ACTH, they are both secreted from the anterior pituitary gland but can also be produced by immune tissues, thereby having an autocrine/paracrine effect on immune cells. Both prolactin and glucocorticoid receptors are thought to be generally immunostimu-latory (Chikanza 1999; Gala, 1991; Hattori, 2009) and are proposed to act as counter measures to glucocorticoids. Many of the effects of glucocorticoid receptors are mediated through glucocorticoid receptor-induced production of insulin-like growth factor-1. NGF is a neurotrophic hormone that is elevated in chronic stress and can regulate the immune response. NGF can function through the hypothalamus to activate the HPA axis and, in addition, NGF can function as an autocrine/paracrine factor to regulate immune cells (Aloe *et al.* 1999). For example, it promotes proliferation and differentiation of T and B lymphocytes and acts as a survival factor for memory B lymphocytes.

Despite their very different cellular sources, glucocorticoid receptor, prolactin, melatonin (Radogna *et al.* 2010) and leptin (La Cava and Matarese 2004) exert remarkably synergistic actions on the immune system. They are proinflammatory signals that support immune cell activation, proliferation, differentiation and the production of proinflammatory cytokines like IL-1, IL-12, TNF-α and of Th1 cytokines like IFN-γ. In contrast, cortisol and catecholamines generally suppress these immune functions in an anti-inflammatory manner, although some specific aspects of immunity may be enhanced by these signals. Timing may be critical factor in these effects, whereby immune suppression is sometimes preceded by a brief period of enhancement.

Psychological stress

Psychological stress has been defined as a constellation of events, comprising a stimulus (stressor) that precipitates a reaction in the brain (stress perception) and activates physiological fight or flight systems in the body (stress response). Psychological stress influences immune function through activation of autonomic nerves innervating lymphoid tissue and by stress hormone-mediated alteration of immune cell functions (Glaser and Kiecolt-Glaser 2005). As stated earlier, the effects of psychological stressors on the immune system are timing dependent. Results from meta-analyses demonstrate consistent effects for certain immune outcomes (Segerstrom and Miller 2004). Acute bouts of stress (minutes to hours) induce rapid changes in the composition of blood leukocytes in peripheral blood, whereby the number of NK cells and, to a lesser extent CD8+ T cells, rapidly increase during acute stressors. In this regard, the effects of acute stress are comparable to those of brief exercise, albeit somewhat smaller. Acute stress also increases NK cell activity and decreases lymphocyte proliferation in response to mitogens. The latter two effects are possibly secondary to the effects of acute stress on blood composition. For example, NK cell activity increases because there are more NK cells in the blood and not because stress makes these cells intrinsically more cytotoxic. Acute stressors have also been found to increase the secretion of SIgA in saliva (Bosch *et al.* 2002) and to cause a transient increase in some plasma cytokines, such as IL-6 (Steptoe *et al.* 2007). These responses likewise mirror what is seen after a brief bout of exercise. Overall, then, acute stress appears to stimulate rather than suppress activity of the immune system.

Effects of prolonged forms of stress (weeks to years), which include psychological disorders such as depression, that are consistently found across studies include reduced NK-cell activity, reduced lymphocyte proliferation to mitogens, reduced responses to vaccination and reactivation of latent herpes viruses (Segerstrom and

Miller 2004). Further, prolonged stress is associated with a moderate elevation of inflammatory markers in plasma, such as cytokines like IL-6 and TNF-α and acute phase proteins like C-reactive protein and fibrinogen (Howren *et al.* 2009). It should be noted that these increases may be secondary to the lifestyle changes that characterise chronically stressed and depressed individuals, such as a lack of exercise and unhealthy dietary behaviours. For example, when individual differences in body mass index are taken into account, the levels of inflammatory cytokines become much more similar to that of healthy, non-stressed individuals.

An important issue is whether effects of stress on immunity have clinical implications. While this issue is as yet unresolved for acute stressors, the effects of chronic stress appear compelling. For example, meta-analysis shows a robust association between stress and wound healing, whereby chronic stress is consistently found to delay the wound repair process (Walburn *et al.* 2009). Vulnerability to infection likewise appears increased. Cohen *et al.* (1991) carried out a well-controlled study (including controls for education, shared housing and personality differences) in which subjects were intentionally exposed to one of five respiratory viruses via nasal drops. The results indicated that psychological stress is associated with an increased risk of infection independent of the possibility of transmission, the strain of administered virus and habitual physical activity. Regrettably, the effects of psychological interventions that aim to mitigate the effects of stress on immunity have been inconsistent. While the occasional study has reported a large effect of interventions like relaxation training, counselling or mindfulness training, such findings are rarely replicated and on average the effects of intervention studies have been very modest (Miller and Cohen 2001).

Besides an effect of psychological states on immunity, there is also good evidence that immune alterations, in particular inflammation, affect mood. An example of this phenomenon is the psychological alterations seen during a common cold, which include lethargy, social withdrawal and moodiness. The features of this psychological state, denoted as 'sickness behaviour', show a remarkable overlap with those seen during clinical depression (Dantzer *et al.* 2008). These and other similarities gave rise to the so-called inflammatory theory of depression, which postulates that inflammatory cytokines may contribute to the development of clinical depression via their effects on mental processes. For example, the incidence of clinical depression is two- to threefold higher among patients with diseases that are characterised by elevated inflammatory activity, such as auto-immune and cardiovascular diseases. Likewise, treatment with cytokines like IFN-γ or IL-2, used in the treatment of some cancers, induces a state of clinical depression in about 40% of the patients (Raison *et al.* 2006). Luckily, and in contrast to what is known about the effects of psychological stress on immunity, the effects of the immune system on psychological functioning is amenable to intervention. For example, the depressogenic (depression-inducing) effects of cytokine treatment can be prevented by prophylactic treatment with antidepressant drugs, and depressed patients with auto-immune and cardiovascular diseases respond equally well to psychotherapy as healthy individuals (Evans *et al.* 2005).

The mechanisms responsible for the effects of immune processes on mood and behaviour have been well-characterised. Brain cells carry receptors for various cytokines, which are transported from the sites of inflammation to the brain, via the blood or via afferent nerves such as the vagus nerve. By activating neurological tissues, these cytokines subsequently affect a broad range of mental functions, such as perception (e.g. pain perception and smell) and mood states (e.g. irritability and feeling blue) that underlie sickness behaviour. The function of sickness behaviours appears to be to promote responses that serve recuperation in ill persons. However, in situations of prolonged inflammatory activity, these neurological effects may become damaging, by impairing cognitive functions and promoting the development of psychopathology (Dantzer et al. 2008; Raison et al. 2006).

Physical stress (exercise)

Elevated levels of stress hormones also occur during strenuous exercise and it is well recognised that acute bouts of exercise cause a temporary depression of various aspects of immune function (e.g. neutrophil oxidative burst, lymphocyte proliferation, monocyte MHC class II expression) that lasts about 3–24 hours after exercise depending on the intensity and duration of the exercise bout (Gleeson and Bishop 1999). Periods of intensified training (overreaching) lasting seven days or more result in chronically depressed immune function and several surveys (described in detail in Chapter 1) indicate that sore throats and flu-like symptoms are more common in endurance athletes than in the general population. The effects of exercise and training on immune function are explored in detail in subsequent chapters.

Sleep

Sleep and the circadian system have a strong influence on immunological processes (Besedovsky et al. 2012). The basis of this influence is a bidirectional communication between the central nervous and immune system that is mediated by neurotransmitters, hormones and cytokines, as well as direct innervations of the immune system by the autonomic nervous system. Many immune functions display prominent rhythms in synchrony with the regular 24-hour sleep–wake cycle, reflecting the synergistic actions of sleep and the circadian system on these parameters. Differentiated immune cells with immediate effector functions, like NK cells and terminally differentiated cytotoxic T cells, peak during the wake period (Besedovsky et al. 2012), thus allowing an efficient and fast combat of invading pathogens and repair of tissue damage, which is more likely to occur during the active phase of the organism. In contrast, undifferentiated or less differentiated cells like naïve and central memory T cells peak during the night, when the more slowly evolving acquired immune response is initiated. Nocturnal sleep, and especially slow wave sleep prevalent during the early night, promotes the release of glucocorticoid receptor and prolactin, while anti-inflammatory actions of cortisol and catecholamines are at the lowest levels. The endocrine milieu during early sleep critically supports the interaction between APC and T cells, as evidenced by an enhanced production of IL-12, a shift of the Th1/Th2 cytokine balance towards Th1 cytokines and an increase in Th cell proliferation and probably also facilitates the migration of naïve T cells to lymph nodes. Thereby, the endocrine milieu during early sleep likely promotes the initiation of Th1 immune responses that eventually supports the formation of long-lasting immunological memories.

Poor quality sleep and prolonged sleep deprivation induce a stress response that invokes a persistent unspecific production of proinflammatory cytokines, best described as chronic low-grade inflammation, and also produce immunodeficiency, which have detrimental effects on health. Both an inadequate amount of nightly sleep and poor sleep quality have been shown to increase the risk of developing common cold symptoms when subjects are experimentally exposed to a dose of human rhinovirus in a nasal spray (Cohen *et al.* 2009).

Diet

It is well established that the general nutritional status of an individual modulates his or her immune function. Both over-nutrition that results in obesity (Nieman *et al.* 1999) and under-nutrition (Scrimshaw and SanGiovanni 1997) affect immune function detrimentally. Particular aspects of the habitual diet, including fat and protein intake, multivitamin and mineral supplements, alcohol consumption and smoking, exert a significant influence on immune function. Deficiencies of specific micronutrients are associated with an impaired immune response and with an increased susceptibility to infectious disease. If a nutrient supplement corrects an existing deficiency in an adult, then it is likely that a benefit to immune function will be seen. Indeed, many human and animal studies have demonstrated that adding the deficient micronutrient back to the diet will restore immune function and resistance to infection (Calder and Kew 2002). What is far less clear is whether increasing the intakes of specific micronutrients above the recommended nutrient intake will improve immune function in a healthy, well-nourished individual. There is also a danger of excessive supplementation of the diet with individual micronu-trients. Excess intakes of some micronutrients (e.g. vitamin E, iron and zinc) impair immune function and increase susceptibility to infection (Calder and Kew 2002). Thus, for many micronutrients, there is a limited range of optimum intake, with levels above or below this resulting in impaired immune function and/or other health problems. The effects of diet and nutritional supplements on immune function are considered in more detail in Chapter 9.

Infectious diseases can affect the status of several nutrients in the body, thus setting up a vicious circle of under-nutrition, compromised immunity and recurrent infection. Under-nutrition is not a problem that is restricted to poor or developing countries. Under-nutrition exists in developed countries, especially among the elderly, premature babies, individuals with eating disorders, alcoholics and patients with certain diseases. Malnutrition was the leading cause of acquired immune deficiency before the appearance of the human immunodeficiency virus (HIV) and poor nutrition is also a major factor contributing to the progression of HIV infection, especially in less developed countries.

CONCLUDING NOTE

This overview of the immune system and the factors affecting it has been given to facilitate the discussions in the chapters that follow on measurement of immune system status and the effects of acute and chronic exercise on immune function. In some places it has been greatly simplified and the complexity of the immune system and its precise coordinated responses should not be underestimated. For further details, the interested reader is recommended to consult the excellent textbooks listed under 'Further reading' at the end of this chapter. You can test your understanding of this chapter by performing the activity described in Group Activity 2.2.

Group activity 2.2

Check your understanding of the organisation of the immune system

The problem

1. Fit the following terms into the diagram below:
   - adaptive immunity
   - antibody
   - B lymphocyte
   - basophil
   - dendritic cell
   - eosinophil
   - granulocytes
   - immunoglobulin (Ig)
   - interferon-gamma (IFN-γ)
   - interleukin 2 (IL-2)
   - interleukin 4 (IL-4)
   - interleukin 5 (IL-5)
   - interleukin 13 (IL-13)
   - macrophage (2 places)
   - monocyte
   - natural immunity
   - natural killer cells
   - neutrophil
   - non-specific immunity
   - plasma cells
   - specific immunity
   - T helper cell (Th)
   - T lymphocyte
   - T suppressor/cytotoxic cell (Tc/s)
   - type-1 T cell (Th1)
   - type-2 T cell (Th2)

---

2. In a different colour, circle the phagocytic cells.
3. In another colour, circle the lymphocytes.
4. Finally, put the following cluster of differentiation (cluster designator) next to the corresponding cell type on your diagram:

CD3+ CD4+ CD8+ CD19+ CD56+

The Organisation of the Immune System

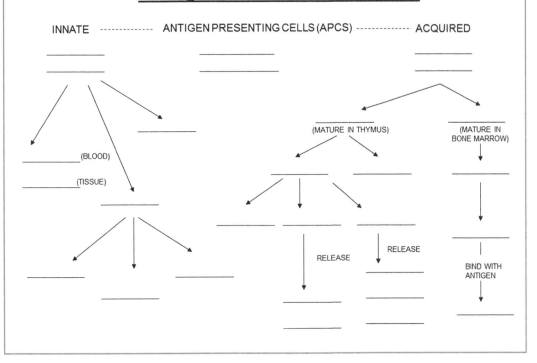

INNATE ----------- ANTIGEN PRESENTING CELLS (APCS) ----------- ACQUIRED

(MATURE IN THYMUS)

(MATURE IN BONE MARROW)

(BLOOD)

(TISSUE)

RELEASE

RELEASE

BIND WITH ANTIGEN

KEY POINTS

- The immune system protects against, recognises, attacks and destroys micro-organisms, cells and cell-parts that are foreign to the body (i.e. non-self). It can be broadly divided into two subsystems, the innate (non-specific, natural) and the acquired (adaptive, specific) immune systems.
- The innate immune system forms the body's first line of defence against invading micro-organisms. It consists of three mechanisms that have the common goal of preventing any foreign agent entering the body: a) physical/structural barriers; b) chemical barriers; and c) phagocytic cells (mainly neutrophils and macrophage/monocytes) and other non-specific killer cells (natural killer cells).
- Neutrophils are the most abundant type of white blood cell or leukocyte. They are the major cell of a subpopulation of leukocytes called granulocytes, so called

because they contain microscopic granules that are released in the killing process. Other types of granulocyte are eosinophils and basophils.

- Other phagocytic cells, monocytes, mature into macrophages in the tissues. Phagocytic cells destroy micro-organisms by engulfing them and releasing toxic substances, including reactive oxygen species and digestive enzymes, on to the micro-organism to kill it and break it up.

- Soluble factors such as complement, acute-phase proteins, lysozyme and cytokines are also important in the innate immune response. Soluble factors help to enhance the innate response, as well as being involved in killing processes directly.

- If an infectious agent gets past the innate host defence mechanisms, the acquired immune response is activated. Following phagocytosis, macrophages and dendritic cells incorporate parts of foreign proteins (antigen) from the digested micro-organism into their own cell surface membrane and present them to T-lymphocytes. Activation of Toll-like receptors on the surface of antigen presenting cells by microbial molecules results in induction of co-stimulatory molecules and T-cell activation.

- There are a number of sub-populations of T-lymphocyte. The presence of an antigen on a macrophage cell surface stimulates the T cells to divide and proliferate into these subpopulations. T-helper (Th) cells coordinate the cell-mediated acquired immune response. They activate T-cytotoxic (Tc) cells and B cells. Tc cells destroy infected cells and are the main effector cells of cell-mediated immunity.

- B cells proliferate into plasma cells. These secrete vast amounts of antibody (or immunoglobulin) specific to the antigen that triggered the immune response. The B cell response is known as the humoral or fluid adaptive immune response.

- Both B cells and T cells 'exhibit' memory, which means that they can mount a rapid response to that specific antigen upon subsequent exposure. This is the rationale behind immunisation programmes.

- Cell-mediated immunity is promoted by the actions of cytokines secreted by Th1 cells, whereas the humoral immune response is activated by cytokines released from Th2 cells.

- Immune function in humans is affected by both genetic and environmental factors. The latter include age, exercise, sex, nutritional status, previous exposure to pathogens, sleep and psychological stress.

- Stress effects on immune function are mostly mediated by the glucocorticoid hormones and catecholamines.

FURTHER READING

Delves, P. J., Martin, S. J., Burton, D. R. and Roitt, I. M. (2011) *Roitt's Essential Immunology*. Oxford: Wiley-Blackwell.

Glaser, R. and Kiecolt-Glaser, J. K. (2005) Stress-induced immune dysfunction: implications for health. *Nature Reviews Immunology* 5: 243–51.

Janeway, C. A. Jr. and Medzhitov, R. (2002) Innate immune recognition. *Annual Review of Immunology* 20: 197–216.

Kindt, T. J., Osborne, B. A. and Goldsby, R. (2006) *Kuby Immunology* (7th ed.). Basingstoke: WH Freeman at Macmillan Press.

Murphy, K. M. (2011) *Janeway's Immunobiology* (8th ed.). New York and London: Garland Science.

Parham, P. (2009) *The Immune System* (3rd ed.). New York and London: Garland Science.

Playfair, J. H. L. and Bancroft, G. (2004) *Infection and Immunity* (2nd ed.). Oxford: Oxford University Press.

Shetty, P. (2010) *Nutrition, Immunity and Infection*. Wallingford: CABI.

Smith, P. D., MacDonald, T. T. and Blumberg, R. S. (2012) *Principles of Mucosal Immunology*. New York and London: Garland Science.

3 The effects of exercise on blood leukocyte numbers

Richard J. Simpson

LEARNING OBJECTIVES

After studying this chapter, you should be able to:

- describe the effects of a single bout of exercise on the total number of leukocytes and their subsets in peripheral blood;
- understand the mechanisms by which discrete leukocyte subsets are selectively deployed into the blood and tissues in response to a single bout of exercise;
- explain some of the factors known to affect the leukocyte response to acute exercise including training status, intensity and duration of the exercise bout, fitness level, age, nutritional status and infection history;
- describe the effects of exercise training on the total number of leukocytes and the composition of leukocyte subtypes in resting blood.

INTRODUCTION

The total number of leukocytes circulating in peripheral blood is strongly influenced by physical exercise. Leukocytosis (an elevated number of white cells in blood) following acute exercise was first reported well over a century ago, with Ralph Larrabee concluding that the increased number of leukocytes observed in four participants after the Boston marathon was due mostly to an influx of polymorphonuclear cells (neutrophils) and that both mechanical and toxic mechanisms were responsible for their exercise-induced mobilisation (Larrabee 1902). Since then, many studies have been conducted to describe the effects of both acute and chronic exercise on the numbers and composition of leukocyte subsets, the kinetics of their response following a single bout of exercise, the impact of intensity, duration and mode of exercise on this response, and the influence that age, training status, nutrition and infection history have on the leukocyte response in both athletes and non-athletes. Many researchers have also attempted to identify the mechanisms responsible for the leukocytosis of exercise and, more recently, how these immunomodulatory effects of performing a single bout of exercise can be harnessed for clinical use. This chapter focuses on the effects of both a single bout of exercise (acute exercise) and regular exercise training (chronic exercise) on the numbers of leukocytes and leukocyte subsets circulating in the blood compartment of healthy people and discusses potential mechanisms and the factors that influence these exercise-induced changes.

Box 3.1 The numbers of circulating leukocytes and subsets are temporarily altered by an acute bout of exercise

- The number of circulating white blood cells (leukocytes) increases during acute exercise. This is referred to as the leukocytosis of exercise.
- The increase in the number of circulating leukocytes during exercise is largely caused by the mobilisation of neutrophils and lymphocytes, with a smaller contribution being made from monocytes.
- During the early stages of exercise recovery (within 30–60 minutes of exercise cessation) there is a rapid reduction in the blood lymphocyte count (lymphocytopenia) that is accompanied by a sustained neutrophilia (elevated blood neutrophil count). This neutrophilia occurs largely from an influx of neutrophils from the bone marrow under the influence of cortisol.
- In response to endurance-based exercise in particular, the blood lymphocyte count may fall 30–50% below pre-exercise values and can remain diminished for up to six hours after exercise.
- At rest, blood leukocyte, neutrophil, lymphocyte and monocyte counts are generally similar in athletes and non-athletes.

THE EFFECTS OF A SINGLE BOUT OF EXERCISE ON CIRCULATING LEUKOCYTE NUMBERS

Elevated numbers of circulating leukocytes are often used in a clinical setting as a sign of the presence of infection and/or inflammation. A typical normal resting blood leukocyte count is in the region of $4–11 \times 10^9$/L but these numbers may increase up to fourfold in response to a single bout of exercise (Figure 3.1). As exercise causes a profound leukocytosis, physical exercise was initially perceived to induce an inflammatory-like state akin to infection. However, it is now known that the leukocytosis that accompanies acute exercise is a transient phenomenon, as the numbers and composition of all leukocyte subsets are usually restored to resting values within 6–24 hours after cessation of exercise. The leukocytosis from exercise is largely caused by the mobilisation of neutrophils and lymphocytes, with a smaller contribution being made from monocytes. During the early stages of exercise recovery (within 30–60 minutes of exercise cessation) there is a rapid reduction in the blood lymphocyte count (lymphocytopenia) that is accompanied by a sustained neutrophilia (elevated blood neutrophil count). In response to endurance-based exercise in particular, the blood lymphocyte count may fall 30–50% below the

Figure 3.1 The effects of exercise intensity and duration on (A) the circulating leukocyte count and (B) the circulating neutrophil and lymphocyte counts. High intensity exercise (80% $\dot{V}O_2$ max) at relatively short duration (37 ± 19 minutes) causes a biphasic leukocytosis, whereby the initial increase in the blood leukocyte count with exercise is followed by a delayed leukocytosis 2.5 hours later. This delayed leukocytosis is driven by a sustained neutrophilia during the recovery phase of exercise, during which time there is a lymphocytopenia. Prolonged exercise (164 ± 23 minutes at 55% $\dot{V}O_2$ max), despite being lower in intensity, produces a much larger leukocytosis, which remains elevated for many hours after completion of the exercise bout. Data are mean ± SEM, n = 18; * indicates significant difference from pre-exercise ($P < 0.05$); † indicates significant difference compared with the 80% $\dot{V}O_2$ max trial. N = neutrophils; L = lymphocytes (data from Robson *et al.* 1999)

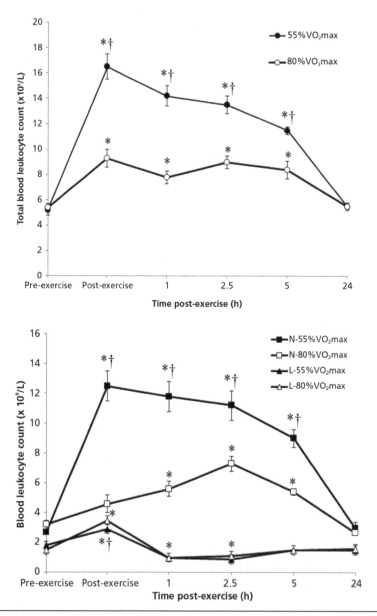

pre-exercise values and can remain diminished for up to six hours after exercise. Although striking changes in the total number of circulatory leukocytes in response to exercise has been well-documented, it is important to note that the total number of leukocytes present in peripheral blood at any given time comprises only one to two per cent of the total number of leukocytes disseminated throughout the entire body.

While the number and composition of certain leukocyte subtypes may not necessarily be indicative of cellular immune presence and function in other tissues, the peripheral circulation has been widely sourced, owing to the relative ease with which blood samples can be obtained from exercising human participants. In modern clinics and research laboratories, total leukocytes and leukocyte subset numbers are typically identified using an automated haematology analyser, which enumerates cells in blood according to their size and granularity. For the detection of more specialised cell subsets, fluorescently tagged monoclonal antibodies are used to bind to a surface receptor on the cell type of interest and quantified using a flow cytometer (see Technique box 3.1). The following sections of this chapter describe the effects of a single bout of exercise on the total number of leukocytes and leukocyte subsets present in the peripheral circulation.

Neutrophils

Neutrophils are the most abundant subset of white cells found in peripheral blood (50–70% of all leukocytes). They are highly responsive to initial infections and play a pivotal role in the inflammatory response to tissue injury and pathogen incursion. Neutrophils are phagocytic cells that help the host to combat rapidly dividing bacteria, yeast and fungal infections, by generating reactive oxygen and nitrogen species, release of proteolytic enzymes and microbicidal peptides from cytoplasmic granules (Shaw *et al.* 2010, 2011; see Chapter 2 for further details). Owing to their shear abundance, neutrophils are highly responsive to acute exercise and they account for the majority of exercise-induced leukocytosis. Very brief (of an order of minutes), high-intensity exercise may cause the neutrophil count to double, while prolonged bouts of endurance exercise may cause neutrophil numbers to increase three- to fourfold after exercise. Neutrophil counts tend to reach peak values during the recovery phase of exercise, although both the magnitude and the kinetics of the neutrophil response are influenced by the intensity and duration of exercise (Robson *et al.* 1999b). After an intensive bout of treadmill-running exercise lasting for around 37 minutes at 80% $\dot{V}O_2$max, neutrophil counts reached peak values three hours after exercise cessation (Robson *et al.* 1999b). In contrast, prolonged exercise lasting around 164 minutes at 55% $\dot{V}O_2$ max, despite causing a substantially greater neutrophilia, caused neutrophil counts to reach peak values immediately after exercise before slowly declining to baseline levels 24 hours later (Robson *et al.* 1999b). Acute exercise tends to mobilise neutrophils with a reduced expression of the low-affinity immunoglobulin G receptor CD16, with the effect being proportional to the intensity of the exercise bout (Peake *et al.* 2004). As CD16 is considered a marker of neutrophil functional capability and viability (Butcher *et al.* 2001), exercise would

Technique box 3.1

Phenotypic analysis and enumeration of lymphocyte subpopulations in whole blood in response to exercise

Whole-blood samples are labelled with monoclonal antibodies (mAbs) that react with specific cell surface markers of interest. Each mAb is conjugated to a particular fluorophore – a fluorescent chemical compound that emits light upon excitation by the flow cytometer's laser(s). The light emission is then collected by the detector filters of the flow cytometer to quantify the number of cells in a population expressing the surface marker of interest. The example in the figure below shows flow cytometry dotplots collected from a four-colour experiment. In this example, a single-cell suspension has been labelled with four separate mAbs that emit light at four different wavelengths. After the cells have been labelled with the mAbs, the red blood cells are lysed and the remaining white blood cells are quantified by the flow cytometer.

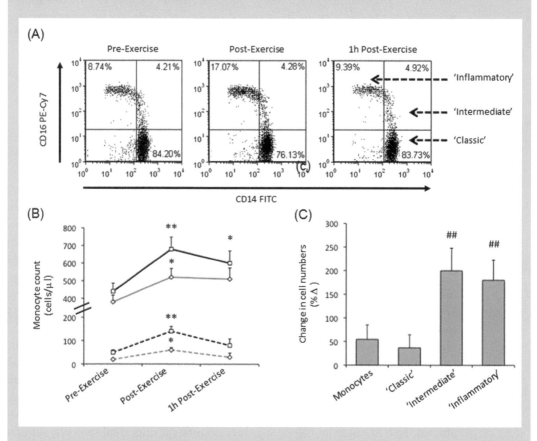

Plots A and D in the figure show the light scatter properties of the cell population. The amount of forward light scatter (FSC) is directly proportional to the size of the cell, while the amount of side scatter (SSC) is directly proportional to the internal complexity of the cell. Each dot in these plots represents a single cell. Lymphocytes, which are relatively small in size and have less internal complexity (granules) can be identified by their light-scatter properties and are electronically 'gated' on the flow cytometer (R1). The number of cells collected in the R1 gate per known volume of blood (after adjusting for any dilutions made with the lysis buffer) can then be used to obtain accurate whole-blood-cell counts. In this example, there has been almost a twofold increase in blood lymphocyte numbers caused by exercise (30 minutes cycling at 15% above the blood lactate threshold). Instructing the flow cytometer to analyse only those events collected in the R1 gate can assess the phenotype characteristics of the lymphocytes. In this example, we are interested in quantifying the CD8+ T cells, which can be identified by the co-expression of the surface antigens CD3 and CD8. To do this, mouse anti-human mAbs against CD3 (conjugated to the fluorophore allophycocyanin; APC) and CD8 (conjugated to the fluorophore peridinin chlorophyll protein complex, PerCP) have been used. Plots B and E show the percentage of all lymphocytes (R1) expressing these antigens. Single-positive, double-positive and double-negative cell populations can be identified by quantifying the dots in each area of the quadrant. In pre-exercise blood (Plot B), 17.9% of all lymphocytes are double positive (express both CD3 and CD8) and are therefore CD8+ T cells. The total number of CD8+ T cells can also be quantified by multiplying the percentage value by the total lymphocyte count. The CD3+/CD8+ cells are then electronically gated (R2) for further phenotypic analysis.

CD8+ T cells can be further stratified in accordance with their stage of differentiation (antigen experience, number of replications, cytotoxic potential) using the surface antigens CD27 and CD28 (Appay et al. 2008). Cells identified as having a 'late' differentiation phenotype do not express CD27 or CD28 (double negative). In plots C and F, changes in the composition of CD8+ subsets in response to exercise can be identified. The 'late' differentiated cells are located in the lower left quadrant, as they did not react with the mouse anti-human CD27 (conjugated to the fluorophore phycoerythrin; PE) or CD28 (conjugated to the fluorophore fluorescein isothiocyanate; FITC) mAbs. In this example, the percentage of 'late' cells among total CD8+ T-cells (R2) changed from 6.1% to 12.1%, owing to exercise. The total number of 'late' cells can readily be calculated by multiplying these percentage values by the total CD3+/CD8+ cell count. This revealed an almost 3.9-fold increase in the number of 'late' CD8+ T-cells from a single bout of exercise.

appear to mobilise neutrophils preferentially at an advanced stage of maturation. This has also been shown in adrenaline infusion studies, which induced a neutrophilia with a larger proportion of the mobilised cells having a segmented nucleus (Fehr and Grossmann 1979), indicating that exercise and/or adrenaline elicits a preferential mobilisation of 'older' neutrophils.

Monocytes and dendritic cells

Monocytes and dendritic cells are the antigen presenting cells found in peripheral blood. Monocytes comprise 5–15% of all leukocytes and can be identified by the surface antigen CD14. They have a half-life of two to three days and are ultimately destined to become tissue-resident macrophages that perform phagocytic and antigen-presenting functions within the immune system. There are three major subpopulations of CD14+ monocytes that can be identified using CD16 as a second surface marker:

- 'classical' monocytes express CD14 at high levels but do not express CD16 (CD14++/CD16-) and make up 70–80% of all monocytes;

- 'proinflammatory' monocytes, which are major producers of TNF-α, express low levels of CD14 and high levels of CD16 (CD14+/CD16++) and make up 8–15% of all monocytes;
- a population that makes up 4–10% of all monocytes, expresses high levels of CD14 but low levels of CD16 (CD14++/CD16+) and, because they produce copious amounts of IL-10 in response to stimulation, are considered to have a role to play in anti-inflammatory immune responses (Skrzeczynska-Moncznik *et al.* 2008).

Blood monocyte numbers increase in response to prolonged bouts (45–100 minutes) of endurance exercise (Booth *et al.* 2010; Lancaster *et al.* 2005a; Simpson *et al.* 2009), short bouts (30–40 seconds) of high-intensity (predominantly anaerobic) exercise (Steppich *et al.* 2000) and acute resistance exercise (Simonson and Jackson 2004), indicating that they are promiscuously responsive to many different types of exercise. Monocyte numbers increase after exercise in a way that alters the composition of their subsets. Monocytes expressing CD16 are preferentially mobilised over 'classical' monocytes (200–300% increase compared with 15–50%), causing a greater relative proportion of CD16+ monocytes post-exercise (Booth *et al.* 2010; Hong and Mills 2008; Simpson *et al.* 2009; Steppich *et al.* 2000). Unlike neutrophils, which continue to increase in number during exercise recovery, monocyte numbers quickly revert back to their original pre-exercise values within a short time after cessation of exercise, although there is some evidence for a delayed monocytosis following 1.5–2.0 hours of recovery after single bouts of endurance-based exercise (Pedersen *et al.* 1990; Shek *et al.* 1995). Changes in the concentration of monocyte subtypes following a single bout of exercise are shown in Figure 3.2.

Dendritic cells in peripheral blood are sparse less than one per cent of all leukocytes) (Haller Hasskamp *et al.* 2005) but are highly prevalent in the tissues and play an important role in regulating adaptive immune responses and maintaining immune self-tolerance (Agrawal *et al.* 2012). Two major subsets of dendritic cells are present in peripheral blood: myeloid (mDCs) and plasmacytoid (pDCs). Once fully mature, mDCs are mostly responsible for stimulating antigen-specific T cells during adaptive immune responses, while pDCs produce high levels of type-1 cytokines (e.g. IFN-γ) and play important roles in host defence against viral infections. There are typically twice as many mDCs compared with pDCs in resting blood, and a recent study showed that both dendritic-cell subset numbers increased in response to a 60-minute training session in elite ice hockey players (Suchanek *et al.* 2010). The relative increase in cell number was greater for pDCs compared with mDCs (171% versus 104%), indicating that pDCs may be more responsive to acute exercise. In contrast, however, Nikel *et al.* (2011) found that mDC numbers increased but pDC numbers decreased after marathon running.

Lymphocytes

Lymphocytes are the most heterogeneous of the blood leukocyte subtypes consisting of T cells, B cells and natural killer (NK) cells. These cell subsets make up 60–80%,

Figure 3.2 Changes in total monocyte and monocyte subset numbers in response to a 60-km cycling time trial (n = 8). 'Classic' (CD14++/CD16–), 'intermediate' (CD14++/CD16+) and 'inflammatory' (CD14+/CD16++) monocytes are identified by the surface expression of CD14 and CD16 (A). Total monocyte numbers increase in response to exercise and remain elevated up to 1 hour post-exercise (B). The numbers of both the 'inflammatory' and 'intermediate' subsets increase after exercise but return to baseline 1 hour later. Although the absolute number of 'classical' monocytes mobilised with exercise is largest, the relative change (from pre- to post-exercise) is greater for those monocyte subsets that express CD16 ('inflammatory' and 'intermediate') (C) causing an altered composition of monocyte subtypes in blood. Data are mean ± SE. Difference from pre-exercise indicated by * ($P < 0.05$) and ** ($P < 0.01$). Difference from total monocytes and 'classic' monocytes indicated by ## ($P < 0.01$) (data from Booth *et al.* 2010)

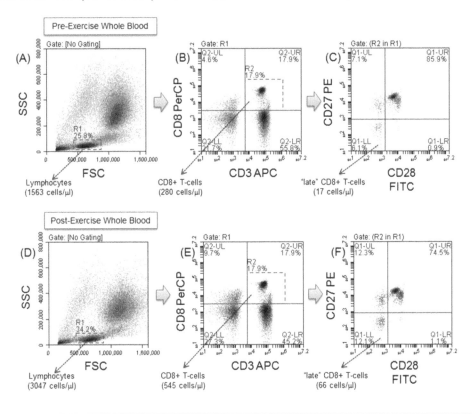

5–15% and 5–20% of the total lymphocyte pool, respectively. Each of these broadly defined lymphocyte subpopulations can be further divided into specialised lymphocyte subtypes that have distinctive phenotype characteristics and functional properties. T cells, in particular, are highly heterogeneous, comprising a various array of specialised subsets that have highly variable cytokine-secretion profiles, effector functions, antigen types and specificities, proliferative capabilities and surface marker expression (see Chapter 2 for further details). Acute exercise elicits a unique biphasic perturbation of the blood lymphocyte count, whereby an increase in lymphocyte number is observed during and immediately after exercise, before rapidly falling below the pre-exercise values during the early stages of exercise recovery, gradually returning to basal levels in the following hours (Shek *et al.* 1995). The effects of exercise on blood lymphocyte and lymphocyte subset numbers are shown in Figure 3.3.

Figure 3.3 The effects of a single bout of exercise on blood lymphocyte and lymphocyte subset numbers. Subjects ran on a treadmill at 65% $\dot{V}O_2$ max for 120 minutes with blood samples collected before exercise, during exercise and during exercise recovery. Total lymphocyte numbers increased (lymphocytosis) during exercise and remained elevated until exercise cessation (A). Within 60 minutes of recovery, the blood lymphocyte count had fallen below pre-exercise values (lymphocytopenia) and remained lowered at 120 minutes post-exercise. The lymphocyte count is restored after 24 hours of recovery. Within the T cell compartment, although the absolute number of CD4+ T cells is greater than CD8+ T-cell numbers, the relative change in CD8+ T-cell numbers (percentage change) is greater (B); data are mean ± SE (from Shek *et al.*(1995)

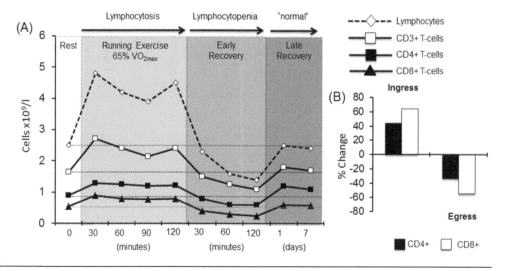

CD4+ and CD8+ T cells

T cells are broadly identified as CD4+ (helper T cells), CD8+ (cytotoxic T cells) or γδ T cells. T cells are highly responsive to acute exercise and, although the absolute number of CD4+ T cells mobilised with exercise is greater than that of CD8+ cells, the relative contribution (percentage change) of the CD8+ T cells is 1.5–2.0 times greater than that of CD4+ cells (Gabriel *et al.* 1991; Shek *et al.* 1995). The same is true for the post-exercise extravasation of T cells, which contributes to the well-documented lymphocytopenia, with the relative egress of CD8+ T-cells being up to three times greater than CD4+ T cells. This selective response of the CD8+ T cells usually causes a decline in the CD4 : CD8 T-cell ratio immediately after exercise, followed by an increase above baseline during the early stages of exercise recovery. However, because CD8 is also expressed on a subset of exercise-responsive NK cells (Campbell *et al.* 2008a), many studies had previously overestimated the CD8+ T cell response to acute exercise by failing to quantify only those CD8+ cells that expressed the T cell marker CD3. Caution should therefore be taken if changes in the CD4+/CD8+ T cell ratio with exercise were determined on cells that were not dual stained for CD3 and CD8 or not, at least, identified by the higher surface expression of the CD8 antigen (Campbell *et al.* 2008a).

More recently, attempts have been made to identify the exercise-responsive subsets of CD4+ and CD8+ T cells. Simpson *et al.* (2007a, 2008) showed that CD4+ and CD8+ T cells with a history of previous antigen exposure (defined by the surface expression of the killer lectin-like receptor G1, KLRG1) are more responsive to acute exercise than antigen-virgin T cells (KLRG1–). Specifically, the absolute number of KLRG1+/CD8+ T cells that were mobilised and subsequently left the blood compartment was two to three times greater than the KLRG1–/CD8+ T cells in response to maximal treadmill-running exercise (Simpson *et al.* 2007a, 2008). CD4+ and CD8+ T cells can be further divided into five distinct subsets according to their expression of the surface antigens CD27, CD28, CCR7 and CD45RA (Appay *et al.* 2008). These surface phenotypes are also indicative of their telomere lengths and, hence, their replicative potential, their ability to secrete cytokines, perform effector functions and also the viral specificity of the antigen-experienced CD8+ T cells (Appay *et al.* 2008). For instance, CD8+ T cells specific to the common latent herpes viruses Epstein Barr virus (EBV) or cytomegalovirus (CMV) are known to have different (although sometimes overlapping) phenotypic characteristics and functional properties compared with T cells specific for influenza or hepatitis (Appay *et al.* 2008). The four most accepted T-cell subtypes in order of their antigen experience (low to high) and ability to undergo multiple rounds of cell division (high to low) are: (1) naïve; (2) central memory; (3) effector memory; and (4) CD45RA+ effector memory cells (EMRA, sometimes referred to as senescent or terminally differentiated cells; Sallusto *et al.* 2004). Campbell *et al.* (2009) showed that effector memory and, particularly, EMRA CD8+ T cells, were mobilised to a greater extent than central memory and naïve CD8+ T cells in response to 20 minutes of cycling exercise. As with total T cell numbers, the mobilisation of the effector memory and EMRA subtypes was governed by the intensity of exercise, as the response was greater following cycling exercise at 85% of maximum aerobic power compared with 35% of maximum aerobic power (Campbell *et al.* 2009).

There is now a clear consensus that T cells with a longer history of antigen exposure and phenotypic characteristics associated with tissue migration and effector functions are preferentially mobilised in response to acute exercise (Simpson 2011). Early studies assumed that exercise mobilised a large number of naïve T cells, owing to the observed influx of cells expressing CD45RA (Ceddia *et al.* 1999; Gabriel *et al.* 1991). Although CD45RA was previously thought to identify naïve T cells (Akbar *et al.* 1988), the receptor was later found to be re-expressed on a subset of effector-memory T cells that had undergone multiple rounds of cell division (Sallusto *et al.* 1999). In essence, it is now clear that the increase in CD45RA+ cells (particularly for the CD8+ T cell subset) mostly represents a mobilisation of EMRA cells and not naïve cells, which actually contribute relatively little to the exercise-induced T-cell lymphocytosis (Campbell *et al.* 2009). The relative response of the CD8+ T cell subsets mobilised and egressed in response to acute exercise are shown in Figure 3.4.

Figure 3.4 Acute exercise elicits a preferential mobilisation of antigen-experienced CD8+ T cell subsets with increased effector functions and tissue migration potential. The surface markers CD28 and killer cell lectin-like receptor G1 (KLRG-1) can be used to identify cells with 'low' (CD28+/KLRG1–), 'medium' (CD28+/KLRG1+) and 'high' (CD28-/KLRG1+) antigen experience, effector functions (i.e. cytotoxicity) and tissue migration potential (A). Comparing the relative mobilisation of these CD8+ T cell subtypes (B) to a single bout of 30 minutes of cycling exercise in healthy adults (n = 16) revealed a stepwise increased ingress (from pre-exercise to post-exercise) and egress (from immediately post-exercise to 1 hour post-exercise) of those cell subsets associated with increased antigen experience, cytotoxic and tissue migration potential. CD8+ T cells are also identified as naïve (NA; CD45RA+/CD62L+), central memory (CM; CD45RA-/CD62L+), effector memory (EM; CD45RA–/CD62L–) and effector memory cells that re-express CD45RA (EMRA; CD45RA+/CD62L–) (C). This model of T-cell differentiation reflects the levels of antigen experience, effector functions and tissue migrating potential of the cell subsets. This phenotypic identification also revealed a stepwise increased mobilisation of those cell subsets associated with increased antigen experience, effector functions and tissue migration potential (D), indicating a preferential mobilisation of specific CD8+ T cell subsets in response to exercise. Data are mean ± SE (Simpson *et al.* unpublished data)

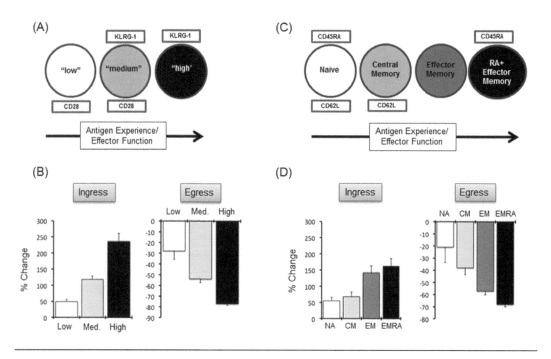

γδ T cells

Gamma delta (γδ) T cells are highly specialised cells of the immune system that recognise lipid and other non-peptide antigens. They are potent cytotoxic cells that aid the host in bacterial elimination, wound repair and delayed-type hypersensitivity reactions. γδ T cells have a high tissue-migrating phenotype and are found to infiltrate epithelial-rich tissue such as skin, intestines and the reproductive tract. They make up 2–15% of the total CD3+ blood T-cell population and are mostly negative for both CD4+ and CD8+ surface antigens. Only two studies to date have examined the effects of acute exercise on the numbers of γδ T cells (Anane *et al.* 2009; Bigley *et al.* 2012) and, as with other cell subsets that show high cytotoxic potential (i.e. CD8+ T cells and NK cells), γδ T cells are also highly responsive to acute exercise. In fact, from a relative standpoint (percentage change from pre-exercise counts), γδ T cells are more responsive to exercise than CD8+ T cells but less responsive than NK cells (Anane *et al.* 2009). Anane *et al.* (2009) showed that the exercise effect of mobilising γδ T cells could be replicated when the participants were infused with varying doses of the β2-agonist isoproterenol. Both exercise (35% and 85% of maximum aerobic power) and isoproterenol infusion increased γδ T cell mobilisation in a dose-dependent manner suggesting that, like many other leukocyte subsets, their mobilisation with exercise is governed by adrenergic mechanisms. Although the absolute number of γδ T cells deployed into the bloodstream is considerably lower than other lymphocyte subtypes, the relative mobilisation (percentage change) for γδ T cells is greater than that of CD4+ and CD8+ T cells but less than that of NK cells (Anane *et al.* 2009)

NK cells and NKT cells

NK cells comprise 5–20% of all blood lymphocytes and account for the majority of the exercise-induced lymphocytosis. NK cells are highly cytotoxic and are capable of distinguishing healthy autologous cells from malignant or virally infected cells without prior antigenic exposure. As such, NK cells can be stimulated by cytokines such as IL-2 and IL-12, allowing them to immediately recognise and destroy target cells. NK cells are identified by a CD3–/CD56+/CD16+ surface phenotype and also have two major subsets based on the level of CD56 expression. NK cells with low expression of CD56 (CD56dim) are highly cytotoxic and stress-responsive, whereas NK cells with higher expression of CD56 (CD56bright) are considered immunoregulatory, as they produce large amounts of cytokines but have low cytolytic activity (Poli *et al.* 2009). NK cells are rapidly mobilised into the blood compartment at the onset of exercise and, depending on the intensity of exercise, their numbers may increase from 50–400% (Gabriel *et al.* 1991, 1994a; Shek *et al.* 1995). Upon cessation of exercise, there is a rapid egress of NK cells that contributes largely to the exercise-induced lymphocytopenia that may take up to 24 or 48 hours to be fully restored. However, in response to very prolonged bouts of exercise (e.g. two hours of cycling) the NK cell count has been reported to be 40% lower than baseline values for up to seven days post-exercise (Shek *et al.* 1995). At rest, approximately 90% of circulating NK cells are CD56dim while the rest are CD56bright; however, these proportions change in response to exercise, owing to the preferential mobilisation of the CD56dim subset (Campbell *et al.* 2009; Timmons and Cieslak 2008).

Recent work has shown a selective mobilisation of NK cells with specific surface receptors. Although there does not appear to be a preferential mobilisation of NK cell subsets defined by their surface expression of KLRG1 or CD57 (Bigley *et al.* 2012; Simpson *et al.* 2008), NK cell subsets expressing CD158a show a preferential deployment (Bigley *et al.* 2012). Although long-considered to be a cellular component of innate immunity, there is mounting evidence in both mice and humans that NK cells possess antigen-specific receptors, proliferate in response to infection and generate long-lived memory cells, all of which are key components of T and B cell responses in adaptive immunity (Sun and Lanier 2011). It was shown recently that NK cells undergo a process of differentiation, with some of them becoming long-lived memory NK cells (Beziat *et al.* 2010). Although T cells with a mature phenotype are more responsive to exercise, it remains to be determined if antigen-experienced memory-like NK cells are also more preferentially mobilised with exercise in a similar manner to CD8+ T cells.

A population of T cells exist that have been referred to as NK-like T cells or simply NKT cells (Peralbo *et al.* 2007). These cells are almost entirely CD3+ and CD8+ but also express the 'NK-cell markers' CD56 and CD161 and respond to glycolipids presented by CD1d (Peralbo *et al.* 2007). NKT cells appear to be preferentially mobilised in response to a single bout of exercise. Bigley *et al.* (2012) reported a greater relative change in CD56+ T cells numbers compared to CD56- T-cell numbers in response to 30 minutes of cycling exercise, although it was not confirmed that these cells expressed CD161 or recognised antigen presented by the MHC-like molecule CD1d. More research work is required to characterise the response of bona fide NKT cells to single bouts of exercise.

B cells

B cells express the surface antigens CD19 and CD20 and account for 5–15% of circulating lymphocytes. Like T cells, B cells are a major cellular component of the adaptive immune system. Owing to the relatively low numbers of these cells present in the circulation, it is not surprising that they contribute relatively little to the exercise-induced lymphocytosis. Although there is a trend for B cell numbers to increase after endurance-based exercise, including 45 minutes of treadmill running at 80% $\dot{V}O_2$ max (Nieman *et al.* 1994) or 30–120 minutes of treadmill running at 65% $\dot{V}O_2$ max (Shek *et al.* 1995), these tend not to reach statistically significant levels. However, B cells are perhaps more sensitive to the intensity and not the duration of exercise because larger increases in B cell numbers have been documented following an exhaustive treadmill running protocol (Fry *et al.* 1992a) and six minutes of maximal rowing exercise (Nielsen *et al.* 1998). As the B cell mobilisation with exercise is relatively small compared with other lymphocyte populations, studies on B cell responses to acute exercise have essentially been neglected since the mid-1990s. This is unfortunate because, like T cells, B cells are also very heterogeneous consisting of both naïve and memory subsets (Bulati *et al.* 2011) but whether or not acute exercise elicits a profound redistribution of discrete B cell subtypes awaits investigation.

Type-1 and type-2 T cells

Cytokines are cell-signalling protein molecules that are secreted by many cells of the immune system and are critical to the development of both pro- and anti-inflammatory immune responses following infection or injury. While some cytokines (i.e. IFN-γ) promote predominantly cell-mediated, or type-1, immune responses, other cytokines (i.e. IL-4) are involved in the activation of humoral, or type-2, immune responses (Mosmann and Sad 1996). The plasma concentrations of many cytokines have been found to change in response to a single bout of exercise, although this provides little information regarding the cell types responsible for their secretion. Almost all nucleated cells produce cytokines that are quickly secreted during an immune response. Therefore, to detect cytokine expression in individual leukocyte subsets, the cells must be stimulated *in vitro* to mimic an immune response (i.e. with a mitogen, lipopolysaccharide or gram-negative bacteria) and the transport of the produced cytokine from the endoplasmic reticulum to the Golgi apparatus must be blocked to prevent its secretion. This allows the cytokine to accumulate in the endoplasmic reticulum where it can be detected following cell permeabilisation and labelling with monoclonal antibodies. This technique has been used to quantify the numbers of type-1 and type-2 T cells in the circulation in response to exercise. Steensberg *et al.* (2001b) reported that the percentage of type-1 CD4+ and CD8+ T-cells expressing IFN-γ and IL-2 was lower immediately after and during the recovery phase of exercise following 2.5 hours of treadmill-running at 75% $\dot{V}O_2$ max, whereas the percentage of type-2 CD4+ and CD8+ T-cells expressing IL-4 remained unchanged. The numbers of CD4+ and CD8+ T-cells were also lowered at these times indicating that exercise may have evoked the preferential egress of T-cells expressing type-1 cytokines (Steensberg *et al.* 2001b). These findings were supported by Lancaster *et al.* (2004) who reported a reduction in both the number and percentage of T cells expressing type-1 cytokines immediately after and during the recovery phase of a prolonged exercise bout. In response to shorter duration exercise (19 minutes at 78% $\dot{V}O_2$ max), Starkie *et al.* (2001c) also reported that the percentage of stimulated T cells expressing IFN-γ and IL-2 was lower immediately after exercise, although the absolute number of type-1 cytokine expressing T cells had increased. The numerical increase in type-1 cytokines was diminished in subjects who received a β-adrenoreceptor antagonist (timolol maleate) two hours before exercise, although this method of adrenergic blockade did not prevent the reduction in the percentage of T cells expressing cytokines (Starkie *et al.* 2001). This indicates that exercise may have altered cytokine production in T cells via catecholamine independent pathways. It is therefore difficult to enumerate type-1 and type-2 cells in response to a single bout of exercise because the exercise bout itself may alter the ability of these cells to express their cytokines.

Although exercise may impair or augment the ability of individual cells to mount a cytokine response following an immune challenge, it is very likely that these apparent changes in cytokine expression with exercise are due to proportional shifts of discrete cell subtypes that have pre-existing cytokine profiles. For instance, CD8+ T cells preferentially mobilised with exercise are known to have a high tissue-migration phenotype (Campbell *et al.* 2009) and cells with this phenotype have, in turn, been shown to express increased levels of type-1 cytokines such as IFN-γ and IL-2 (Matsui *et al.* 2003). Indeed, Ibfelt *et al.* (2002) concluded that the decreased percentage of CD8+ T-cells expressing IFN-γ after exercise was due to a decrease in the number and proportion of memory (CD45RO+) cells that constitutively express increased levels of type-1 cytokines. However, a more recent study reported an increased number of lymphocytes and monocytes expressing both type-1 and type-2 cytokines immediately after exercise in cells that were not stimulated with an immunogenic agent (Zaldivar *et al.* 2006). This may indicate that exercise primes effector leukocytes to express an array of cytokines in preparation for their migration to bodily areas that require enhanced immune surveillance following physical stress.

MECHANISMS INVOLVED IN THE LEUKOCYTE RESPONSE TO ACUTE EXERCISE

Ever since Larrabee (1902) first reported that exercise induced a pronounced leukocytosis, three pertinent questions regarding this phenomenon emerged: (1) what are the mechanisms that underpin the leukocyte response to exercise; (2) where in the body are these cells coming from; and (3) what are the evolutionary and/or clinical implications for rapidly mobilising large numbers of leukocytes in response to a single bout of exercise. A great deal of effort has been made over the last three decades to help answer these questions. In terms of mechanisms, early studies had purported that homeostatic proliferation and exercise-induced hypovolaemia as a result of fluid loss from the blood plasma as possible reasons. Although infection may cause some cells of the immune system (i.e. lymphocytes) to proliferate, the increased leukocyte count after exercise is too rapid to be an effect of increased rates of cell division, which can take as long 48–72 hours to occur. Moreover, neutrophils are largely responsible for the exercise-induced leukocytosis and, as they are already terminally differentiated, are incapable of homeostatic proliferation. Fluid loss from blood plasma, despite causing a degree of haemoconcentration, is also unlikely to fully account for the leukocytosis of exercise. For instance, plasma volume rarely decreases by more than 15% after prolonged exercise whereas the blood leukocyte count may increase up to 400% (Shek *et al.* 1995).

The mechanisms responsible for the mobilisation of discrete leukocyte subtypes are now known to be multi-factorial and involve the demargination of leukocyte reservoirs contained within the blood vessels, lung, spleen and the liver and the actions of catecholamine and glucocorticoid hormones (see Box 3.2). The recruitment of leukocytes into the blood also appears to be highly selective in that only those cells that would be considered useful in response to a 'flight or fight' situation are markedly deployed in response to exercise. Here, we discuss a number of potential mechanisms involved in the leukocyte response to a single bout of exercise.

Leukocyte demargination

The intravascular pool of leukocytes is composed of one compartment that is circulating and another that is marginated (adhered) to the vascular endothelium

---

Box 3.2 Mechanisms contributing to the leukocytosis of exercise

- There are several mechanisms that are responsible for the increase in the numbers of leukocytes in the circulation during exercise
- Fluid loss from blood plasma causes a small degree of haemoconcentration: plasma volume typically decreases by 5–15% after exercise at 50–90% $\dot{V}O_2$ max and this will result in an equivalent concentration of the numbers of cells (both erythrocytes and leukocytes) per litre of blood. Since the blood leukocyte count may increase up to 400% after prolonged exercise (Shek *et al.* 1995), this haemoconcentration obviously only plays a minor role.
- In the early stages of acute exercise, leukocytes that were adhered to blood vessel walls, particularly those blood vessels in the lungs, spleen and the liver (referred to as the marginated pool of leukocytes) become detached and enter the circulating pool as a result of increased blood flow (shear stress) and the actions of catecholamines (adrenaline and noradrenaline), which reduce adhesion-molecule expression on the cell surface of leukocytes and endothelial cells making them 'less sticky'. This effect can account for up to a 100% increase in the circulating leukocyte count and will account for most of the leukocytosis observed after short-term high intensity exercise (greater than 90% $\dot{V}O_2$ max).
- Further increases (up to 400%) in the blood leukocyte count may occur during prolonged exercise (e.g. a marathon race), mainly as a result of influx of neutrophils from the bone marrow. In fact, the number of circulating lymphocytes may start to fall below pre-exercise levels when exercise duration exceeds two to three hours.
- The recruitment of leukocytes into the blood also appears to be highly selective in that only those cells that would be considered useful in response to a 'flight or fight' situation are markedly deployed in response to exercise.

(Berkow and Dodson 1987) that lines the entire circulatory system. The pulmonary vascular bed and, to a lesser extent, the spleen and liver, harbours a large reservoir for the marginated pool of leukocytes that can be mobilised by exercise or catecholamines. Circulatory leukocytes become marginated when they move closer to the vessel walls where the blood flow is considerably slower than in the main axial stream. This allows them to adhere to the vessel walls, presumably in preparation for rolling adhesion and potential activation and migration to the tissues that may require their presence (i.e. sites of infection). The size of the marginal pool that lines the blood vessel walls is estimated to be equal to that of the circulatory pool (Athens *et al.* 1961); hence, a complete demargination would double the number of circulating leukocytes (Figure 3.5). However, marginal pools in the lung, spleen, liver and other organs also contribute to the leukocytosis of exercise, with the lung marginated pool of lymphocytes estimated to be ten times larger than the circulating pool (Hogg and Doerschuk 1995). Therefore, a demargination of leukocytes from the pulmonary, hepatic or splenic reservoirs, in combination with a release of leukocytes from the blood vessel walls, might explain why the total leukocyte count can increase three- to fourfold after a single bout of prolonged exercise.

Figure 3.5 Leukocyte demargination in response to a single bout of exercise increases the blood leukocyte count. Around 50% of all leukocytes in resting blood are adhered to the blood vessel walls. These are referred to as marginated leukocytes. Increases in cardiac output, shear stress and catecholamines with exercise cause leukocyte demargination that increases the circulating leukocyte count. A complete demargination of leukocytes from the vessel walls into the circulation would result in a twofold increase in the total circulating leukocyte count

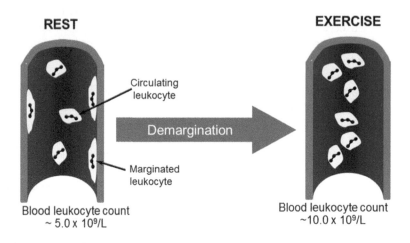

Although catecholamines and glucocorticoids are involved in the leukocytosis of exercise (discussed further in this chapter), the increased mechanical forces associated with elevations in cardiac output, vascular vasodilation and blood flow can demarginate leukocytes by detaching them from the endothelium and into the circulatory pool. This, in combination with greater levels of shear stress within the capillary structures that contain marginated leukocytes, can also sever leukocyte–endothelial cell interactions and force more leukocytes into the peripheral circulation. An increase in lymphatic flow with exercise could also contribute to the expansion of the circulatory leukocyte pool, owing to the increased emptying of lymph into the blood via the thoracic duct. Thus, haemodynamic factors appear to be responsible for the majority of the leukocyte demargination that occurs with exercise, particularly for neutrophils and most monocytes. However, this mechanism of leukocyte recruitment may not be sufficient to deploy adequate numbers of lymphocytes and monocytes, as certain lymphocyte and monocyte subtypes appear to have a greater reliance on catecholamine-mediated mechanisms (Dimitrov *et al.* 2010).

Sources and destinations of the leukocytes mobilised by exercise

Although the vast majority of leukocytes that enter the blood with exercise come from the marginal pools, the tissues and organs that deliver these cells to the blood are not fully understood. Owing to the substantial size of their marginated leukocyte reservoirs, it would appear that the lung, spleen and liver are major contributors, while other tissues that contain large numbers of white cells such as the lymph nodes, intestines, bone marrow, thymus gland, and even skeletal muscle, may also be responsible for deploying certain leukocyte subsets into the circulation. It is highly probable that the mechanisms and tissues responsible for the mobilisation of leukocytes into the circulation will vary depending on the type of cell that is deployed. For instance, neutrophil recruitment may enter the circulatory pool from the marginated pool or the bone marrow, while lymphocyte demargination may occur from the spleen under the influence of adrenaline and noradrenaline.

Most granulocytes mobilised with exercise are believed to come from the vascular and pulmonary marginated pools, especially those that rapidly enter the blood during the onset of exercise. However, following more prolonged and/or intensive exercise bouts, the leukocyte count may continue to rise during exercise recovery. This delayed leukocytosis is mostly attributable to a delayed neutrophilia and appears to be influenced by cortisol as, not only do plasma cortisol levels reach peak values during the recovery phase of very prolonged exercise, infusion of exogenous glucocorticoids for several hours also induces a delayed neutrophilia (Tonnesen *et al.* 1987). It has been suggested that an increased release of neutrophils from the bone marrow contributes to the delayed neutrophilia (Allsop *et al.* 1992), resulting in a greater proportion of immature neutrophils among the total circulating pool. It is possible that certain monocyte subtypes are also released into the circulation from the bone marrow during exercise recovery. Although monocyte numbers tend to return to baseline values during the early stages of exercise recovery (i.e. 30–60 minutes post-exercise), a delayed monocytosis has been observed after 1.5–2.0 hours of recovery following 60 minutes of cycling exercise at 75% $\dot{V}O_2$ max (Pedersen *et al.* 1990). Similarly, Shek *et al.* (1995) reported a delayed monocytosis two hours after completing a bout of treadmill running exercise at 65% $\dot{V}O_2$ max lasting two hours. Although B cells also mature in the bone marrow, their numbers in the peripheral circulation increase only marginally with exercise and, like other lymphocyte subsets, B cell numbers tend to decrease during the early stage of exercise recovery (Shek *et al.* 1995).

The spleen is considered to harbour an extensive reservoir of exercise-responsive lymphocytes (Baum *et al.* 1996) and acute exercise models in splenectomised humans have revealed a blunted mobilisation of T cells and NK cells into the periphery when compared with healthy age-matched controls (Nielsen *et al.* 1997). As splenectomised individuals mobilise about one-third of all the T cells and NK cells that are mobilised by healthy subjects, despite exhibiting similar plasma catecholamine levels and cardiac outputs to exercise (Nielsen *et al.* 1997), this would indicate that the spleen is a major source of the lymphocytes deployed into the blood with exercise. As you will learn in the next section of this chapter, catecholamines play a major role in the leukocytosis and lymphocytosis of exercise; however, when both adrenaline and noradrenaline were infused into both healthy and splenectomised individuals, a similar recruitment of NK cells into the blood was observed (Schedlowski *et al.* 1996), suggesting that NK cells are mobilised via spleen-independent β2-adrenoreceptor (β2-AR) mechanisms. Taken together, these studies indicate that NK cell mobilisation with exercise may involve both shear stress-induced demargination and β2-AR mechanisms, and that shear stress (associated with increased cardiac output and blood flow that is markedly greater during exercise than with catecholamine infusion) is required to elicit a pronounced demargination of NK cells from the spleen. Indeed, subjects who received an intravenous injection of the β2-antagonist propranolol immediately prior to performing an acute bout of exercise still exhibited a lymphocytosis, although this response was blunted compared with the control condition (Foster *et al.* 1986). As cardiac output and catecholamine concentrations were similar between the propranolol and control conditions (Foster *et al.* 1986), this would also indicate that both shear stress and catecholamine mechanisms are involved in exercise-induced lymphocytosis. It is interesting to note that the total leukocytosis was unaffected by propranolol infusion (Foster *et al.* 1986), suggesting that haemodynamic stress and not β2-AR mechanisms may be largely responsible for the demargination of neutrophils and other granulocytes with exercise.

Although lymphocytes are widely disseminated throughout the body, the phenotypic characteristics of those lymphocyte subsets deployed by exercise (i.e. mature, differentiated, high tissue migration potential) indicate that they are unlikely to come from the primary lymphoid organs such as the thymus or bone marrow (Campbell *et al.* 2009; Simpson *et al.* 2007a; 2008). Conversely, secondary lymphoid organs such as the spleen and intestinal Peyer's patches, in addition to tertiary lymphoid tissue such as the skin and mucosal epithelium of the gastrointestinal and pulmonary tracts, are likely to be a source of lymphocyte recruitment into the blood. It is also unlikely that the lymph nodes contribute much toward the mobilised lymphocytes, as most lymphocytes that enter the blood with exercise do not express the lymph node homing receptor CD62L (Hong *et al.* 2004; Simpson *et al.* 2008). Moreover, naïve T cells and central memory T cells, which preferentially circulate among the blood and lymph nodes, are mobilised in relatively fewer numbers with exercise, compared with those lymphocytes that preferentially migrate to the peripheral tissues such as effector memory and EMRA T cells (Campbell *et al.* 2009).

A single bout of exercise elicits a large deployment of leukocytes from the marginated pools into the circulation; however, on cessation of exercise, many of these leukocyte subsets eventually return to resting levels (neutrophils, monocytes) or even retract below the baseline values (lymphocytes). It is not fully understood what happens to cause these large numbers of immune cells to leave the blood after exercise. They may simply return to their pre-exercise destinations or be deployed to other tissues and organs throughout the body that require increased immune surveillance after exercise. As with the leukocytosis, it is likely that the fate of the mobilised cells will differ among the specific leukocyte subtypes. When normal blood flow is restored, many of the demarginated leukocytes that entered the circulatory pool will simply remarginate by adhering to the vascular endothelium or re-joining the marginated pool of the lung, spleen and liver. Some neutrophils and monocytes may infiltrate skeletal muscle, particularly if the exercise bout caused a significant amount of muscle damage (Tidball 2002) or migrate toward the intestines to compensate for a lack of blood flow to this tissue during exercise. The lung and upper airways are also likely to attract a greater amount of leukocyte trafficking, owing to the increased ventilation rates associated with exercise, drying of the mucosal surfaces and possible exposure to airborne pathogens and environmental air pollutants (Gomes *et al.* 2011).

Catecholamines and glucocorticoids

The mechanisms that underpin exercise-induced leukocytosis are fairly well characterised and appear to be largely governed by increased sympathetic nervous system activity and the resulting secretion of catecholamines (i.e. the hormone adrenaline and the neurotransmitter noradrenaline) (Anane *et al.* 2009; Atanackovic *et al.* 2006). Moreover, the corticotrophin-releasing hormone, adrenocorticotrophic hormone (ACTH) and cortisol make up the hypothalamic–pituitary–adrenal (HPA) axis and any activation of the HPA axis also has a profound effect on leukocyte trafficking. While activation of the sympathetic nervous system, especially those activities that induce a strong noradrenaline response (high-intensity exercise), causes a profound leukocytosis within minutes of the stressor being applied, activation of the HPA axis and the resulting secretion of cortisol causes an increase in leukocyte (neutrophil) numbers that is most evident within a few hours after cessation of the stressor (i.e. during the recovery phase following a bout of exercise) (Dhabhar 2009). The involvement of the sympathetic nervous system and HPA axis on leukocyte mobilisation is also evident in other forms of acute stress, such as public speaking tasks (Bosch *et al.* 2005; Schedlowski *et al.* 1993) or parachute jumping (Schedlowski *et al.* 1993). For the most part, these types of acute psychological stress elicit the same biphasic response of the total blood leukocyte count that is akin to exercise, suggesting that the effects of exercise on leukocyte trafficking are largely governed by an activation of the sympathetic nervous system and HPA axis.

This contention is supported by a large number of studies that have used catecholamine and glucocorticoid infusion models in resting humans (Figure 3.6). Similar to acute stress and exercise, leukocytes are rapidly deployed into the bloodstream in response to intravenous infusion with catecholamines (Dimitrov *et al.* 2010) or synthetic β-agonists (isoproterenol) (Anane *et al.* 2009) and the use of non-selective β-blockers such as propranolol, enables the blocking of this response (Schedlowski *et al.* 1996). These studies provide strong evidence that the mobilisation of leukocytes with exercise is largely influenced by the release of catecholamines that bind to adrenoreceptors expressed on the surface of the exercise-responsive cells. It is not surprising, therefore, that the cell types that show the greatest response to exercise (in terms of being mobilised into the blood compartment) also express predominantly high affinity β2-AR compared with those cell types mobilised in relatively fewer numbers. For example, CD8+ T cells, in addition to being more responsive to exercise, are more sensitive to β2-AR upregulation *in vitro* compared with CD4+ T cells (Wahle *et al.* 2001). Moreover, because β2-AR expression also increases with leukocyte activation and differentiation, this has been proposed as basic evolutionary mechanism that allows for the rapid redistribution of cytotoxic

Figure 3.6 The percentage change in the numbers of lymphocyte subsets in response to 16 minutes of low (35% maximum power) or high (85% maximum power) intensity cycling exercise (A) in healthy subjects (n = 11). The mobilisation of NK cells, γδ T cells and CD8+ T cells was replicated by infusing resting subjects (n = 12) with low (20 ng/kg/minute) and high (40 ng/kg/minute) concentrations of the β-agonist isoproterenol (B), indicating that lymphocyte mobilisation with exercise is dependent, at least partially, on catecholamine- mediated mechanisms (data from Anane *et al.* 2009)

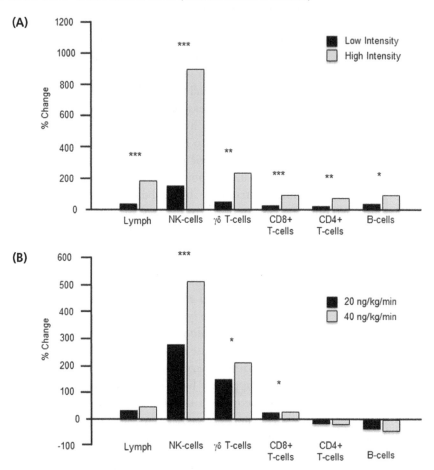

effector cells to increase immunosurveillance requirements at sites of potential injury during and after an acute stressor (Dimitrov *et al.* 2010).

Those leukocyte subtypes that preferentially egress from the blood during exercise recovery are highly responsive to glucocorticoids. For instance, monocytes stimulated with cortisol or post-exercise serum *in vitro* show an increased expression of CCR2 and an increased migratory response toward monocyte chemotactic protein-1 (MCP-1) (Okutsu *et al.* 2008). These effects were blocked by the glucocorticoid receptor antagonist RU486, indicating that monocytes exit the blood compartment after exercise via glucocorticoid receptor and CCR2-dependent mechanisms (Okutsu *et al.* 2008). The same group reported similar results for the extravasation of blood lymphocytes (Okutsu *et al.* 2005). Peripheral blood mononuclear cells were stimulated *in vitro* with cortisol or autologous serum obtained before and after an acute bout of exhaustive cycling exercise. Both cortisol and post-exercise serum were found to augment CD4+ and CD8+ T-cell CXCR4 expression, which was subsequently blocked by RU486 (Okutsu *et al.* 2005). T-cell migration toward CXCL12 was also markedly elevated by cortisol and post-exercise plasma stimulation, indicating that endogenous cortisol may be involved in the lymphocytopenia of exercise via CXCR4 signalling pathways (Okutsu *et al.* 2005).

The biphasic response of blood leukocytes following exercise and acute stress has been metaphorically likened to a military operation (Dhabhar 2009). During a period of acute stress or exercise, secreted catecholamines (i.e. adrenaline and noradrenaline) deploy the body's 'soldiers' (leukocytes) to exit the 'barracks' (spleen, lung, marginated pool and other organs) and enter the 'ramparts' (blood vessels and lymphatics) (Dhabhar 2009). This causes a profound increase in the total number of circulating leukocytes, with the mobilisation of granulocytes and lymphocytes accounting for the vast majority of the blood leukocyte response. As those leukocyte subtypes that have high cytotoxic and/or effector functions (i.e. NK cells, non-classical monocytes, γδ T cells, etc.) appear to be preferentially deployed to the 'ramparts', it is mostly 'armed' soldiers that are moved in preparation for battle with a would be enemy (i.e. tissue injury or invading microorganisms). Thus, the mobilisation of leukocytes from the barracks to the ramparts not only increases strength in numbers but also increases virility by deploying only those cells that are efficient fighters. As the exercise bout continues, activation of the HPA axis and the release of glucocorticoid hormones (i.e. cortisol) elicits the extravasation of leukocytes from the blood to take up their positions at potential 'battle stations', such as the skin, lung, gastrointestinal and urinary-genital tracts, mucosal surfaces and lymph nodes, in preparation for potential immune responses that may be required, owing to the stressor (Dhabhar 2009).

Adhesion molecules

In addition to an increased expression of high-affinity β2-AR, the selective recruitment of leukocytes with exercise appears to be influenced by the expression profile of adhesion molecules on the surface of the cell (Shephard 2003). Adhesion molecules are ubiquitously expressed on many cells throughout the body and play a critical role in cell-to-cell binding and, in particular, the trafficking of leukocytes between blood vessels and tissues (Figure 3.7). In general, the leukocyte subtypes that are preferentially mobilised with exercise tend to have a higher surface expression of the integrins (Gannon *et al.* 2001; Shephard 2003; Simpson *et al.* 2006a; van Eeden *et al.* 1999). Integrins such as LFA-1 (CD18/CD11a) or Mac-1 (CD18/CD11b) mediate the attachment of the cell to the surrounding tissues and extracellular matrix. They are therefore important for cell transmigration (from the blood to the tissue) and for signal transduction and activation. van Eeden *et al.* (1999) reported that the expression of CD11b on total granulocytes was more than doubled immediately after maximal treadmill running. Similarly, monocyte

Figure 3.7 The multistep process of leukocyte extravasation from the bloodstream. The initial phase of leukocyte (lymphocytes are used as an example here) extravasation involves tethering and rolling of the cell along the endothelium, a process that is mediated by selectins and their ligands. L-selectin (CD62L) on the cell surface binds to its ligand CD34 on the endothelium, which facilitates a weak transient contact between the lymphocyte and the endothelial cells (A). The lymphocyte then rolls along the endothelium in the direction of blood flow until the cell becomes activated by a chemokine (B). This increases the avidity of LFA-1 for its endothelial ligand ICAM-1. When these receptors bind, the rolling arrests and the lymphocyte becomes firmly attached to the endothelium resisting the forces of blood flow. Diapedesis then occurs as the lymphocyte squeezes through adjacent endothelial cells into the interstitial space before subsequently migrating along the chemokine concentration gradient into the tissues

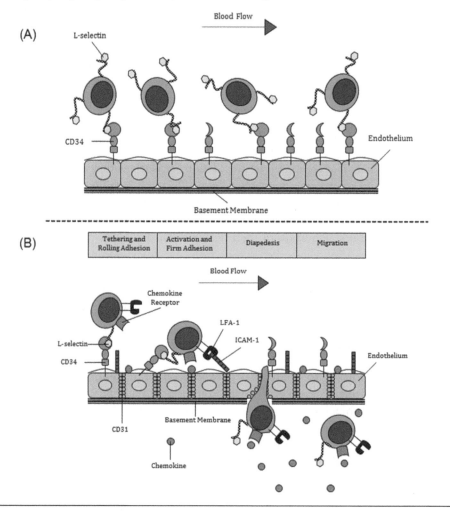

expression of CD11b was elevated after acute exercise, particularly on the classical and intermediate subtypes (Hong and Mills 2008), while Simpson et al. (2006a) showed that CD8+ T cells and NK cells mobilised with exercise had a heightened expression of the adhesion molecules CD18 (β2 integrin), CD54 (intracellular adhesion molecule-1, ICAM-1) and CD53, indicating that the mobilised lymphocytes had a mature, previously activated phenotype. Similar adhesion molecule profiles have been observed in lymphocyte subtypes mobilised in response to acute psychological stress tasks and (β-agonist infusion (Dimitrov *et al.* 2010; Goebel and Mills 2000).

Some adhesion molecules also function as homing receptors that are believed to provide leukocytes with an 'address' for tissue-specific migration (Sackstein 2005). For example, L-selectin (CD62L) facilitates the attachment and rolling of leukocytes to activated endothelium by binding to GlyCam-1 on high endothelial venules, or CD34 and MadCAM-1 expressed by endothelial cells, and is a known T-cell homing receptor for lymph nodes (see Shephard 2003 or Sackstein 2005 for a more detailed review on the role of adhesion molecules in lymphocyte trafficking). Although highly expressed on naïve T cells, CD62L is also expressed on neutrophils, monocytes and B cells and is generally considered to be a marker of an immature immune cell (Shephard 2003). Neutrophils, monocytes and lymphocytes mobilised with exercise tend to express very low levels of this receptor (Gannon *et al.* 2001; Hong *et al.* 2004; Hong and Mills 2008; Nielsen and Lyberg 2004; Simpson *et al.* 2007a; van Eeden *et al.* 1999), adding to the evidence that exercise preferentially deploys mature, previously activated immune cells. However, during the recovery phase of exercise when the neutrophil count may continue to rise, it is likely that a mobilisation of immature neutrophils from the bone marrow is contributing at least partially to this response (Allsop *et al.* 1992). The preferential mobilisation of lymphocytes expressing no or very low levels of CD62L would indicate that the lymph nodes are not major contributors to the lymphocytosis of exercise (Simpson 2011).

Although catecholamines are known to be potent stimulators of leukocyte deployment into the blood, it appears that this response is linked to a specific adhesion molecule and chemokine receptor expression profile. Dimitrov *et al.* (2010) analysed adhesion molecule and chemokine receptor expression of 14 leukocyte subsets in response to adrenaline infusion in humans. Those cell subsets that have heightened cytotoxic/effector properties, namely EMRA CD8+ T cells, γδ T cells, NK cells, NKT cells, CD56dim cytotoxic NK cells, and proinflammatory (CD14+/CD16++) monocytes, were rapidly and preferentially deployed into the blood after infusion with physiological concentrations of adrenaline (Dimitrov *et al.* 2010). These cells exhibited a CD62L-/CD11a[bright]/CXCR3[bright] surface phenotype that was strongly associated with the adrenergic-induced leukocytosis and they also had the strongest adherence to activated endothelium *in vitro* (Dimitrov *et al.* 2010). The adherence of these cells to the endothelium was reversed by adding physiological concentrations of adrenaline (Dimitrov *et al.* 2010), indicating that the release of catecholamines during exercise rapidly severs the attachment of leukocytes from the endothelium to allow the demargination and release of these potent cytotoxic/effector cells into the bloodstream.

It is important to note that the leukocytes mobilised into the blood with exercise may constitutively express certain surface adhesion molecules (and indeed other receptors) that are not necessarily altered at the individual cell level (Simpson *et al.*

2006a; Turner *et al.* 2011). Therefore, terms such as 'increased/decreased expression' or 'upregulation/downregulation' are misnomers, as they suggest that an increased de novo synthesis or a shedding/internalisation of the receptor has occurred on the individual cell. It is more likely that exercise causes a selective recruitment of specific leukocyte subsets that have pre-existing differences in surface adhesion molecule expression, thus altering their proportions among a total cell population and are often misinterpreted as 'expression changes'. For instance, the percentage of all lymphocytes expressing the T-cell marker CD3 may be 70% at rest, before decreasing to around 50% immediately after exercise. This does not mean that exercise has caused a 'downregulation' of CD3 expression in individual cells but rather evoked a preferential mobilisation of lymphocyte subsets that do not constitutively express CD3 (i.e. NK cells) into the blood. In fact, the total number of CD3+ T cells in the blood will be markedly elevated when the percentage values are multiplied by the total lymphocyte count (see Technique box 3.1). The same is true when the mean fluorescent intensity of the receptor is used to quantify expression, as exercise could simply mobilise a greater number of cells that have a lower or higher number of pre-existing receptors on the surface. Unfortunately, proportional shifts within a cell type that are dramatically altered with exercise have often been misinterpreted as changes occurring at the individual cell level.

Exercise-responsive leukocytes have similar properties

All leukocyte subtypes that are preferentially mobilised with exercise appear to have similar traits, regardless of their lineage. These can be categorised into three major components:

- cytotoxic/effector functions;
- tissue migration potential; and
- expression levels of adrenoreceptors and glucocorticoid receptors and the ability to respond to catecholamines and cortisol.

Cytotoxic/effector functions

It is clear that the vast majority of exercise responsive leukocytes have high cytotoxic/effector properties. For instance, potent cytotoxic cells such as NK cells, CD8+ T cells and γδ T cells, and non-lymphocyte cells that have high effector functions (including CD16+ monocytes) are highly stress responsive when compared with other leukocyte subtypes that have limited cytotoxic/effector functions and are mobilised in relatively fewer numbers (CD4+ T cells, B cells, classical monocytes). Even within CD8+ T cells, there is a stepwise preferential mobilisation of those subsets in order of their cytotoxic function, migratory potential and history of prior antigen exposure (Campbell *et al.* 2009; Simpson *et al.* 2010). There is also an increase in the number of cells constitutively expressing both type-1 and type-2 cytokines such as IFN-γ and IL-4 (Zaldivar *et al.* 2006) and intracellular granules that are important for cell-mediated cytotoxicity such as perforin and granzyme-b (Wang *et al.* 2009). NK cell killing (Miles *et al.* 2002; Shek *et al.* 1995; Wang *et al.* 2009), neutrophil and monocyte phagocytosis (Nieman *et al.* 2011b) and lymphocyte activation (Bishop *et al.* 2005a; Vider *et al.* 2001) also tend to increase after a single bout of exercise, possibly owing to a redistribution of effector subsets into the blood.

Tissue migration potential

Leukocytes mobilised into the circulation with exercise exhibit phenotype characteristics associated with tissue migration. While those leukocytes deployed with exercise or acute-stress tend to express mostly integrins and intercellular adhesion molecules (Simpson *et al.* 2006a) and a range of chemokine receptors (CXCR2, CXCR3 and CXCR5) that have ligands for activated endothelium (Bosch *et al.* 2003), selectins are expressed at lower levels (Hong *et al.* 2004; Simpson *et al.* 2007a). This adhesion molecule and chemokine receptor profile of the mobilised cells is associated with high tissue migration potential and are less likely to be mobilised from or to the primary (i.e. bone marrow, thymus) and even some secondary (i.e. lymph nodes), lymphoid organs. It can generally be said, therefore, that exercise elicits a preferential deployment of leukocytes at an advanced stage of maturation.

Expression levels of adrenoreceptors and glucocorticoid receptors and the ability to respond to catecholamines and cortisol

The leukocyte subtypes deployed by exercise are also highly responsive to β-agonist infusion (Dimitrov *et al.*, 2010) and have a greater surface expression of β2-AR. This may indicate a selective deployment of specific leukocyte subtypes that have high cytotoxic and tissue-migration properties via catecholamine and adrenoreceptor-mediated mechanisms. Moreover, those leukocyte subtypes (particularly monocytes and lymphocytes) that preferentially egress from the blood (either by remargination or transmigration to the peripheral tissue) during post-exercise recovery are highly responsive to glucocorticoids, indicating that leukocyte trafficking between the blood and tissues is strongly influenced by both sympathetic nervous system and HPA axis activation.

Taken together, the idiosyncrasies that exist across all leukocyte subsets mobilised with exercise would indicate that the response is highly regulated (particularly for lymphocytes and monocytes) and is not merely due to a non-specific 'washing out' of leukocytes from the marginal pools. As those cells with potent effector/cytotoxic functions and tissue migratory potential are preferentially deployed under the influence of catecholamines, glucocorticoids and their receptors, it would appear that the exercise-induced leukocytosis is a protective evolutionary component of the 'flight or fight' response, whereby specific immune cells are deployed to vulnerable areas in preparation for immune challenges that may be imposed by the actions of the stressor (Dhabhar 2009).

Exercise-induced lymphocytopenia: apoptosis or extravasation?

Although the actions of glucocorticoids, adhesion molecules and chemokine receptors are accepted governing factors of leukocyte egress from the blood compartment during post-exercise recovery, why the blood lymphocyte count would often fall below the baseline values and why exercise would require around 40–60% of circulatory lymphocytes to follow the demarginated lymphocytes out of the bloodstream left exercise immunologists puzzled. Moreover, although many of the exercise effects on immune cell mobilisation and extravasation can be replicated using acute psychological stress or β-agonist infusion models, the acute stress-induced lymphocytopenia appears to a phenomenon that is unique to exercise. The lymphocytopenia of exercise is mostly due to a decline in the numbers of NK cells and CD8+ T cells within 30–60 minutes after cessation of exercise (Gabriel *et al.* 1991) and, because changes in NK cell function (i.e. antibody-dependent cell-mediated cytotoxicity) closely parallel changes in blood NK cell numbers (Pedersen and Ullum 1994; Shek *et al.* 1995), exercise-induced changes in lymphocyte numbers may be an important mediator of apparent changes in lymphocyte 'activity'. This retraction of the blood NK cell numbers and, ultimately, NK cell function, was believed to be a major contributing factor to the so-called 'open-window' of post-exercise immune suppression (Pedersen and Ullum 1994), which triggered a number of investigations aimed at identifying a mechanism for this phenomenon.

Following the initial report by Mars *et al.* (1998) that acute exercise dramatically increased lymphocyte apoptosis levels in the blood, cell death was considered a possible mechanism (Mooren *et al.* 2002, 2004; Steensberg *et al.* 2002). Although some studies have reported an increased percentage of apoptotic lymphocytes immediately after exercise (Mooren *et al.* 2002, 2004; Steensberg *et al.* 2002), the total number of apoptotic cells may remain unchanged despite an increased presence of apoptotic stimuli (Steensberg *et al.* 2002). Moreover, the levels of apoptosis reported in these studies are usually very small (less than five per cent) (Mooren *et al.* 2002; Simpson *et al.* 2007b; Steensberg *et al.* 2002) and unlikely to account for the 40–60% reductions in the blood lymphocyte count seen after exercise (Simpson 2011). Indeed, other studies have documented a lymphocytopenia in response to acute exercise without any concomitant evidence of an increased number of apoptotic lymphocytes (Simpson *et al.* 2007b; Steensberg *et al.* 2002). As lymphocytes do not appear to undergo apoptosis in the blood, it is unlikely that cell death is a major contributor to exercise-induced lymphocytopenia.

A more accepted mechanism for this lymphocytopenia is a selective extravasation of specific lymphocyte subsets, leaving the blood compartment to enter the peripheral tissues (Kruger *et al.* 2008; Simpson *et al.* 2006a). Indeed, it is known that lymphocytes that preferentially egress from the peripheral blood compartment (i.e. CD8+ T cells, NK cells) have a heightened expression of certain cell surface activation and adhesion molecules that facilitate their transmigration (Simpson *et al.* 2006a), allowing them to pass through adjacent endothelial cells and into the tissues. Animal studies indicate that the extravasated lymphocytes migrate to peripheral tissues, such as the lungs and intestinal Peyer's patches, following exercise (Kruger *et al.* 2008, 2009), presumably as part of an increased immunosurveillance response to acute stress. Indeed, adrenergic mechanisms are purported to play a role as adrenaline infusion partially mimicked the T cell migratory responses to exercise (Kruger *et al.* 2008). Moreover, glucocorticoids appear to stimulate CD4+ and CD8+ T cell migration toward CXCR4 ligands *in vitro* (Okutsu *et al.* 2005). However, the role of cortisol in exercise-induced lymphocytopenia is somewhat perplexing. While cortisol infusion in humans also elicits a lymphocytopenia, this tends to induce a selective decline in the numbers of naïve T cells that display a lymphoid-homing phenotype (Dimitrov *et al.* 2009), which is in contrast to the highly differentiated cells with a tissue migratory phenotype that preferentially egress from the blood with exercise (Campbell *et al.* 2009; Simpson *et al.* 2007a; 2008; Turner *et al.* 2010). In our studies, the proportions of KLRG1+, CD57+ and CD28null CD8+ T cells was lower than baseline at one hour post-exercise, indicating that the exercise-induced lymphocytopenia is due to a preferential egress of T cells with an effector-memory or terminally differentiated phenotype (Simpson *et al.* 2008; 2007a). This was investigated in more detail by Turner *et al.* (2010), who reported a 60% decrease in late differentiated effector/memory cells, compared with a 29% decrease in naïve T cells within one to two hours after a 60-minute treadmill-running protocol.

While acute exercise elicits the preferential extravasation of highly-differentiated T cells and cytotoxic NK cells, the homing destinations of these cells are not known. It is also not known what happens to these cells when they reach the peripheral tissues following their egress from the blood. It is possible that they may simply recirculate or undergo selective apoptosis (Simpson 2011). Furthermore, although the blood lymphocyte count normally returns to resting values within 6–24 hours after cessation of exercise, the cell types and tissues responsible for this restoration of the blood lymphocyte count are not fully understood.

FACTORS AFFECTING THE LEUKOCYTE RESPONSE TO ACUTE EXERCISE

Several factors influence the magnitude and time course of leukocytosis during exercise. These include the intensity and duration of the exercise bout; single versus repeated bouts of exercise, training status, age, nutritional status and infection history.

Exercise intensity and duration

The exercise responses of almost all leukocyte and lymphocyte subsets are influenced by both the intensity and the duration of exercise. It is known that prolonged endurance exercise causes a more pronounced and sustained increase in total leukocyte and neutrophil counts compared to high-intensity exercise protocols of short duration. Robson *et al.* (1999b) reported that prolonged exercise (164 ± 23 minutes) at 55% $\dot{V}O_2$ max elicited a much larger leukocytosis compared with shorter-duration exercise (37 ± 19 minutes) at 80% $\dot{V}O_2$ max (Figure 3.1). However, exercise duration may only augment leukocytosis if the exercise bout is very prolonged (in excess of 60 minutes), with the intensity of exercise being more influential during exercise bouts of shorter duration. For instance, Gimenez et al. (1986) reported that total leukocyte and lymphocyte counts were larger at 100% $\dot{V}O_2$ max compared with submaximal exercise and that cells enumerated after 45 minutes of submaximal exercise were similar to the cell counts observed after 15 minutes. Similarly, Shek et al. (1995) reported that total leukocyte and neutrophil counts observed after 60 minutes of cycling exercise at 65% $\dot{V}O_2$ max were similar to those observed at 30 minutes (Figure 3.2). However, after 120 minutes of exercise, total leukocyte and neutrophil numbers were almost twice as large as the cell counts observed at 30 and 60 minutes of exercise and persisted for up to 120 minutes after cessation of the exercise bout (Shek et al. 1995). Monocyte numbers, although increasing rapidly in response to short-duration, high-intensity exercise (Steppich et al. 2000), also tend to rise with increasing exercise duration that may persist during exercise recovery (Shek et al. 1995). Although, while CD14++/CD16– classical monocyte numbers in blood may persist for up to one hour after prolonged exercise (92.1 ± 6.8 minutes of strenuous cycling), both CD14+/CD16++ and CD14++/CD16+ numbers return to near resting values (Booth et al. 2010).

While the leukocytosis due to exercise (governed mostly by a neutrophilia) is positively associated with exercise intensity during exercise bouts of short duration (less than 60 minutes), this response is substantially larger during prolonged exercise bouts at a lower intensity. In contrast, the lymphocytosis with exercise appears to be influenced by intensity more than duration. Kendall et al. (1990) reported that lymphocyte proportional shifts and numerical changes were strongly affected by the intensity of exercise and that these eclipsed any effects of exercise duration. Moreover, total lymphocyte counts, although rising at the onset of exercise, tend to plateau after 15 minutes of exercise for durations lasting 45 minutes to 2.5 hours (Gabriel et al. 1992c; Gimenez et al. 1986; Shek et al. 1995), while neutrophil and monocyte numbers may continue to rise after 60 minutes of exercise (Shek et al. 1995). The egress of blood lymphocytes during exercise recovery (Campbell et al. 2009) and the lymphocytopenia associated with exercise (Simpson et al. 2007b) is also more pronounced following high- compared with moderate-intensity exercise. It is not known, however, if exercise-induced lymphocytopenia would be amplified in response to prolonged versus shorter duration exercise of the same intensity, as no study to date has asked this research question using a within-subjects experimental design. The effects of exercise intensity on the mobilisation of blood lymphocytes and their subsets are shown in Figure 3.8.

Repeated bouts of exercise

Athletes are often required to perform multiple training sessions per day, which could cause more profound changes in blood leukocyte trafficking. The 'open-window' hypothesis proposed by Pedersen and Ullum (1994) suggests that immune function is stimulated during high-intensity exercise, quickly followed by a period of immunodepression that may last for 3–72 hours (the 'open window') depending on the intensity, duration and type of activity performed. They propose that it is during

Figure 3.8 The magnitude of lymphocyte mobilisation with exercise is intensity-dependent. Healthy subjects (*n* = 13) rested quietly in the laboratory (control) or exercised at low (35% of maximum power) and high (85% of maximum power) intensity on a cycling ergometer for 16 minutes. Total lymphocyte (A), CD4+ T cell (B), CD8+ T cell (C), NK cell (D) and B cell (E) numbers did not change in the control condition. Exercise increased the numbers of all lymphocyte subsets in the circulation, with the high-intensity protocol eliciting a greater response than the low-intensity exercise protocol. Data are mean ± SE (from Campbell *et al.* 2009)

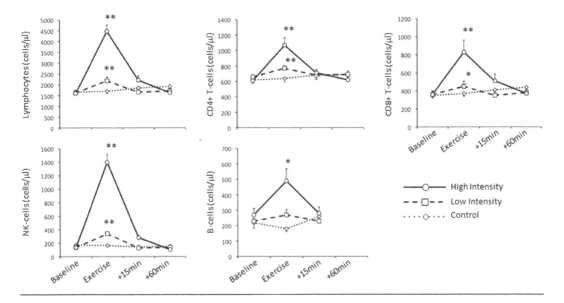

this time that the individual will be most susceptible to opportunistic infection. This theoretical framework further proposes that, if an additional bout of exercise is performed during the 'open window', the initial stimulating effects of exercise will be followed by a more severe and prolonged decline in immunity. Researchers have attempted to test this hypothesis by asking subjects to complete multiple exercise bouts in a single day and/or over a number of consecutive days. Healthy subjects who performed a 60 minutes bout of cycling exercise at 65% $\dot{V}O_2$ max each day for five consecutive days were found to have an impaired mobilisation of T cells and NK cells after the fifth day of exercise compared to the third and first days (Hoffman-Goetz *et al.* 1990). Suzuki *et al.* (1996) examined blood neutrophil responses to a 60-minute bout of exercise (70% $\dot{V}O_2$ max) performed daily for seven days. The magnitude of the exercise-induced changes tended to decrease with each exercise bout, although they were not reported to be statistically significant. However, the number of segmented (mature) neutrophils in resting blood progressively declined, indicating that repeated bouts of exercise placed additional demands on the bone marrow to replenish the blood neutrophil count (Suzuki *et al.* 1996). In a study in trained hill-runners, we found that running 24.5 km over mountainous terrain (1,126 metres total ascent/descent) each day for four consecutive days resulted in a progressive decline in the magnitude of the exercise-induced leukocytosis (Simpson *et al.* 2006b). This was predominantly due to a reduced neutrophilia, as lymphocyte, CD4+, CD8+ and NK cell responses to exercise did not change across the four days. This response was probably caused by a steady increase in the average completion time (2.25–2.5 hours) and reduction in mean heart-rate responses observed across the four exercise bouts. Despite the arduous nature of this exercise protocol, total leukocyte, lymphocyte and lymphocyte subset numbers returned to baseline values within 24 hours after each exercise bout (Simpson *et al.* 2006b).

In response to multiple exercise bouts performed on the same day, Ronsen *et al.* (2001) found that total leukocytes, neutrophils, lymphocytes, CD4+ T-cells, CD8+ T cells and NK cells were significantly elevated after a second bout of cycling exercise (75 min at 75% VO_2max) compared to an identical bout that was completed around 4 h earlier. Although exercise caused a lymphocytopenia, this was not exacerbated by performing the second exercise bout (Ronsen *et al.*, 2001b). Exercise bouts of shorter duration also show similar effects. Elite rowers who performed three bouts of six-minute 'all out' exercise at six-hour intervals over two consecutive days had elevated leukocyte, neutrophil and CD14+ monocyte counts after the second and third bouts compared with the first (Nielsen *et al.* 1996). Cell concentrations of lymphocytes, CD4+ T cells, CD8+ T cells and NK cells were also elevated after the third bout compared with the first (Nielsen *et al.* 1996). This occurred despite similar heart rates and catecholamine responses to exercise being observed during the subsequent exercise bouts. Taken together, these studies indicate that a 'carry-over' effect on the immune system exists when multiple exercise bouts are performed on a single day (Ronsen *et al.* 2001b). In contrast, Rohde *et al.* (1998) found that the absolute numbers of NK cells, CD4+ cells, CD8+ cells and monocytes were found to be similar immediately before and immediately after three exercise bouts performed at 71% VO_2 max for 60, 45 and 30 minutes with two hours' recovery between each bout. Although consistent with the studies of Nielsen *et al.* (1996) and Ronsen *et al.* (2001b), total leukocyte numbers, driven by a sustained neutrophilia, continued to increase with each bout of exercise (Rohde *et al.* 1998).

In summary, the effects of repeated exercise bouts on immune cell trafficking are relatively understudied. What we know at present is that multiple bouts of exercise performed on the same day appear to be associated with an amplified mobilisation of many leukocyte subtypes, particularly neutrophils and, to some extent, monocytes. If more than two exercise bouts are performed, or if the exercise bouts are of long duration, then lymphocyte mobilisation may also be amplified during subsequent bouts. Unfortunately, repeated bout studies are associated with a number of experimental confounders that can cloud their interpretation. These include differences in cardiovascular responses, catecholamines, glucocorticoids and carbohydrate availability, all of which may exist from one bout to the next. More controlled studies are required to determine the impact of repeated bouts of long duration exercise performed over multiple days as this is likely to have important implications for the military and athletes competing in stage events and adventure races. It should be noted that the effects of multiple exercise bouts on leukocyte redistribution is not necessarily indicative of immune cell function. For instance, repeated exercise bouts have been shown to alter immune cell function including NK cell activity and T-cell proliferation even when leukocyte redistribution was not affected. The impact of multiple exercise bouts on leukocyte function is addressed in Chapter 8.

Training status

The effects of training status on blood leukocyte numbers following a single bout of exercise have been assessed in two different ways: by using a cross-sectional experimental design that compares leukocyte numbers before, during and after exercise between trained and untrained participants; or by longitudinally comparing the leukocyte response to a single bout of exercise in the same subjects before and after a period of exercise training. In response to an 18-minute incremental submaximal cycling protocol, Moyna *et al.* (1996) reported no effects of fitness level on the number of leukocytes, neutrophils, monocytes, eosinophils, lymphocytes, NK cells or CD3+, CD4+ and CD8+ T cells in blood during and after the exercise. Kendall *et al.* (1990) also found no effect of training status (stratified by $\dot{V}O_2$ max and weekly energy expenditure) on the percentage of lymphocyte subsets present in peripheral blood after multiple bouts of cycling exercise at various intensities and durations. However, the absolute number of NK cells, CD4+ T cells and CD8+ T cells mobilised into the blood with exercise did vary among the fitness groups, with CD8+ T cell mobilisation being higher in subjects of low fitness (Kendall *et al.* 1990). The inconsistencies between the studies of Moyna *et al.* (1996) and Kendall *et al.* (1990) could be attributable to differences in exercise duration, as Kendall *et al.* (1990) found that training status differences only existed in response to the exercise protocols of longer duration. Similarly, lymphocyte mobilisation in response to acute exercise was blunted after six weeks of aerobic training compared with baseline exercise responses and controls (Soppi *et al.* 1982). Strength training status also appears to alter the leukocytosis to a single bout of exercise, with untrained participants exhibiting a more pronounced leukocytosis to resistance exercise compared to their trained counterparts (Potteiger *et al.* 2001). However, six months of strength training did not influence the number of lymphocytes or lymphocyte subsets mobilised in response to a single session of resistance exercise (Miles *et al.* 2003).

Taken together, it would appear that training status does not alter the composition of broad leukocyte or lymphocyte subsets after acute exercise, but the absolute number of leukocytes redistributed by acute exercise may be affected by training. More often than not, the numbers of neutrophils and monocytes mobilised into the blood does not appear to be affected by training status, although lymphocyte mobilisation may be reduced in those with superior training status. As the relative intensity of exercise (heart rate or $\%\dot{V}O_2$ max) is usually controlled, it is assumed that the levels of mechanical stress that could result in leukocyte demargination are similar between the trained and untrained participants in these studies. As such, any impairments in leukocyte and lymphocyte redistribution after acute exercise are most likely caused by a reduction in leukocyte β2-AR density and sensitivity with training, possibly caused by repeated exposure to high concentrations of catecholamines (Butler *et al.* 1982). Moreover, glucocorticoid receptor sensitivity also appears to be reduced with training (Duclos *et al.* 2003), which may account for reduced numbers of extravasated lymphocytes during exercise recovery in trained subjects. This may indicate an adaptation of the HPA axis to repeated increases in glucocorticoids that are secreted during exercise. Although plasma concentrations of adrenaline, noradrenaline and cortisol may change in response to a single bout of exercise after a period of exercise training, an impaired leukocytosis has still been documented, despite similar exercise-induced concentrations of catecholamines and glucocorticoids between trained and untrained participants or after an exercise training intervention. This indicates that the effects of training status on leukocyte redistribution after a single bout of exercise are most likely to involve alterations in the sensitivity and density of β2-AR and glucocorticoid receptors as opposed to changes in the secretion of catecholamines and glucocorticoids. Another possibility is an impaired ability for demarginated leukocytes to adhere to endothelial ligands in trained individuals. Mills *et al.* (2006) reported that peripheral blood mononuclear cell adhesion to human umbilical venous endothelial cells *in vitro* was lower after acute exercise in trained but not untrained subjects.

Age

There is evidence to indicate that leukocyte redistribution in response to a single bout of exercise is altered with age. Ceddia *et al.* (1999) reported that the leukocytosis was lower in older compared with younger subjects after a graded exercise test, despite both groups achieving similar relative exercise responses, including maximal respiratory exchange ratio, age-predicted maximum heart rate and time to exhaustion. The numbers of neutrophils, monocytes and lymphocytes mobilised into the circulation were also lower in the older participants (Ceddia *et al.* 1999). Cannon *et al.* (1994) also documented a blunted mobilisation of neutrophils in older subjects compared with the young, following a bout of muscle-damaging exercise. Conversely, neutrophil responses to downhill running exercise were not age-related in a group of trained runners (Sacheck *et al.* 2003), indicating that impairments in exercise-induced neutrophilia with age may only be evident in relatively untrained individuals.

Ageing is associated with a profound decline in total circulating T-cell numbers (Provinciali *et al.* 2009). Although the relative change in T-cell numbers does not differ between young and older participants in response to a single bout of exercise (when the percentage change from baseline is determined) (Mazzeo *et al.* 1998; Simpson *et al.* 2008), the absolute number of T cells mobilised is often lower in older participants (Ceddia *et al.* 1999; Mazzeo *et al.* 1998; Figure 3.9). Despite the mobilisation of total T cells being similar between the age-groups, older individuals had an impaired mobilisation of CD4+ T cells, especially those expressing the surface marker CD45RA (expressed on both naïve and EMRA T cells) (Ceddia *et al.* 1999). Mazzeo *et al.* (1998) reported that the relative response of T cells to acute exercise is similar between young and old, although it can be clearly seen in this study that the absolute number of T cells mobilised was substantially less in the old. This appeared to affect both CD4+ and CD8+ T cells (Mazzeo *et al.* 1998). In contrast, NK-cell

Figure 3.9 Ageing is associated with an impaired mobilisation of total circulating leukocytes (A), neutrophils (B), lymphocytes (C) and monocytes (D) in response to acute exercise. Young (mean age: 22.4 ± 0.7 years; n = 14) and elderly (mean age: 65.3 ± 0.8 years; n = 33) subjects completed a maximal treadmill exercise test. Although $\dot{V}O_2$ max was lower in the elderly, maximal respiratory exchange ratio, age-predicted heart rate and time to fatigue were not different, indicating that both groups achieved relative maximal exercise intensity. Difference from pre-exercise indicated by * ($P < 0.05$) and group x exercise interaction effects indicated by # ($P < 0.05$). Data are mean ± SE (from Ceddia et al. 1999)

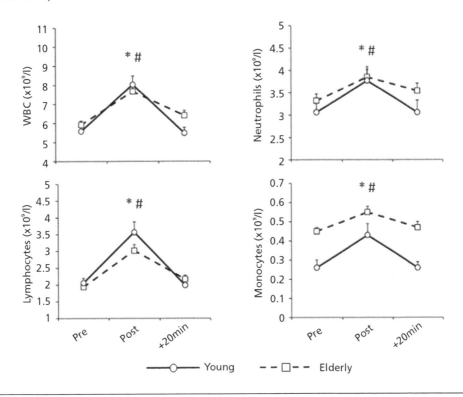

mobilisation with exercise does not appear to be affected by age (Mazzeo et al. 1998; Simpson et al. 2008).

A number of factors could be involved in the impaired exercise-induced mobilisation of leukocytes with age. As circulating T-cell numbers are known to decline with age, it could be assumed that T-cell numbers in marginal pools are also lowered. This, coupled with the known age-related reductions in cardiac output and blood flow during exercise (Poole et al. 2003), is likely to result in less leukocyte demargination in older subjects. An age-related impairment in the binding of catecholamines to β2-ARs is also a possibility. Although both young and older subjects exhibit similar catecholamine responses to exercise (Kastello et al. 1993), β2-AR sensitivity (but not density) is altered with age (Feldman et al. 1984). This would suggest that older individuals have a higher threshold for catecholamine-induced leukocyte demargination compared with the young. For a more detailed review on the effects of ageing on leukocyte number and function, see Simpson et al. (2012) In addition to age, differences in the leukocyte response to a single bout of exercise are also apparent between males and females. For a detailed account on the influence of sex differences on these responses see Gillum *et al.* (2011) and Gleeson *et al.* (2011).

Nutritional status

The impact of nutritional status on the immune response to acute exercise has been studied extensively. Nutritional status and leukocyte responses to acute exercise are only briefly addressed here; see Chapter 9 for a detailed discussion of this topic. Of all the macronutrients, carbohydrate availability has the most pronounced effect on exercise-induced leukocytosis. Ingestion of carbohydrate during exercise has been shown to prevent falls in blood glucose and insulin levels, to lower HPA axis activity (cortisol secretion) and to reduce the release of IL-6 into the plasma from exercising muscles. Consequently, the leukocytosis to exercise is markedly reduced when adequate carbohydrate is available during exercise. Conversely, exercising in a state of glycogen depletion or low carbohydrate intake is associated with enhanced leukocytosis, exacerbated lymphocytopenia, increased cortisol and adrenaline secretion and elevated IL-6 release. The response of all leukocyte and lymphocyte subsets to exercise appears to be altered by both acute (i.e. sports drinks taken during exercise) and chronic (i.e. carbohydrate loading) carbohydrate ingestion (Lancaster *et al.* 2005b; Nieman *et al.* 1997). The International Society of Exercise and Immunology currently recommends that 60 g of carbohydrate are ingested every hour during heavy exertion to dampen immune and inflammatory responses (although not necessarily immune dysfunction) (Walsh *et al.* 2011a).

The mechanism by which carbohydrate availability alters the leukocyte response to acute exercise is believed to be via indirect pathways that alter the factors responsible for leukocytosis, as opposed to altering the leukocytes themselves. When muscle glycogen and blood glucose levels start to decline during exercise, there is an increased secretion of catecholamines and cortisol to facilitate gluconeogenesis. Therefore, adequate carbohydrate intake before and during exercise helps to maintain muscle glycogen and plasma glucose above critical levels, thus blunting catecholamine and cortisol-induced leukocytosis.

Intake of certain micronutrients may also alter the leukocyte response to acute exercise. Two weeks of vitamin C supplementation prior to an acute bout of endurance exercise resulted in a blunted neutrophilia without altering neutrophil function (Davison and Gleeson 2006); however, supplementation with vitamin C in combination with carbohydrate does not appear to exert any additional effects above carbohydrate ingestion on the leukocyte response to acute exercise (Davison and Gleeson 2005). Overall scepticism remains on whether or not micronutrient ingestion (especially in those individuals who are not already deficient) can alter leukocyte responses to acute exercise and ultimately modulate immune function. This is mostly because of the large number of exercise studies that report no differences on many indices of immunity between supplementation and placebo trials for a wide range of vitamins and minerals and also 'immune enhancing' supplements including probiotics, β-glucan, ginseng, glutamine and bovine colostrum, to name but a few (Walsh *et al.* 2011a).

Infection history

The influence of infection history on the cellular immune response to acute exercise in otherwise healthy people has only recently been investigated (Bigley *et al.* 2012; Turner *et al.* 2010). Cytomegalovirus (CMV), a highly prevalent latent β-herpes virus that infects 40–70% of the otherwise healthy adult population (Bate *et al.* 2010), appears to exert strong influences on the exercise response of blood lymphocytes. NK cells and CD8+ T cells predominantly control CMV infection and individuals with a latent CMV infection have greater numbers of effector memory and EMRA CD8+ T cells compared with the non-infected (Derhovanessian *et al.* 2011). As effector memory and EMRA cells are preferentially mobilised with exercise (Campbell *et al.* 2009), Turner *et al.* (2010) hypothesised that latent CMV infection would be associated with an amplified CD8+ T-cell response to exercise. They showed that the mobilisation and egress of CD8+ T cells after exercise was substantially greater in healthy subjects with a latent CMV infection compared with their non-infected counterparts (Figure 3.9). The amplified response of the CD8+ T cells was attributed to the preferential mobilisation of intermediate (CD27–/CD28+) and late-stage differentiated (CD27-/CD28-) cells in those with CMV (Turner *et al.* 2010). These findings were corroborated by Bigley *et al.* (2012), who reported an amplified mobilisation and egress of antigen-experienced CD8+ T cells (identified by their surface expression of KLRG1) in those infected with CMV after an acute bout of cycling exercise. In contrast to CD8+ T cells, Bigley *et al.* (2012) also showed that the exercise-induced mobilisation of NK cells was impaired in people with CMV, indicating that latent CMV infection has contrasting effects on CD8+ T cells and NK cells. The exercise response of CD4+ T cells, γδ T cells, neutrophils or monocytes does not appear to be influenced by latent CMV infection (Bigley *et al.* 2012; Turner *et al.* 2010), although it is not known whether these responses are directly attributable to CMV or are secondary to a greater presence of exercise-responsive CD8+ T cell subsets in people with CMV. For instance, many CMV-negative individuals also have an elevated frequency of effector memory and EMRA cells (Derhovanessian *et al.* 2011) that could also cause them to exhibit an amplified exercise response.

This work has shown that latent CMV infection has a major confounding effect on the lymphocyte response to acute exercise. It remains to be determined whether other prevalent viral infections are also influential in this response. While Epstein-Barr serostatus does not appear to influence T-cell or NK-cell responses to exercise (Bigley *et al.* 2012), other common viruses that infect humans and establish latency, such as herpes simplex virus (HSV), varicella-zoster virus (VZV), roseolovirus or parvovirus B19 may also have a role to play and should be investigated. Other viruses associated with chronic illness (such as HIV or hepatitis) can also influence the exercise response of certain leukocyte subtypes and these are addressed in more detail in Chapter 13.

THE EFFECTS OF EXERCISE TRAINING ON CIRCULATING LEUKOCYTE NUMBERS

Many studies have investigated the effects of exercise training on the total number of blood leukocytes and their subsets in resting blood (defined as blood samples collected no less than 24 hours following the last exercise session). Most of these studies are cross-sectional in design and have compared leukocyte counts between trained and untrained individuals, while others have adopted a longitudinal design to examine the effects of an exercise training intervention on resting blood leukocyte counts in athletes or previously untrained subjects. The majority of research in this area have focused on aerobic or endurance-based exercise but there is also a substantial amount of literature devoted to strength and resistance exercise training.

Studies in athletes

Resting total leukocyte numbers tend to be similar between athletes and healthy age-matched controls (Bain *et al.* 2000). The same is true for the numbers of most leukocyte subtypes (neutrophils, monocytes, eosinophils), although it has been reported that marathon runners have lower lymphocyte numbers than controls (Bain *et al.* 2000). When groups of athletes are compared, those who participate in predominantly aerobic or endurance events tend to exhibit lower blood leukocyte counts. Horn *et al.* (2010) collected full blood counts on 2,247 elite-level Australian athletes across a wide-range of sporting disciplines over a ten-year period (Table 3.1). They reported that total leukocyte, monocyte and neutrophil counts were lowest among cyclists and triathletes. Specifically, 17% of all cycling and 16% of all triathlete resting blood samples were considered to be neutropenic (less than $2.0 \times 10^9/L$), while 5% of all athletes across all sports were neutropenic. Only 2% of athletes across all sports were lymphopenic (less than $1.0 \times 10^9/L$) or monocytopenic (less than $0.2 \times 10^9/L$) (Horn *et al.* 2010). The lowest lymphocyte counts were found in male canoeists and female volleyball players and cricketers (Horn *et al.* 2010).

Leukocyte numbers in resting blood may also change in response to a period of exercise training. Gleeson *et al.* (2000) observed lower resting NK-cell numbers in elite swimmers following a 12-week period of intensified training. Baj *et al.* (1994) reported decreased CD3+ and CD8+ T cell numbers in competitive cyclists following a six-month period of intensive training (approximately 500 km/week). Bury *et al.* (1998) examined blood leukocyte profiles in professional Belgian soccer players before, during and after a full season. They reported no change in total leukocyte counts but did observe declines in neutrophil and CD4+ T cell counts (Bury *et al.* 1998). A similar study in Portuguese soccer players had contrasting results. Rebelo *et al.* (1998) reported that total leukocyte, neutrophil and CD8+ T cells counts were elevated at the end of the season compared with pre-season values, with the increased CD8+ T cell numbers also caused a decrease in the CD4+/CD8+ T cell ratio. The composition of broad T-cell subsets may also change with training. Rebelo *et al.* (1998) also reported a decrease in CD8+ T cells expressing CD57 (considered to be

Table 3.1 Total leukocyte and leukocyte subtype counts in male and female elite athletes; blood samples were obtained in the resting state in healthy athletes (presenting without illness); cycling and triathlon were the two sports with the lowest leukocyte, neutrophil and monocyte counts

SPORT	ATHLETES	TOTAL LEUKOCYTES (x 10^9/L)		NEUTROPHILS (x 10^9/L)		LYMPHOCYTES (x 10^9/L)		MONOCYTES (x 10^9/L)	
	(n)	Mean	95% ref. range	Mean	95% ref. range	Mean	95% ref. range	Mean	95% ref. range
Males	113	6.3	3.9–10.2	3.5	1.7–7.1	1.9	1.2–3.1	0.39	0.22–0.70
Athletics	101	6.6	4.3–10.3	3.7	1.9–7.2	1.9	1.1–3.2	0.41	0.22–0.74
Basketball	173	5.7	3.7–8.8	2.8	1.5–5.5	2.0	1.2–3.3	0.36	0.20–0.65
Cycling	195	6.1	3.7–10.1	3.4	1.6–6.9	1.9	1.1–3.2	0.39	0.22–0.71
Rowing	127	6.7	4.3–10.3	3.4	1.8–6.5	2.2	1.4–3.7	0.44	0.24–0.79
Swimming	165	6.9	4.1–11.7	3.7	1.7–8.0	2.0	1.1–3.5	0.42	0.23–0.75
Soccer	48	5.9	3.5–9.9	2.9	1.3–6.4	2.0	1.2–3.5	0.35	0.18–0.69
Triathlon	32	6.4	4.2–9.8	3.5	1.7–7.0	1.9	1.0–3.5	0.37	0.21–0.66
Winter sports	66	6.2	3.8–10.1	3.5	1.6–7.6	1.9	1.1–3.0	0.33	0.18–0.62
Females	99	6.5	3.9–10.7	3.6	1.7–7.4	1.9	1.2–3.2	0.37	0.20–0.69
Athletics	101	5.9	3.5–9.8	2.9	1.3–6.5	2.0	1.1–3.6	0.33	0.18–0.63
Basketball	108	6.4	4.0–10.3	3.6	1.8–7.1	2.0	1.2–3.3	0.36	0.20–0.66
Cycling	114	6.5	4.2–10.2	3.2	1.6–6.3	2.4	1.4–4.0	0.35	0.19–0.66
Rowing	80	6.3	3.9–10.4	3.6	1.8–7.2	1.9	1.1–3.2	0.39	0.22–0.71
Swimming	33	5.9	3.8–9.2	2.9	1.5–5.4	2.1	1.3–3.3	0.33	0.18–0.60
Soccer	38	6.4	4.2–9.8	3.6	2.0–6.6	1.9	1.1–3.4	0.34	0.18–0.63
Triathlon	113	6.3	3.9–10.2	3.5	1.7–7.1	1.9	1.2–3.1	0.39	0.22–0.70
Winter sports	101	6.6	4.3–10.3	3.7	1.9–7.2	1.9	1.1–3.2	0.41	0.22–0.74

Source: modified from Horn *et al.* (2010)

a marker of terminal differentiation) at the end of the soccer season. Cosgrove *et al.* (2012) reported that the proportions of differentiated (KLRG1+/CD57-) CD8+ T cells and 'transitional' (CD45RA+/CD45RO+) CD4+ and CD8+ T cells increased over a six-month training period in preparation for an Ironman® triathlon, during which subjects trained on, average, for 8–11 hours per week.

It appears that athletes who are exposed to prolonged periods of exercise training may experience alterations in the total number and composition of various immune cells. The total number of certain leukocyte subpopulations may occasionally fall below clinical lower limits (particularly endurance athletes), although the vast majority of athletes have total and differential leukocyte counts within normal ranges (Bain *et al.* 2000; Horn *et al.* 2010). Changes in the composition of leukocyte and lymphocyte subtypes could be attributed to a number of reasons, including increased exposure to external pathogens, increased levels of oxidative stress, the release of inflammatory mediators or the reactivation of latent viruses (Cosgrove *et al.* 2012). It is also possible that these subtle changes in cell composition with training have no underlying clinical consequences. Whether or not alterations in the number and composition of specialised leukocyte subtypes can serve as prognostic biomarkers of illness in athletes remains to be determined.

Studies in non-athletes

In young healthy adults, resting blood leukocyte, granulocyte, monocyte, lymphocyte, CD4+ T cell, CD8+ T cell, B cell and NK cell numbers tend to be similar between aerobically trained and untrained participants (as determined by $\dot{V}O_2$ max values) (Moyna *et al.* 1996). As such, the effects of exercise training on the numbers and composition of blood leukocytes in non-athletes have focused mostly on the elderly and the obese. Although most longitudinal studies have found no effects of exercise training on blood neutrophil counts in otherwise healthy elderly people (Walsh *et al.* 2011b; Woods *et al.* 1999), some cross-sectional studies indicate that regular exercise training is associated with lower blood neutrophil numbers in elderly men (de Gonzalo-Calvo *et al.* 2011; Michishita *et al.* 2008). In a study of overweight women who had completed six weeks of regular aerobic exercise training, Michishita *et al.* (2010) found that exercise training lowered blood neutrophil counts, with these changes being associated with percent change in insulin sensitivity and body mass index. Indeed, regular aerobic exercise has been associated with lower numbers of circulating leukocytes, lymphocytes and monocytes in overweight/obese women (Johannsen *et al.* 2010). Johannsen *et al.* (2012) randomised 390 sedentary overweight/obese postmenopausal women to either a non-exercise control group or one of three exercise groups with various degrees of weekly energy expenditure. The exercise intervention lasted six months and was performed at 50% $\dot{V}O_2$ peak. An exercise dose-dependent decrease in total leukocyte and neutrophil counts was observed in response to the exercise training intervention compared with the control group. As elevated leukocyte and neutrophil counts are considered inflammatory markers, it was concluded that exercise training might help to reduce the low-grade inflammation that has been associated with obesity (Johannsen *et al.* 2012). See Chapter 12 for further information on the anti-inflammatory effects of exercise.

Although NK cell function may change with exercise training in the elderly (discussed more in Chapter 4), NK cell numbers appear to be similar between trained and untrained people (Nieman *et al.* 1993a). Similarly, a period of exercise training, although increasing NK cell function, has no effect on total NK cell numbers (Woods *et al.* 1999). Total monocyte numbers tend to be unaffected by exercise training in the elderly, although 12 weeks of endurance/strength training in older adults reduced blood counts of the proinflammatory monocyte subset (Timmerman *et al.* 2008). Another study consisting of a 12-week exercise training intervention composed of both strength and endurance exercise did not alter total monocyte numbers in elderly subjects compared with non-exercising controls but did elevate the number of monocytes expressing the co-stimulatory molecule CD80 (Shimizu *et al.* 2011).

In healthy people, CD4+ T cells are numerically superior to CD8+ T cells and an inverted CD4 : CD8 ratio is indicative of memory CD8+ T cell inflation, presumably owing to excessive homeostatic proliferation of CD8+ T cells (Simpson *et al.* 2012). The CD4 : CD8 T-cell ratio decreases with age and those with a ratio below 1.0 are said to be in the 'immune risk profile' category, which has been associated with morbidity and mortality in the elderly (Simpson *et al.* 2012). However, both cross-sectional and longitudinal exercise training studies have failed to find any effects of exercise on resting CD4 : CD8 T cell ratio in older adults (Simpson and Guy 2010). Exercise may, however, alter the composition of CD4+ and CD8+ T cell subsets. Spielmann *et al.* (2011) showed that the age-related accumulation of senescent (KLRG1+/CD57+) CD4+ and CD8+ T cells and reduction in naïve T cells was blunted in individuals with higher $\dot{V}O_2$ max scores, indicating that aerobic exercise training may contribute to the negation of immunosenescence and the associated immune risk profile. Shimizu *et al.* (2008) found increased numbers and percentages of CD4+ T cells expressing the co-stimulatory molecule CD28 (a receptor that typically decreases with age) after a six-month supervised aerobic exercise programme in elderly males and females aged 61–76 years. Other longitudinal studies have, however, failed to report any effect of exercise training on CD28+ T-cell numbers in older adults (Kapasi *et al.* 2003; Raso *et al.* 2007).

KEY POINTS

- A single bout of exercise elicits a profound leukocytosis that is mostly caused by an increase in the numbers of circulatory neutrophils (neutrophilia), lymphocytes (lymphocytosis) and, to a lesser extent, monocytes (monocytosis). The neutrophil count (and, consequently, the total leukocyte count) may continue to rise for a number of hours after cessation of prolonged (over 60 minutes) exercise, while the lymphocyte count typically falls below the pre-exercise values (lymphocytopenia) during exercise recovery. Monocyte numbers usually return to pre-exercise values within the early stages of exercise recovery. Among lymphocytes, the relative change in numbers of NK cells is largest, followed by γδ T cells, CD8+ T cells, CD4+ T cells and B cells.

- Exercise duration exerts a stronger influence on the blood neutrophil and total leukocyte count, while changes in the number of lymphocytes are mostly dependent on the intensity of exercise. Monocyte numbers are strongly influenced by the intensity of exercise but prolonged endurance exercise may also cause a sustained monocytosis.

- The mechanisms for increased leukocyte numbers during exercise are believed to be caused by a demargination of leukocytes from the marginal pools of the blood vessels, splenic, pulmonary and hepatic reservoirs as a result of increased blood flow and cardiac output. The release of catecholamines (i.e. adrenaline, noradrenaline) and glucocorticoids (i.e. cortisol) also play a role as they bind to receptors expressed by the exercise responsive leukocytes. It appears that neutrophils and some monocytes are dependent on shear-stress mechanisms for their demargination, while lymphocytes and some specialised monocyte subtypes are mostly dependent on the actions of catecholamines. The release of cortisol during exercise is believed to cause the sustained leukocytosis as additional neutrophils are recruited from the bone-marrow, while cortisol also facilitates the extravasation of lymphocytes that can result in a lymphocytopenia.

- The leukocyte subtypes that are preferentially mobilised into the circulation during a single bout of exercise tend to have similar characteristics. These include increased cytotoxic/effector function capabilities, increased tissue migration potential, a greater expression of adrenoreceptors and glucocorticoid receptors and an increased ability to respond to catecholamines and cortisol. This indicates that the leukocyte response to exercise (and other stressors) is highly regulated (particularly for lymphocytes and monocytes) and not merely due to a non-specific 'washing out' of leukocytes from the marginal pools.

- There are many factors that can influence the leukocytosis to a single bout of exercise. Untrained individuals tend to have a smaller leukocytosis to exercise (particularly for lymphocytes) that may be due to exercise training induced reductions in the sensitivity, and to a lesser extent the density, of β2-ARs and glucocorticoid receptors.

- The absolute number of leukocytes mobilised into blood after a single bout of exercise is usually less in older people. This could be from lowered leukocyte reservoirs in the marginal pools and/or less shear-stress, owing to the reductions in cardiac output that occur with age. Altered sensitivity to catecholamines with ageing may also play a role.

- Repeated bouts of exercise may exert a 'carry-over' effect on leukocyte redistribution from one exercise bout to the next; however, this appears to be dependent on a number of factors, including the intensity/duration of exercise and the recovery time between the bouts.

- Infection history appears to have a strong influence on exercise-induced leukocyte redistribution. Latent CMV infection has a striking effect on the numbers of CD8+ T cells and NK cells mobilised into the circulation during exercise, but has no influence on CD4+, $\gamma\delta$ T cell, neutrophil or monocyte numbers.

- Carbohydrate availability strongly influences the leukocyte response to a single bout of exercise. Exercising in state of glycogen depletion increases plasma cortisol and IL-6 concentrations, which, in turn, increases total leukocyte numbers. This effect is reversed when exercise is performed following a period of carbohydrate loading or if adequate amounts of exogenous carbohydrate are consumed during exercise.

- Resting blood leukocyte and leukocyte subset counts tend to be similar among athletes and healthy controls, although athletes participating in endurance events (i.e. marathon running, cycling, triathlon) tend to have lower numbers of blood leukocytes. A minority of athletes may also have total cell counts below the clinically normal range. Leukocyte numbers in resting blood may also change in response to a period of exercise training, particularly within the lymphocyte compartment.

- In young healthy adults, resting blood leukocyte, granulocyte, monocyte, lymphocyte, CD4+ T cell, CD8+ T cell, B cell and NK cell numbers tend to be similar between aerobically trained and untrained participants. However, there is evidence to suggest that exercise training may alter the composition of specific leukocyte subtypes in the elderly and the obese.

- The number of leukocytes in the circulation at any given time is less that two per cent of the total number of white cells in the body. It is therefore difficult to ascertain whether the number and composition of leukocytes in the circulation is indicative of systemic immune compromise or activation. Moreover, it remains to be determined whether changes in the number and composition of leukocytes in the blood compartment have any clinical ramifications in both athletes and non-athletes.

FURTHER READING

Campbell, J. P., Riddell, N. E., Burns, V. E., Turner, M., van Zanten, J. J., Drayson, M. T. and Bosch, J. A. (2009) Acute exercise mobilises CD8+ T lymphocytes exhibiting an effector-memory phenotype. *Brain, Behavior and Immunity* 23: 767–75.

Foster, N. K., Martyn, J. B., Rangno, R. E., Hogg, J. C. and Pardy, R. L. (1986). Leukocytosis of exercise: role of cardiac output and catecholamines. *Journal of Applied Physiology* 61: 2218–23.

Horn, P. L., Pyne, D. B., Hopkins, W. G. and Barnes, C. J. (2010) Lower white blood cell counts in elite athletes training for highly aerobic sports. *European Journal of Applied Physiology* 110: 925–32.

McCarthy, D. A. and Dale, M. M. (1988). The leucocytosis of exercise: A review and a model. *Sports Medicine* 6: 333–63.

Shephard, R. J. (2003) Adhesion molecules, catecholamines and leucocyte redistribution during and following exercise. *Sports Medicine* 33: 261–84.

4 Effects of exercise on innate immune function

Michael Gleeson

After studying this chapter, you should be able to:

- describe the effect of acute exercise on neutrophil functions, including chemotaxis, phagocytosis, degranulation, oxidative burst and microbicidal capacity;
- describe the effect of acute exercise on monocyte and macrophage innate immune functions including phagocytosis, oxidative burst, Toll-like receptor expression;
- describe the effect of acute exercise on natural killer cell cytolytic activity;
- understand the mechanisms of innate immune system modulation by acute exercise;
- discuss the impact of exercise intensity, duration and fitness of subjects on the innate immune response to exercise;
- identify the effect of exercise training on innate immune cell functions;
- appreciate the *in vitro* methods used to measure innate immune cell functions.

█ **INTRODUCTION**

The ability to defend ourselves against invading micro-organisms depends on a number of mechanisms including physical barriers (e.g. skin), innate immunity (front-line defences such as neutrophils) and acquired immunity (e.g. antibodies). If the infectious agent is able to circumvent the physical barriers of the human body, an immune response is essential to prevent damage to the host. Invading microbes may be totally eliminated by the innate immune system. However, the innate immune system may be unsuccessful in eliminating the micro-organism but it still has an important 'holding' effect, which gives acquired mechanisms time to respond. During the early stages of invasion, the pathogen replicates to establish an infection, while the host defence attempts to clear foreign bodies. This early exchange between pathogen and innate mechanisms is often crucial in determining whether a clinical infection is established.

Innate immunity is our first line of defence against infectious pathogens. As explained in Chapter 2, the major difference between innate immune responses and adaptive responses is that innate responses do not strengthen upon repeated exposure (there is no memory function). In addition, innate responses are less specific in terms of pathogen recognition. So, whereas innate responses recognise classes of pathogens (e.g. Gram-negative bacteria) through Toll-like receptors (TLRs), lymphocytes exhibit exquisite specificity for epitopes of individual pathogens (e.g. the influenza virus).

The innate branch of the immune system includes both soluble factors and cells. Soluble factors include complement proteins, which mediate phagocytosis, control inflammation and interact with antibodies, interferons, which limit viral infection, and antimicrobial peptides like defensins, which limit bacterial growth. Major cells of the innate immune system include neutrophils, which are first-line defenders against bacterial infection, dendritic cells, monocytes and macrophages, which perform important phagocytic, regulatory and antigen presentation functions, and natural killer (NK) cells which recognise altered host cells (e.g. those that have become virally infected or transformed). However, many host cells, not just those classified as innate immune cells, can initiate responses to pathogenic infection. It should be emphasised that, while partitioning the immune system into innate and adaptive systems makes the system easier to understand, in fact, these branches are inextricably linked with each other. For example, the innate immune system helps to develop specific immune responses through antigen presentation, whereas cells of the adaptive system secrete cytokines that regulate innate immune cell function. This chapter focuses on the influence of acute and chronic exercise on cellular and soluble components of innate immunity.

EFFECT OF ACUTE EXERCISE ON INNATE IMMUNE CELL FUNCTIONS

Immunological integrity depends on, among other things, the number of immuno-competent cells and also on the functional capabilities of these cells. If we are to understand further the mechanisms through which exercise can alter the immune response, it is paramount that we determine whether this occurs by altering cell numbers, cell function, or both. The effect of a single bout of exercise on circulating numbers of innate immune leukocytes (neutrophils, monocytes/macrophages and natural killer cells) are described in Chapter 3; this chapter focuses on how exercise affects innate immune cell functions.

Neutrophils

Neutrophils constitute 50–60% of the circulating blood leukocyte pool. They have an important role in non-specific host defence against a variety of microbial pathogens, including bacteria, viruses and protozoa. Neutrophils are attracted to areas of infection (chemotaxis) and kill microbes by ingestion (phagocytosis) followed by enzymatic attack and digestion within intracellular vacuoles, using granular hydrolytic enzymes and reactive oxygen species (ROS) in a process called the oxidative or respiratory burst (see Chapter 2). Various neutrophil functions, including chemotaxis, phagocytosis and oxidative burst, can be quantified in the laboratory (see Technique box 4.1). Disorders of neutrophil function and neutropenia are associated with recurrent infections. An impaired or depleted neutrophil function could possibly be an important contributing factor to the increased susceptibility to infection of athletes (Pyne 1994). The effects of acute exercise and training on various neutrophil functions (adherence, chemotaxis, phagocytosis, degranulation and respiratory burst) have been reviewed by Ortega (2003), Pyne (1994) and Peake (2002).

Technique box 4.1

Measurement of phagocyte functions

Phagocytosis by neutrophils and monocytes

Substrates for phagocytosis include bacteria, sheep red blood cells and yeast particles; these can be studied in the opsonised and unopsonised states. Flow cytometry allows identification of both the number of cells participating in phagocytosis and the phagocytic activity per cell. Measures of phagocytosis can be coupled to measures of oxidative burst or to measures of bacterial killing.

Oxidative burst activity of neutrophils and monocytes

The oxidative (respiratory) burst activity of phagocytes (neutrophils and monocytes) can be separately assessed via flow cytometry. A key aspect of phagocyte function is their ability to generate reactive oxygen species (ROS) that aid in the destruction of ingested foreign organisms. We can assess the production of ROS from neutrophils in response to stimulation via flow cytometry. Neutrophils are activated with a stimulatory agent (e.g. LPS, PMA or *Escherichia coli*) in the presence of a compound called dihydrorhodamine (DHR). Upon contact with ROS generated by the activated neutrophil the non-fluorescent DHR is oxidised to the highly fluorescent compound rhodamine 123. The fluorescence intensity of the rhodamine 123 is proportional to the intensity of the neutrophil oxidative burst, thus allowing the investigator to quantify the amount of ROS generated following neutrophil activation. Experimental conditions should allow for both increased and decreased oxidative burst to be measured. Flow cytometry allows identification of both the number of cells participating in oxidative burst and the activity per cell. The same principle can be applied to the monocyte population in the blood sample.

Chemotactic response of neutrophils or monocytes

Chemotaxis is the movement of these cells towards particular stimuli. Stimuli used include leukotriene B4, bacterial cell-wall peptides such as formyl-methionyl-leucyl-phenylalanine (fMLP), interleukin-8 and autologous serum.

Chemotaxis

Since neutrophils exert their main functions in tissues outside the blood circulation, they are dependent on the ability to emigrate into the surrounding tissues by diapedesis and to move to the required location when guided by chemical attractants (a process called chemotaxis). Most reports indicate that neutrophil adherence to the endothelium (which is the first stage in diapedesis) is not affected by acute exercise of a moderate (Ortega *et al.* 1993b) or exhausting nature (Lewicki *et al.* 1987; Rodriguez *et al.* 1991), although Lewicki *et al.* (1987) observed an attenuation of this function during acute exercise in trained individuals. Neutrophil adherence at rest has been reported to be lower (Lewicki *et al.* 1987) or unaltered (Ortega *et al.* 1993a) in trained individuals compared with controls. Neutrophil chemotaxis may be enhanced by acute moderate exercise (Ortega *et al.* 1993b) or unchanged by single bouts of exhaustive exercise (Rodriguez *et al.* 1991), while being higher (Ortega *et al.* 1993a) or no different (Hack *et al.* 1992) in trained versus untrained individuals.

Phagocytosis

To improve the efficiency of their arsenal, neutrophils usually engulf the pathogen. Neutrophils achieve this process, known as phagocytosis, by extending pseudopodia (finger-like extensions of cytoplasm) out around the pathogen. Fusion of these extensions results in trapping of the pathogen within intracellular vacuoles, where the neutrophil can begin to attack the pathogen (see Figure 2.5). The ability to engulf foreign material has been used to assess neutrophil function *in vitro*. Most studies indicate that the phagocytic activity of neutrophils is increased during acute exercise (Hack *et al.* 1992; Lewicki *et al.*, 1987; Ortega *et al.* 1993b), although others have not reported such enhancement (Gabriel *et al.* 1994; Rodriguez *et al.* 1991). The phagocytic ability of granulocytes, of which most are neutrophils, has been reported to increase in response to 2.5 hours of exercise at 75% $\dot{V}O_2$ max (Nieman *et al.* 1998a). Data collected before and after a marathon show a shift in phagocytic activity of neutrophils: the percentage engaging in phagocytosis was increased, while the phagocytic capacity of the activated neutrophils was reduced (Chinda *et al.* 2003). This is consistent with data from Blannin *et al.* (1996a), which showed an increase in the percentage of neutrophils that are phagocytically active following acute exercise (Blannin *et al.* 1996a). These authors investigated the effects of long-term (over ten years) endurance training and submaximal exercise on the phagocytic activity of circulating neutrophils. The ability of stimulated blood neutrophils isolated from well trained cyclists ($n = 8$; $\dot{V}O_2$ max: 61.0 ± 8.8 ml.kg^{-1}.min^{-1}; age: 38 ± 4 years) and age-matched sedentary controls ($n = 8$; $\dot{V}O_2$ max: 37.4 ± 6.6 ml.kg^{-1}.min^{-1}) to ingest nitroblue tetrazolium was assessed at rest and following a standardised submaximal bout of exercise on a cycle ergometer. The circulating neutrophil phagocytic capacity was approximately 70% lower in trained individuals at rest compared with the control subjects (Figure 4.1). Acute submaximal exercise increased this variable in both groups but circulating phagocytic capacity remained substantially lower in the trained subjects compared with the controls (Figure 4.1). Circulating phagocytic

Figure 4.1 Effect of moderate exercise on the circulating phagocytic capacity of the blood in trained and untrained subjects matched for age and body mass. Acute exercise increases the circulating phagocytic capacity of blood, some of which will be due to a neutrophilia (data from Blannin *et al.* 1996a); † = $P < 0.05$; †† = $P < 0.01$ trained compared with untrained; * = $P < 0.05$; ** = $P < 0.01$ significant difference compared with corresponding resting value

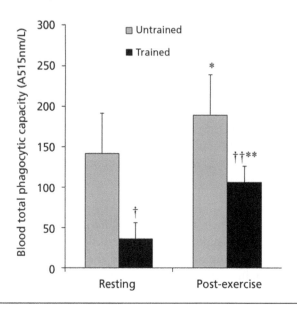

capacity is a function of the neutrophil count, the percentage of neutrophils that are phagocytically active and the phagocytic capacity of individual neutrophils. These data show the neutrophil count and the percentage of phagocytically active cells are increased by moderate exercise (Blannin *et al.* 1996a). Although neutrophil phagocytic activity is only one parameter that contributes to immunological status, prolonged periods of endurance training may lead to increased susceptibility to opportunistic infections by diminishing this activity at rest.

Degranulation

Following phagocytosis, neutrophils digest micro-organisms by releasing granular lytic enzymes (a process called degranulation) and generating reactive oxygen species (a process called the oxidative or respiratory burst) as described in Chapter 2. Degranulation appears to be induced by exercise, since elevated plasma concentrations of elastase (Blannin *et al.* 1996b; Robson *et al.* 1999b) and myeloperoxidase (MPO; Suzuki *et al.* 2003) have been reported following various exercise protocols, although this could simply reflect the simultaneous neutrophilia (Suzuki *et al.* 1999). Blannin *et al.* (1996b) investigated the effects of acute exercise and endurance training on the neutrophil degranulation response to submaximal exercise in 14 previously sedentary individuals. The effect of exercise training on plasma elastase concentration and stimulated neutrophil degranulation was assessed on blood taken before and up to

2.5 hours after cycling for 30 minutes at 70% V̇O₂ max and compared with untrained controls. Acute exercise significantly elevated plasma elastase levels (83.1 ± 12.0 compared with 56.0 ± 9.2 µg/L at rest) and this response was reduced by training. Stimulated neutrophil degranulation, measured by elastase release per neutrophil in response to bacterial stimulation, was unaltered during exercise but was significantly suppressed 2.5 hours after exercise (Figure 4.2). Training attenuated the bacterially stimulated release of elastase per volume of blood in resting and 2.5-hour post-exercise blood samples. The reduced degranulation response to bacteria following acute exercise may be attributable to desensitisation after the exercise stimulus, as neutrophils can enter a refractory period following activation. It is unlikely that depletion of neutrophil granules is the explanation for the reduced stimulated degranulation observed in the study because an acute bout of exercise does not appear to affect total neutrophil elastase content (Blannin *et al.* 1997; Bishop *et al.* 2003). Bishop *et al.* (2002) have also observed an attenuation of stimulated neutrophil degranulation after acute exercise. It appears, therefore, that acute exercise leads to an increase in spontaneous neutrophil degranulation but the ability of the neutrophil to degranulate when stimulated is lowered by acute exercise bouts.

Figure 4.2 Effect of 30 minutes of exercise at 70% V̇O₂ max on the stimulated neutrophil degranulation response (data from Blannin *et al.* 1996b); data (mean ± SD, $n = 14$) are expressed as release of elastase (fg) per neutrophil; * indicates a significant difference compared with rest ($P < 0.05$)

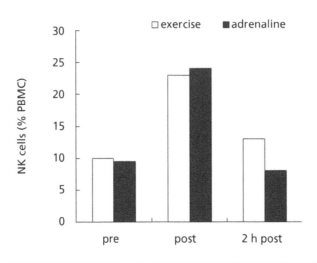

Oxidative burst

The other part of the neutrophil's arsenal, the production of reactive oxygen species (called the oxidative or respiratory burst), has been reported to be attenuated by acute exercise (Hack *et al.* 1992; Pyne 1994). Furthermore, Macha *et al.* (1990) have demonstrated that the generation of H_2O_2 by stimulated neutrophils is attenuated during acute exercise by a plasma borne inhibitor. This is in contrast to the increased production of hydrogen peroxide (H_2O_2) and hydrochlorous acid (HOCl) by stimulated neutrophils reported by Smith et al. (1990) during acute exercise. This ambiguity may be a consequence of an intensity-dependent effect on neutrophil function, since cycling at 50% $\dot{V}O_2$ max and 80% $\dot{V}O_2$ max has been reported to enhance and attenuate the oxidative burst of neutrophils (Dziedziak 1990). Furthermore, the respiratory burst continues to decrease in the hours following intense exercise, whilst being enhanced during recovery from moderate intensity exercise (Pyne et al. 1994). The severity of the bout appears to be the key factor, as evidence shows that neutrophil oxidative burst activity is significantly lowered during a marathon race (Chinda et al. 2003; Suzuki et al. 2003). The mechanism for these effects could be via the actions of adrenaline, as adrenaline decreases neutrophil respiratory burst in vitro by elevating cyclic adenosine monophosphate (Tintinger et al. 2001). However, elevated levels of interleukin (IL)-6 following exercise could be another important mechanism that regulates neutrophil respiratory burst (Peake 2002), which would also be in keeping with the different results found at moderate and high intensities. Since superoxide anion (O_2^-) production has been shown to be increased 24 hours after acute exercise (Hack et al. 1992), and the increase in the oxidative burst during exercise appears to be attenuated one week after a prolonged endurance run (Gabriel et al. 1994b), the effects of acute exercise on the respiratory burst activity of neutrophils can potentially be long-term in nature. Neutrophils from trained individuals have been reported to have a lower respiratory burst activity compared with untrained individuals (Smith et al. 1990), although Hack et al. (1992) did not observe such a difference.

Microbicidal capacity

The combined effect of release of lytic enzymes (degranulation) and the production of reactive oxygen species by neutrophils is the generation of a hostile environment for the destruction of 'foreign bodies'. Killing capacity or microbicidal activity (assessed by measuring the percentage of viable intracellular micro-organisms) has been shown to be unaffected (Lewicki et al. 1987; Ortega et al., 1993b) or enhanced (Rodriguez et al. 1991) by acute exercise. Resting neutrophil bactericidal activity was reported to be similar in trained and untrained subjects (Lewicki et al. 1987), although this capacity was attenuated by acute exercise in trained individuals. The apparent contradictions in the effects of acute and chronic exercise on neutrophil functions probably arise from the differences in age, gender and initial fitness levels of the subjects, the exercise protocols used and the various parameters of neutrophil function studied.

> **Group activity 4.1**
>
> **Discuss a paper on the effects of a sporting activity on innate immunity**
>
> *The problem*
>
> Read this paper: Takahshi, I. *et al.* (2007). Effects of rugby sevens matches on human neutrophil-related non-specific immunity. *British Journal of Sports Medicine* 41: 13–18.
>
> *Points for discussion within your groups*
>
> Terminology: The following terms were used in the paper; what are they/what do they mean?
>
> - serum myogenic enzymes
> - neutrophilia
> - chemiluminescence response
> - SOA (serum-opsonic activity)
> - phagocytic activity
> - reactive oxygen species production
>
> What was the aim of the study?
> What were the KEY findings of the study? (Give no more than three bullet points.)
> Are the observed changes in neutrophil numbers and function likely to be beneficial or harmful to host defence? Are they likely to alter susceptibility to upper respiratory tract infections?
> What are the practical implications of these findings?
> What are the main limitations of the study and what information that the authors do not tell us would be useful to know?

Monocyte/macrophage phagocytic function

Phagocytic function

Brief exhaustive exercise, insulin and dexamethasone all appear to reduce phagocytic activity of monocytes when incubated with opsonised zymosan particles (Bieger *et al.* 1980). In contrast, the phagocytic function of monocytes has been shown to increase following 2.5 hours of exercise at 75% $\dot{V}O_2$ max (Nieman *et al.* 1998a). For macrophages, their function appears to change dependent on the exercise intensity; moderate acute exercise enhances many macrophage functions (adherence, chemotaxis, phagocytosis, microbicidal activity), while acute exercise to exhaustion appears to have no effect on macrophage functions (Ortega 2003). The functional changes in monocytes and macrophages after acute exercise might be due to the actions of cortisol.

Monocyte Toll-like receptor expression and function

A new and potentially important finding is that following a prolonged bout of strenuous exercise the expression of some TLRs on monocytes is decreased. You may recall from Chapter 2 that TLRs enable antigen-presenting cells to recognise pathogens and control the activation of the adaptive immune response. Following recognition of their specific ligand (e.g. bacterial lipopolysaccharide binds to TLR4 and zymosan binds to TLRs 2 and 6), TLRs expressed by antigen-presenting cells regulate the production of several cytokines including IL-6, IL-8, IL-12 and tumour necrosis factor alpha (TNF-α), as well as the expression of accessory signal molecules (CD80, CD86) and major histocompatibility (MHC) II class II proteins, which are required for the activation of naïve T lymphocytes. Thus, TLRs, through the recognition of highly conserved microbial patterns and the subsequent induction of inflammatory, innate and adaptive immune responses, play a fundamental role in host defence. A study by Lancaster et al. (2005b) found that following 90 minutes of cycling at 65% $\dot{V}O_2$ max in the heat (35 degrees Celsius) the monocyte expression of TLRs 1, 2 and 4 (but not TLR9) was substantially decreased (Figure 4.3) with little or no recovery by two hours post-exercise. Furthermore, the induction of monocyte CD86 and MHC class II expression by known TLR ligands was significantly lower in samples obtained following exercise compared with pre-exercise. Monocyte expression of TLRs 1, 2, 3 and 4 was also found to be reduced for several hours following exercise in temperate conditions (Oliveira and Gleeson 2010). These effects may represent an important mechanism through which exercise stress impairs both innate and adaptive (acquired, specific) immune function since the stimulation of TLRs is essentially the first important event in the activation of the adaptive immune response.

Monocyte cytokine production

Several studies have examined monocyte cytokine production after acute exercise and found that while spontaneous cytokine levels in CD14+ cells change little (Rivier et al. 1994; Starkie et al. 2000), acute exercise reduces TLR ligand-stimulated IL-6 (Figure 4.4), IL1-β and TNF-α production (Lancaster et al. 2005b; Starkie et al. 2001a) perhaps as a consequence of reduced TLR expression. Further studies regarding the effects of acute exercise on monocyte TLR signalling may clarify these observations.

Monocyte phenotype

In response to acute exercise, there is a preferential mobilisation of CD14+/CD16+ expressing monocytes (Steppich et al. 2000; Hong and Mills 2008) that exhibit a proinflammatory phenotype relative to CD14+/CD16– classical monocytes. Indeed,

Figure 4.3 Effect of exercise on Toll-like receptor (TLR) expression on CD14+ monocytes. Peripheral blood samples were obtained from 11 healthy volunteers before, immediately after and following 2 hours of resting recovery from 90 minutes of exercise at 55% W_{max} in the heat (34°C). Samples were labelled with specific TLR monoclonal antibodies or isotype controls for TLR 1 (A), TLR 2 (B), TLR 4 (C) and TLR 9 (D) and examined by flow cytometry. All data represent the mean ± SEM; † denotes a statistically significant difference ($P < 0.05$) from pre-exercise (data from Lancaster *et al.* 2004)

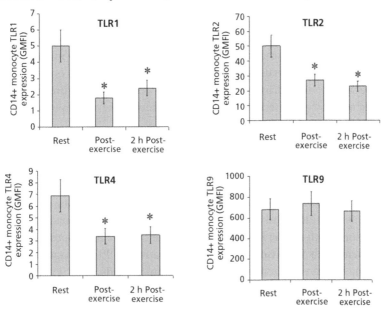

Figure 4.4 Effect of exercise on intracellular IL-6 expression in lipopolysaccharide-stimulated CD14+ monocytes. Peripheral blood samples were obtained from 10 healthy volunteers before, immediately after and following 2 hours of resting recovery from 90 minutes of exercise at 55% W_{max} in the heat (34°C). Samples were incubated with either LPS (TLR4 ligand) or with culture media only (unstimulated) for 6 hours, following which monocyte intracellular IL-6 expression was examined by flow cytometry. All data represent the mean ± SEM; * denotes a statistically significant ($P < 0.01$) difference from pre-exercise (data from Lancaster *et al.* 2004)

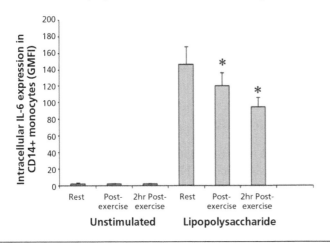

it may be that these marginated cells have a more mature inflammatory function for entry into tissues and are knocked off the blood vessel endothelium in response to exercise. Interestingly, the percentage of these CD14+/CD16+ cells is reduced in recovery; perhaps indicating remarginalisation or tissue recruitment (Simpson *et al.* 2009). The extent to which reductions in monocyte TLR expression during exercise reflect a true decrease, as opposed to monocyte population shifts, is unclear. In an attempt to reconcile this, Simpson *et al.* (2009) examined cell surface proteins on monocyte subpopulations in response to acute exercise. They found that TLR4 and HLA.DR (major histocompatibility molecule II important in antigen presentation) expression were altered on total CD14+ monocytes but also on individual monocyte populations, indicating that changes in cell surface expression are not solely influenced by exercise-induced changes in monocyte subpopulations in blood.

Macrophage functions

Because monocytes are relatively immature, exercise-induced changes in their function may not reflect actual tissue macrophage function, which is central to inflammation and immune responses. For this, studies have been performed in animals to understand the influence of exercise on tissue macrophage number and function. Both moderate and intense acute exercise have potent stimulatory effects on chemotaxis (Okutsu *et al.* 2008; Ortega *et al.* 1997), phagocytosis (Ortega *et al.* 1996), reactive oxygen species production (Woods *et al.* 1993, 1994) and anti-tumour activity (Davis *et al.* 1998; Woods *et al.* 1993, 1994). However, not all functions are enhanced by exercise. Prolonged exercise-induced reductions in macrophage MHC class II expression (Woods *et al.* 1997) and antigen presentation capacity (Ceddia *et al.* 1999, 2000) have been reported in mice and exhaustive (but not moderate) exercise reduces the ability of murine macrophages to restrict viral replication at eight hours post-exercise (Davis *et al.* 1997) as illustrated in Figure 4.5. Some effects may be dose-dependent as exhaustive exercise was shown to decrease alveolar macrophage anti-viral function, an effect that was correlated to increased susceptibility to herpes simplex virus (HSV)-1 infection (Kohut *et al.* 1998a, 1998b) and related to increased release of adrenal catecholamines but not corticosterone (Kohut *et al.* 1998a). Thus, it appears that exercise, perhaps dependent on dose with respect to some functions, can affect tissue macrophage and, in some studies, disease outcomes in animals. Whether these same effects can be generalised to humans is presently unknown.

Natural killer cell cytotoxic activity

Activation of NK (CD3−CD16+CD56+) cells does not require recognition of an antigen−MHC class II combination. NK cells may serve as a 'front line of defence' before a specific response can be mounted by T and B cells. The effects of intense exercise on NK-cell function appear to be biphasic, with an initial enhancement followed by a delayed suppression (Kappel *et al.* 1991b; Pedersen 1991; Nieman *et*

Figure 4.5 The ability of alveolar macrophages from mice to restrict viral replication at 8 hours post-exercise was significantly decreased (* $P < 0.05$) after exhaustive (exh) running (2.5–3.5 hours at a running speed of 18–36 metres/minute to fatigue) but not after moderate (mod) exercise (running speed of 18 metres/minute for 30 minutes) compared with the control (no exercise) treatment (data from Davis *et al.* 1997)

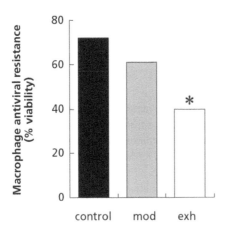

al. 1993b), as illustrated in Figure 4.6. NK-cell cytotoxicity is a major functional measure of NK activity and can be quantified in the laboratory (see Technique box 4.2). Many authors have shown NK cytolytic activity to be higher at the end of moderate and intense exercise (Pedersen *et al.* 1988; Roberts *et al.* 2004), which may be partly due to the large increase in the NK population produced by exercise

Figure 4.6 Changes in natural killer cell activity (expressed as lytic units per litre of blood) after 45 minutes of running at 80% $\dot{V}O_2$ max; * denotes a statistically significant ($P < 0.05$) difference from pre-exercise (data from Nieman *et al.* 2003b)

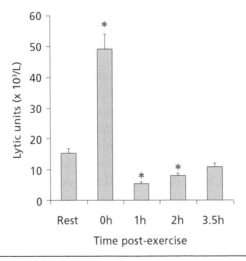

Technique box 4.2

Measurement of natural killer cell functions

Natural killer (NK) cell cytolytic activity is measured as the killing of tumour cells known to be specific targets for NK cells. Killing of the target cells results in lysis of the target cells. The K562 cell line is often used as a target for human NK cells. The assay is normally conducted at several ratios of killer to target cell (e.g. 100 : 1; 50 : 1; 25 : 1; 5 : 1). Typically, the assay time is quite short – about four hours. There are a number of ways to measure target-cell killing. Classically, target cells are preloaded with radioactive chromium (^{51}Cr) and the release of ^{51}Cr into the medium as a result of target cell death is determined by a gamma counter. One advantage of this assay is that background counts can be low, giving a high level of sensitivity. However, the use of ^{51}Cr requires suitable precautions. There are alternative methods for determining NK cell activity. It is possible to label target cells fluorescently and to determine target-cell killing using flow cytometry.

Alternatively, target cell death has been determined as the appearance of lactate dehydrogenase in the medium; this is released from dead target cells. If this approach is used, a number of controls are required, because there may be spontaneous release of lactate dehydrogenase from both killer cells and target cells. This assay must also be done in serum-free medium, because serum contains lactate dehydrogenase. Whatever approach is used, the data can be expressed in various ways, such as per cent target-cell killing at each killer to target cell ratio or 'lytic ratio', which is the ratio required to kill a particular percentage (e.g. 25% or 50%) of target cells.

(Roberts *et al.* 2004). Immediately after a single bout of moderate or exhaustive exercise, there is a 50–100% increase in human peripheral blood NK cytolytic activity (Gannon *et al.* 1995; Woods *et al.*, 1998). The exercise-induced increase in NK cytolytic activity is largely due to an increase in the absolute number and percentage of blood NK cells (Gannon *et al.*, 1995). NK cytolytic activity expressed on a per-cell basis does not appear to change much after acute exercise unless the bout was intense and prolonged, in which case it can be depressed for several hours (Nieman *et al.* 1993b; Figure 4.7), possibly indicating an enhanced period of susceptibility to infection.

An attenuation of the NK cytolytic activity has also been reported a few hours after an intense bout of exercise (Kappel *et al.* 1991b; McFarlin *et al.* 2004; Pedersen 1991). A proposed mechanism for the delayed reduction in NK-cell function is an elevated level of prostaglandins released from the relatively numerous monocytes observed 1.5–2.0 hours after intense exercise, since this effect is abolished *in vitro* and *in vivo* by indomethacin (which inhibits prostaglandin synthesis) and is also blocked if the monocytes are removed from the culture (Pedersen 1991). Furthermore, adrenaline infusion to recreate plasma concentrations similar to those observed after one hour of exercise at 75% $\dot{V}O_2$ max also induced a delayed monocytosis, suppressed NK activity with a two-hour delay, which was blocked by indomethacin and removal of monocytes (Kappel *et al.* 1991b; Figure 4.8). This illustrates how adrenaline can

Figure 4.7 Changes in blood natural killer (NK) cell numbers (circles), total NK cell activity (NKCA; triangles) and NKCA per NK cell (squares) after 45 minutes of treadmill running at 80% $\dot{V}O_2$ max (data from Nieman *et al.* 1993b)

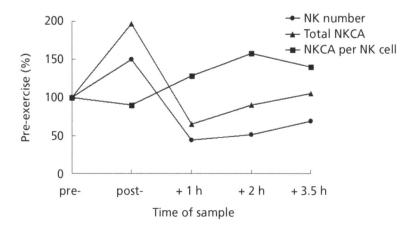

Figure 4.8 Changes in the percentage of natural killer (NK) cells and NK cell activity (NKCA) per NK cell after 1 hour cycling at 75% $\dot{V}O_2$ max (light columns) or intravenous infusion of adrenaline to give plasma levels similar to those observed after the exercise (data from Kappel *et al.* 1991b)

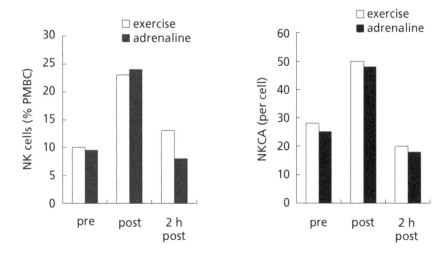

have more long-term influences on immunity, even though its plasma half-life is relatively short. Since intense exercise can induce a delayed neutrophilia, and neutrophils can suppress NK-cell activity (Pedersen *et al.* 1988), an increased circulating neutrophil count may contribute to the attenuation of NK-cell function in the hours following intense exercise. However, since a five-hour infusion of cortisol, which induced a neutrophilia, had no effect on NK-cell numbers or activity

(Tonnesen *et al.* 1987), the influence of neutrophils on NK cells is probably minimal. More recently McFarlin *et al.* (2004) have postulated that the post-exercise fall in NK cytolytic activity might be due to an exercise-induced change in the Th1/Th2 balance (see Chapter 2). An important Th1 cytokine is IL-2, which appears to stimulate NK cells. IL-2 release is suppressed by corticosteroids and reduced plasma levels and decreased *in vitro* production of IL-2 by lymphocytes after a bout of vigorous exercise have been reported (Shephard *et al.* 1994).

Only a few studies have examined whether NK cells mobilised into the circulation in response to exercise have altered sensitivity to stimulating agents like IL-2 or interferon-α (Fiatarone *et al.* 1989; Woods *et al.* 1998); however, like unstimulated NK cytolytic activity, these effects are likely mediated by distributional shifts in NK-cell subsets and may not necessarily be interpreted as altered NK-cell function on a per-cell basis.

MECHANISMS OF CHANGES IN INNATE IMMUNE FUNCTION DURING EXERCISE

The stress hormones adrenaline and cortisol are involved in many of the changes in innate immunity outlined above. Adrenaline and cortisol are involved in the production of the leukocytosis by demargination and bone marrow release. In addition to changing the number of circulating cells, these changes in population may introduce cells with different functional capacity. Furthermore, the stress hormones, and cortisol in particular, appear to regulate innate immune cell function. Moderate intensity exercise, which is often associated with enhanced immune cell function, increases the clearance of cortisol and lowers its secretion. In contrast, high intensity, exhaustive exercise, which can induce depression of innate immune cell functions, is associated with increased secretion of cortisol. *In vitro* studies help to explain the influence of exercise intensity on changes in leukocyte function because low physiological concentrations of cortisol appear to improve function, while very high physiological to pharmacological concentrations are typically immunosuppressive (Ortega 2003).

In addition to the hormones that have been discussed, other immunological regulators appear to be influenced by exercise. It is noteworthy that there are many similarities between the response to acute strenuous exercise and the acute inflammatory response to infection, including leukocytosis, moderate fever and an increase in cytokines, influencing leukocyte function. The complex functions of cytokines and their responses to exercise are discussed in more detail in Chapter 12.

The exercise-induced mediators of the changes in neutrophil function remain to be clarified. One candidate, the rapid immunological amplifier complement (described in Chapter 2), has been shown to be activated by prolonged (Dufaux and Order 1989) and short intense exercise (Camus *et al.* 1994; Dufaux *et al.* 1991). Complement increases adherence of C3b-coated microbes to phagocytic cells and therefore aids in phagocytosis, and fragments C3a and C5a stimulate the respiratory burst in neutrophils and the production of many different mediators which enhance the immune response such as chemotactic factors. It appears that severe exercise of a prolonged or brief exhaustive nature can activate complement, possibly by inducing proteolytic reactions (Dufaux and Order, 1989; Dufaux *et al.*, 1991). It has been suggested that only severe exercise of the kind described will activate complement, but an acute phase inflammatory response (known to be mediated by activated complement) has been reported to occur one day after a single submaximal bout of eccentric exercise (Gleeson *et al.* 1995c). Activated complement has a range of biological functions: it facilitates adherence of complement-coated micro-organisms to phagocytic cells and therefore enhances phagocytosis; it can directly (and indirectly via mediators) establish an acute inflammatory response at the site of a microbial invasion; and it can insert membrane attack complexes into bacteria, possibly resulting in lysis.

An increase in circulating IL-6 occurs during prolonged exercise. Bente Pedersen's group have demonstrated that the IL-6 appearing in the circulation during exercise is produced and released from exercising muscle (Steensberg *et al.* 2000). Rises in circulating IL-6 increases the secretion of cortisol, IL-1ra and IL-10 (Steensberg 2003; Steensberg *et al.* 2003) and, thus, the post-exercise increase in IL-6 is almost certainly involved in some of the immune changes induced by exercise. For example, elevated IL-6 released from energy challenged muscle has been implicated in the shift in the T helper-1/T helper-2 balance following exercise (Steensberg *et al.* 2003) and changes in neutrophil function (Suzuki *et al.* 2003). Further details of the biological roles of IL-6 and the effects of exercise on IL-6 can be found in Chapter 12.

ACUTE EFFECTS OF EXERCISE ON SOLUBLE FACTORS

Soluble factors of the innate immune system include complement proteins, which mediate phagocytosis, control inflammation and interact with antibodies, interferons, which limit viral infection, and antimicrobial peptides like defensins, which limit bacterial growth. Unaccustomed, long duration and/or intense exercise has been shown to elicit aspects of an acute-phase response (Weight *et al.* 1991; Meyer *et al.* 2001). This response, which ultimately serves to protect the body and restore homoeostasis, can be initiated by a wide variety of stimuli, including microbial invasion, chemical/physical trauma and ischaemic necrosis. C reactive protein, α1 antitrypsin and complement proteins are classified as acute-phase proteins. Traditionally, an acute-phase protein has been defined as a protein that either increases (positive acute-phase protein) or decreases (negative acute-phase protein) in concentration in response to homoeostatic disturbance in which cell damage and/or tissue death has occurred. This response is a generalised systemic reaction closely linked to inflammation and forms part of the innate immune response.

Most studies investigating the response of acute phase proteins to physical activity have examined prolonged bouts of running (Weight *et al.* 1991; Semple *et al.* 2004), short-term maximal and submaximal exercise (Meyer *et al.* 2001; Dufaux *et al.* 1991) or the changes in acute-phase proteins over extended periods (Mattusch *et al.* 2000). The focus of these investigations has been proinflammatory mediators, with anti-inflammatory proteins receiving less attention. Exercise that causes muscle damage generally results in elevated levels of C-reactive protein and complement proteins, which peak around 24 hours post-exercise, whereas chronic exercise training may reduce resting concentrations of some inflammatory markers. Few studies have investigated this response in exercise that involves less mechanical loading – that is, less eccentric damage – such as cycling. However, one such study by Semple *et al.* (2006) evaluated the concentrations of proinflammatory (C-reactive protein, complementary proteins C3 and C4) and anti-inflammatory (α1 antitrypsin, C1 esterase inhibitor [C1-INH]) acute phase proteins in elite cyclists at two time points during a three-week cycle tour. The authors found increases in two of the three proinflammatory (C-reactive protein, C4) and both of the anti-inflammatory (C1-INH, α1 antitrypsin) acute-phase proteins, indicative of an acute phase/inflammatory response, occurred at the mid-point of the tour and they observed that resting concentrations of some acute phase proteins in elite cyclists were lower than in sedentary subjects. The acute phase/inflammatory response is classified as an integral component of non-specific/innate immunity. Further studies are needed to shed light on how this response affects adaptive immunity as evidence is mounting to support a close link between the two systems.

THE EFFECT OF EXERCISE INTENSITY, DURATION AND SUBJECT FITNESS ON THE INNATE IMMUNE RESPONSE TO EXERCISE

Since many of the immunological changes to acute exercise appear to arise in response to stress hormones, factors such as exercise intensity, duration and subject fitness, which influence stress hormone secretion, will affect the immune response. Both leukocyte numbers and functions are affected by catecholamines, which are elevated by acute exercise in an intensity dependent manner. Subject fitness has a bearing on the relative intensity of a bout and will, therefore, alter the immunological outcome to an acute exercise bout (e.g. Blannin *et al.* 1996a). Furthermore, exercise-induced elevations in cortisol affect the leukocyte count and function and this hormone is effected by the intensity and duration of exercise.

Mild to moderate exercise (less than 50% $\dot{V}O_2$ max) seems to reduce cortisol concentrations, owing to an enhanced elimination and a suppressed secretion, whereas more intense exercise (greater than 60% $\dot{V}O_2$ max) increases cortisol (Galbo 1983). However, if the bout is sufficiently prolonged, even relatively moderate intensities can elicit increases in cortisol because it is released to increase gluconeogenesis and maintain blood glucose concentrations. Exercise intensity and duration both contribute to the metabolic stress of the bout and thus influence fuel depletion. Since evidence suggests that skeletal muscle can release IL-6 when fuel provision becomes challenged (Steensberg *et al.* 2000) and this cytokine is known to have immunological actions (Steensberg *et al.* 2003), factors such as intensity, duration and subject fitness that can influence metabolic demand will effect the immunological outcome.

EFFECTS OF EXERCISE TRAINING ON CELLULAR INNATE IMMUNE FUNCTION

Neutrophils

Regular exercise training does not appear to appreciably alter blood leukocyte counts, including those of neutrophils. However, there are a few reports that exercise training reduces blood neutrophil counts in those with chronic inflammatory conditions (e.g. people who are obese) or neutrophils in sites of chronic inflammation (Michishita *et al.* 2010), raising the possibility that such exercise acts in an anti-inflammatory fashion in those with elevated inflammation. This effect could be beneficial or deleterious, depending on the context. While there is little known about the influence of exercise training on neutrophil function, regular exercise, especially heavy, intense training, may attenuate neutrophil respiratory burst (Hack *et al.* 1994; Pyne *et al.* 1995). This could reflect a sustained effect of previous acute exercise as attenuation of respiratory burst has been documented to last several days post-exercise (Suzuki *et al.* 1999).

Monocytes/macrophages

In people, both longitudinal exercise training and cross-sectional studies have shown that physically active subjects exhibit reduced blood monocyte inflammatory responses to lipopolysaccharide, lower TLR4 expression and a lower percentage of CD14+/CD16+ inflammatory monocytes (Gleeson *et al.* 2006; Sloan *et al.* 2007; Timmerman *et al.* 2008). The extent to which these effects on the relatively small blood monocyte pool contribute to the anti-inflammatory effect of exercise training is unknown. In contrast, animal studies have demonstrated that exercise training can increase induced inflammatory responses of peritoneal macrophages (Kizaki *et al.* 2008; Sugiura *et al.* 2002), indicating a possible difference between the effects of training on blood monocytes when compared with differentiated tissue macrophages. Animal studies have the potential to shed additional light on the source of the anti-inflammatory effect of regular exercise, especially in populations that exhibit elevated inflammation. Indeed, two studies have shown that exercise training, with or without a low-fat diet, reduces visceral adipose tissue (e.g. macrophage infiltration and pro-inflammatory cytokine gene expression) and systemic inflammation in high-fat, diet-fed mice (Vieira *et al.* 2009a, 2009b). Regular exercise may also reduce macrophage infiltration into other sites of chronic inflammation including growing tumours (Zielinski *et al.* 2004) and could be interpreted as a benefit, given the tumour-supporting role of these cells. In contrast, reduced infiltration of macrophages into sites of chronic infection could lead to higher morbidity, although this has not been demonstrated. In fact, macrophages appear to play a definitive role in mediating the beneficial effects of regular moderate exercise, as it relates to intranasal infection with HSV-1 in mice Murphy *et al.* (2004).

Dendritic cells

There are two reports from the same group demonstrating an effect of exercise training on rat dendritic cells. Liao *et al.* (2006) reported that dendritic cell numbers increased after training, with no difference in co-stimulatory molecule (CD80 or CD86) expression, while Chiang *et al.* (2007) found that MHC class II expression, mixed leukocyte reaction and IL-12 production were increased in dendritic cells from exercise trained rats. Given the importance of dendritic cells in early immune regulation, this is an area ripe for investigation.

Natural killer cells

Despite much research regarding the effects of exercise training on NK-cell numbers and function, there appears to be much controversy regarding their effect. Several cross-sectional studies or interventions with limited subject numbers have reported modest increases in NK cytolytic activity after moderate exercise training in previously sedentary subjects (McFarlin *et al.* 2005; Nieman *et al.* 1990b, 1995; Pedersen *et al.* 1989; Shephard and Shek 1999a). In two of the larger trials, one study (Fairey *et al.* 2005) found that 15 weeks of moderate exercise training increased NK cytolytic activity compared with sedentary controls, while another 12-month trial found no change in NK cytolytic activity in 115 post-menopausal women (Campbell *et al.* 2008b). However, intense training has been shown to alter NK-cell subsets and reduce NK cytolytic activity (Gleeson *et al.* 1995b; Suzui *et al.* 2004; Rama *et al.* 2013). Studies in animals have demonstrated that regular exercise can increase *in vivo* cytotoxicity (MacNeil and Hoffman-Goetz 1993; Jonsdottir *et al.* 2000), although the specific contribution of NK cells in mediating this exercise effect is unclear.

KEY POINTS

- For strenuous exercise lasting less than one hour, there is an immediate leukocytosis consisting mainly of neutrophils and lymphocytes, which begin to recover, leaving a developing neutrophilia peaking between two to three hours post-exercise. If the exercise is more prolonged, however, these events superimpose upon each other.
- The initial leukocytosis appears to be produced by demargination of leukocytes, owing to increased shear stress and catecholamines. In contrast, the neutrophilia observed at the end of prolonged exercise or hours after brief, intense exercise is produced by release of neutrophils from the bone marrow induced by elevated plasma cortisol.

- The various aspects of neutrophil function appear to respond to exercise independently of each other. The number of neutrophils engaging in phagocytosis is increased by acute exercise but their phagocytic capacity is lowered. Exercise induces a slight degranulation of neutrophils, which may be responsible for the attenuated degranulation response to bacterial stimulation that is seen for several hours after exercise. Finally, the effect of exercise on neutrophil respiratory burst activity appears to be dependent on the intensity of the bout; moderate work rates elicit enhanced respiratory burst but severe exercise bouts compromise neutrophil respiratory burst.
- Functional changes are brought about by a variety of bloodborne factors produced by exercise. Activation of complement and increased circulating concentrations of catecholamines, cortisol and IL-6 are important regulators of innate immune function during and following exercise.
- Exercise training affects some aspects of innate immunity. Regular exercise training does not appear to appreciably alter blood leukocyte counts, including those of neutrophils. However, there are a few reports that exercise training reduces blood neutrophil counts in those with chronic inflammatory conditions (e.g. people who are obese) or neutrophils in sites of chronic inflammation raising the possibility that such exercise acts in an anti-inflammatory fashion in those with elevated inflammation.
- Both acute and chronic exercise can alter circulating monocyte and NK cell subsets.
- Modest increases in NK cytolytic activity may occur after moderate exercise training in previously sedentary subjects.

FURTHER READING

Ceddia, M. A. and Woods, J. A. (1999) Exercise suppresses macrophage antigen presentation. *Journal of Applied Physiology* 87: 2253–8.

Field, C. J., Gougeon, R. and Marliss, E. B. (1991) Circulating mononuclear cell numbers and function during intense exercise and recovery. *Journal of Applied Physiology* 71: 1089–97.

Gleeson, M., McFarlin, B. and Flynn, M. (2006) Exercise and Toll-like receptors. *Exercise Immunology Review* 12: 34–53.

Nieman, D. C., Buckley, K. S., Henson, D. A., Warren, B. J., Suttles, J., Ahle, J. C., Simandle, S., Fagoaga, O. R. and Nehlsen-Cannarella, S. L. (1995) Immune function in marathon runners versus sedentary controls. *Medicine and Science in Sports and Exercise* 27: 986–92.

Peake, J. M. (2002) Exercise-induced alterations in neutrophil degranulation and respiratory burst activity: possible mechanisms of action. *Exercise Immunology Review* 8: 49–100.

Shephard, R. J. and Shek, P. N. (1999) Effects of exercise and training on natural killer cell counts and cytolytic activity: a meta-analysis. *Sports Medicine* 28: 177–95.

5 Effects of exercise on acquired immune function

Nicolette C. Bishop

LEARNING OBJECTIVES

After studying this chapter, you should be able to:

- understand how acute exercise affects T cell functions, including cytokine production, proliferation and migration;
- understand how acute exercise affects B cell antibody production;
- appreciate the mechanisms of acquired immune system modulation by exercise;
- recognise the influence of exercise intensity, duration and fitness level on the acquired immune response to exercise;
- identify the effect of exercise training on acquired immune cell functions;
- appreciate the *in vivo* methods used to measure immune function.

ACQUIRED IMMUNITY REVISITED

A more detailed description of acquired immunity can be found in Chapter 2 but, here, we briefly revisit the key features of this aspect of the immune system before looking at the influencing effects of exercise.

Acquired immunity (also known as adaptive or specific immunity) is designed to combat infections by preventing colonisation of pathogens and destroying invading micro-organisms. With only a few exceptions, it is initiated by the presentation of antigen within the peptide-binding groove of major histocompatibility complex class II molecules on antigen-presenting cells to T helper (CD4+) lymphocytes. CD4+ T cells form a key part of the cell-mediated immune response, since they orchestrate and direct the subsequent response. Helper T-cell clones can be divided into two main phenotypes (there are others): type-1 (Th1) and type-2 (Th2) cells, according to the cytokines that they produce and release. Th1 cells play an important role in defence against intracellular pathogens (e.g. viruses) and Th2 cells are involved in protection against extracellular parasites and stimulation of B-cell antibody production (although some antigens can activate B cells independently of CD4+ cells). Although cytotoxic T cells (CD8+) can also be classified into type-1 (Tc1) and type-2 (Tc2) cells according to their cytokine profiles, the functional significance of these cells is, at present, unclear.

ACUTE EXERCISE AND T-CELL FUNCTIONS

As described in Chapter 2, T cells play a fundamental role in the orchestration and regulation of the cell-mediated immune response to pathogens. One important consequence of a defect in T-cell function is an increased incidence of viral infections (Fabbri *et al.* 2003). With this in mind, it has been suggested that the apparent increased susceptibility of sportsmen and women to upper respiratory tract infections may be due to exercise-induced decreases in T-cell function. The effect of acute exercise on cell-mediated immune function has been most commonly been assessed using a variety of *in vitro* methods relating to specific T-cell actions, such as cytokine production and proliferation (see Technique box 5.1).

Technique box 5.1

Measurement of antigen-stimulated cytokine production by leukocytes

To measure stimulated cytokine production from leukocytes, blood samples are incubated for a predetermined time (usually between 4 hours and 48 hours, depending on the particular cytokine being examined) with a specific activating agent. The choice of which activating stimulus is used primarily depends on the cell type from which one wishes to examine cytokine production. For example, if one wishes to examine monocyte cytokine production, lipopolysaccharide (a structural component of specific bacteria that is recognised by specific receptors present on the monocyte cell surface) might be used. On the other hand, to examine lymphocyte cytokine production, we might use pharmacological activators such as phorbol myristate acetate and ionomycin. Following completion of the incubation period, samples can either be examined flow cytometrically for the expression of cytokines within individual cells (using fluorescence-labelled antibody to a specific cytokine) or the concentration of a specific cytokine in the cell culture media can be determined by an enzyme-linked immunosorbent assay (ELISA). Explanations of ELISA can be found in Technique box 2.1 in Chapter 2. Flow cytometry is described in Chapter 3.

T cell cytokine release

The release of cytokines by activated Th (CD4+) cells largely determines whether the subsequent immune response to an antigen challenge will be T cell-mediated (e.g. IL-2 and IFN-γ; a Th1 response) or favour B-cell antibody production (e.g. IL-4; a Th2 response). Prolonged strenuous physical activity decreases the proportion of circulating Th1 cells but has little effect on the proportion of circulating Th2 cells

(Steensberg *et al.* 2001b). It is not clear whether these changes are caused by cell death (apoptosis) or changes in the distribution of cells between the circulation and the tissues. It is likely that both these mechanisms play a role.

Box 5.1 Exercise affects the Th1/Th2 balance and impairs interferon-γ production by Th1 cells

Similar to physical fitness, fitness of the immune system requires training. Animals that have been raised under sterile conditions have a poor immune system and fail to thrive. 'Immune training' is normally provided by contact with live microorganisms or by immuni- sation. Increasing evidence has suggested that moderate amounts of activity can decrease the frequency of infections while excessive, exhausting exercise can lead to the opposite, a situation that has been described by a J-curve (see Chapter 1). Following prolonged, exhausting exercise, a transient partial suppression of several immune functions can be shown and it has been suggested that this period provides a window for invasion of microbes. On the basis of data showing that endotoxin-inducible interferon-gamma (IFN-γ) production is virtually abrogated for a short period following excessive exercise, it has been hypothesised that the rigorous regulatory blockade of one of the ways of IFN-γ induction may be critically involved in causing the transient immunosuppression following exhaustive exercise stress.

It is important to recognise that alterations in the proportion of circulating T cells capable of releasing type-1 and type-2 cytokines do not necessarily reflect actual cytokine release when stimulated by mitogen or antigen. Having said this, several studies have found that the release of T-cell cytokines when stimulated *in vitro* does indeed follow a similar pattern. For example, one hour of cycling at 75% $\dot{V}O_2$max markedly decreased IL-2 production from stimulated T cells compared with resting values (Tvede *et al.* 1993), yet IL-4 production by stimulated lymphocytes was unaffected by 18 minutes of incremental exercise consisting of six minutes at 55%, 70% and 85% $\dot{V}O_2$max in active and sedentary males and females (Moyna *et al.* 1996). The effects of exercise on T-cell cytokine production are described further in Chapter 12.

T-cell proliferation

Given the frequency of viral infections in some athletes it is tempting to argue that an impaired Th1 response indicates reduced host defence against intracellular pathogens such as viruses. However, cytokine production is just one step of the multi- stage process that ultimately leads to lymphocyte proliferation (cell division) and cytotoxicity. These pathways require many other co-stimulatory signals, including specific antigen encounters, without which the cells may enter a dormant state of inactivity or 'anergy'. Assuming that the required co-stimulatory signals are present, T cells will proliferate *in vivo* in response to an antigen challenge to produce a clone of functional effector cells specific to the antigen that caused the initial response. This function is modelled *in vitro* using a mitogen (a substance that triggers cell division) or an antigen to stimulate the cells and is widely used to assess the general ability of cells to respond to a challenge.

Numerous studies in the literature report that lymphocyte proliferation decreases during and after exercise (Walsh *et al.* 2011a). For example, significant decreases in mitogen-stimulated T-cell proliferation have been observed following incremental treadmill test exercise to exhaustion in trained men (Fry *et al.* 1992a), strenuous resistance exercise in women before and after a period of training (Miles *et al.* 2003), following both 2.5 hours of treadmill running and 2.5 hours of cycle ergometry at 75% $\dot{V}O_2$max in trained male and female triathletes (Henson *et al.* 1999) and after a 90-minute shuttle-running protocol design to mimic the activity patterns of a football match (Bishop *et al.* 2005b). Like many other measures of the immune response to exercise, the magnitude of the response appears to depend upon the duration and intensity of the exercise. For example, 45 minutes of treadmill running at 80% $\dot{V}O_2$max was associated with a 50% fall in lymphocyte proliferation at one hour post-exercise, whereas only a 25% decrease in the proliferation response was observed after performing the same exercise at 50% $\dot{V}O_2$max (Nieman *et al.* 1994; Figure 5.1).

Figure 5.1 Absolute (A) and adjusted per T cell (B) changes in concanavalin A-stimulated lymphocyte proliferative responses to a 45-minute treadmill run at 80% $\dot{V}O_2$ max (high intensity) and 50% $\dot{V}O_2$ max (moderate intensity); * indicates a significant difference from pre-exercise values, $P < 0.05$ (data from Nieman *et al.* 1994)

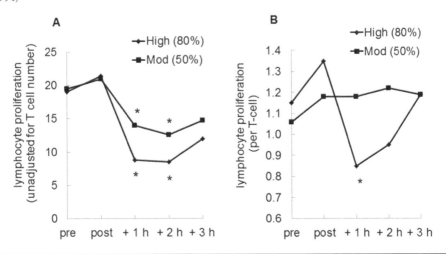

Mitogen versus antigen stimulation

While intense exercise is associated with transient decreases in mitogen-induced lymphocyte proliferation, we should remember that lymphocyte responses are antigen-specific and assessment of cell responses to mitogens such as the plant lectins, phytohaemagglutinin (PHA), concanavalin A (Con A) and pokeweed mitogen (PWM), *in vitro* will not necessarily provide an exact model for the *in vivo* situation. Whereas PHA will only activate a high percentage of circulating T cells, PWM can also activate B cells and Con A can activate NK cells. This could result in unrealistically large changes in lymphocyte function. Furthermore, responses to PHA may lack the sensitivity to detect subtle but highly relevant alterations in the activity of T-cell populations involved in defence against common pathogens. In support of this, performance of 90 minutes of soccer-specific intermittent exercise resulted in a differing pattern of proliferative responses to PHA, influenza and tetanus toxoid; with relative responses to PHA highest and relative responses to tetanus toxoid lowest (Bishop *et al.* 2005b; Figure 5.2). It could be argued these differences could be related to the dose of mitogen and antigen used. However, an earlier pilot study had previously determined the concentration of PHA and each antigen to use to give a comparable amount of proliferation at rest.

Figure 5.2 Relative change in proliferative response to phytohaemagglutinin (PHA), influenza and tetanus toxoid stimulation following 90 minutes of soccer-specific intermittent exercise. Responses relative to the first (resting) sample were highest when cells were stimulated with the T-cell-specific mitogen PHA and lowest in response to the antigen tetanus toxoid (data from Bishop *et al.* 2005b)

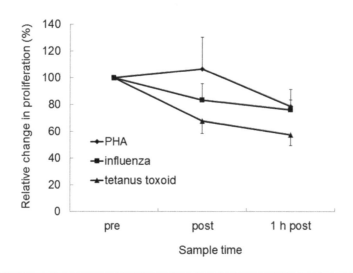

Effect of alterations in circulating lymphocyte populations

There is an additional need for caution when it comes to the interpretation of proliferative response to exercise. As we have seen in Chapter 3, acute exercise is associated with marked changes in the circulating numbers of lymphocytes and lymphocyte subsets. Proliferation assays tend to use a constant number of peripheral blood lymphocytes or a fixed amount of whole blood. While this is appropriate for samples taken at rest, the proportions of the different lymphocyte subsets in those samples will have changed after exercise. For example, there is a greater influx of NK cells into the circulation relative to T cells following exercise. This is important because NK cells do not respond to PHA, the most common mitogen used to assess T-cell proliferation in lymphocyte cultures. Given that after exercise there will a greater proportion of NK cells relative to T cells in a fixed number of total lymphocytes or fixed volume of blood, it is perhaps not surprising that 'T-cell' proliferation decreases after exercise. That is to say that a post-exercise decrease in proliferation to PHA in culture may simply reflect the smaller proportion of cells in the culture that can respond to that mitogen, rather than any impairment of the ability of individual T cells to proliferate.

The significance of the presence of NK cells in proliferation cultures has been highlighted by Green *et al.* (2002) Changes in proliferation in response to a one-hour intensive treadmill run were assessed in cultures containing a fixed number of lymphocytes except in half of the cultures the NK cells were removed using magnetic microbeads. Interestingly, immediately after the run, PHA-stimulated proliferative responses were significantly lower in the cell culture that contained NK cells compared with the one containing the same number of lymphocytes but from which the NK cells had been removed (Figure 5.3).

Figure 5.3 Phytohaemagglutinin-stimulated proliferation in (A) mixed lymphocyte and monocyte cultures with (B) in natural killer cell-depleted cultures. Samples were taken during an exercise trial when subjects completed 60 minutes of treadmill running between 6 a.m. and 7 a.m. and in a resting control session; * indicates a significant difference between the exercise and control condition, $P < 0.05$ (data from Green *et al.* 2002)

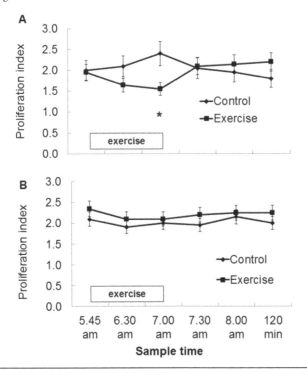

Other than depleting cultures of NK cells, one other way employed by researchers to overcome the problem of disproportionate changes in numbers of lymphocyte subsets in response to exercise is to mathematically adjust the proliferation data for changes in circulating numbers of T cells. Reporting proliferation on a 'per T cell' basis in this way tends to have the resulting effect that only decreases in proliferative responses following longer and more intensive exercise remain. For example, in the study by Nieman *et al.* (1994) described above, proliferation was assessed in response to Con A (a T- and NK-cell stimulant). Adjusting the data for changes in circulating T cell numbers alone resulted in a 21% fall in proliferative responses at one hour post-exercise in the higher-intensity exercise trial, compared with the 50% fall observed in the unadjusted data. Moreover, the post-exercise fall on the moderate intensity exercise trial was abolished when the data were adjusted in this way, with values remaining close to pre-exercise values throughout the exercise (Figure 5.1B). Further support for a genuine reduction in T-cell proliferation with intensive exercise comes from the study of Bishop *et al.* (2005b), where proliferation was assessed in cultures using a fixed number of T cells, rather than a fixed number of total lymphocytes. Here, PHA-stimulated T-cell proliferation fell significantly after performance of 90 minutes of a football-specific intermittent exercise on two consecutive days (Figure 5.4).

Figure 5.4 Proliferative response in a fixed number of T cells to the T-cell-specific mitogen phytohaemagglutinin following 90 minutes of soccer-specific intermittent exercise on 2 consecutive days; * indicates a significant difference compared with pre-exercise on day 1 ($P < 0.05$) (data from Bishop *et al.* 2005b)

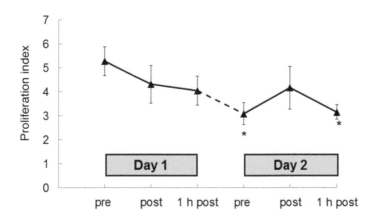

There is an argument that the post-exercise decline in lymphocyte responsiveness is at least partly related to an increase in cell death rates in culture. This has primarily been provided by a study that used carboxyfluorescein diacetate succinamidyl ester (CFSE) labelling of lymphocyte populations to quantify cell division in response to PHA on an individual cell basis (Green and Rowbottom 2003). It was found that samples taken midway through a 60-minute treadmill run at 95% of the ventilatory threshold demonstrated a 60% decrease in the number of responsive CD4+ and CD8+ cells in culture. This was mirrored by a 65% increase in cell death (apoptosis) in those samples. Cell mitosis rates were unchanged. These data therefore suggest that the exercise decreased the ability of cells to survive in culture, with little effect on the ability of the cells to divide. While this may simply reflect the difficulties of modelling *in vivo* situations in isolated cells *in vitro*, it could also indicate a cortisol-mediated stimulation of apoptosis or the exercise-induced mobilisation of a subpopulation of cells susceptible to apoptosis into the circulation. Certainly, a 60% increase in the percentage (but not actual number) of apoptotic lymphocytes has been reported two hours after a strenuous 2.5-hour treadmill run (Steensberg *et al.* 2002).

T-cell migration and homing

We have seen how acute exercise can affect T-cell functions and speculated on the consequences of this for host defence, particularly against common viral pathogens. In addition, there is now some evidence to suggest that prolonged exercise leads to an alteration in the migratory or homing properties of T cells (i.e. the capacity of these cells to move to where they are needed to 'fight infection'). Airway epithelial cells produce several chemical attractants (chemokines) and proinflammatory cytokines when infected with human rhinovirus. These result in increased airway inflammation, which is thought to trigger or exacerbate cold symptoms. Following a two-hour treadmill run at 60%, there was a decrease in the ability of CD4+ and CD8+ cells and their memory and naïve subpopulations to migrate towards supernatants released from human rhinovirus-infected human bronchial epithelial cells (Bishop *et al.* 2009; Figure 5.5). Such reductions in migration may transiently deprive the lung of immune surveillance by T cells specific for respiratory pathogens, which may give rise to the apparent increased incidence of respiratory infection in athletes.

In vivo cell mediated immunity

The previous sections illustrate that the majority of studies in the literature have used *in vitro* measures to assess exercise-induced changes in T-cell function. However, this always raises the issue of how well such measurements of isolated circulating lymphocytes truly reflect the situation that would occur if an individual who had performed an acute bout of strenuous exercise came into contact with a pathogen. Furthermore, it should be considered that, at any one time, the majority of lymphocytes are not circulating in the blood and so any observed changes in peripheral blood lymphocytes may not necessarily reflect changes that may occur in cells located in lymph nodes and other tissues throughout the body. *In vivo* methods to measure the effects of exercise on the T-cell response (cell-mediated response) to specific antigens provide a strong approach to this problem and are described more fully in Technique box 5.2.

Figure 5.5 Percentage of CD4+ cells migrating towards the supernatant from human rhinovirus-infected human bronchial epithelial cells compared with control (uninfected cell) supernatant. Values are expressed as a percentage of the pre-exercise response; * indicates a significant decrease in CD4+ cell migration at 1 hour post-exercise compared with control at that time (data from Bishop *et al.* 2009)

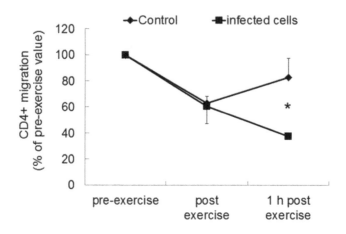

One study that assessed cell-mediated immune function *in vivo* injected trained triathletes with seven previously encountered (recall) antigens, including tetanus, diphtheria and group C streptococcus intradermally following a half-Ironman race (Bruunsgaard *et al.* 1997b). The resultant delayed-type hypersensitivity (DTH) skin response was assessed 48 hours later by measuring the size (diameter) of the resulting skin indurations in millimetres. It was found that the response in these triathletes after the race was significantly smaller than that of a group of non-exercising triathletes and also a group of non-exercising moderately trained men. However, while the use of recall antigens in this way allows assessment of pre-existing immunological memory, a limitation is that it does not provide information about the effects of exercise on the primary (induction) response to a novel antigen. Furthermore, assessing DTH in this way typically gives rise to highly variable responses, another limitation which is likely caused, at least in part, by the lack of control over the timing and dose of the initial exposure. A recent study (Harper Smith *et al.*, 2011) dealt with these limitations by assessing both the *in vivo* induction and memory (recall) responses to a topically applied novel antigen, diphenylcyclopropenone (DPCP). It was found that two hours of running on a treadmill at 60% $\dot{V}O_2$ peak before initial sensitisation to DPCP reduced the subsequent induction response to DPCP four weeks later, compared with controls that had been sensitised to DPCP after resting quietly in the laboratory (Harper Smith *et al.* 2011). The recall *in vivo* T-cell-mediated immune response was assessed in a separate group of previously sensitised participants who had received several monthly DPCP challenges to boost the response until reaching a plateau. Participants then received two further DPCP challenges, in a crossover

Technique box 5.2

Measurement of *in vivo* acquired immune functions

Antigen-stimulated antibody production

In vivo methods involve challenging experimental subjects more commonly with antigenic (immune-stimulating but not sickness-causing) or less commonly with pathogenic (immune-stimulating and possibly sickness-causing) stimuli and assessing subsequent antigen-driven responses (Walsh *et al.* 2011a). Such responses include the circulating antibody response to injection of either a novel antigen, such as keyhole limpet haemocyanin, or a previously encountered antigen, such as influenza vaccine or tetanus toxoid. The generation of an antigen-specific immunoglobulin response reflects a functionally important end product of the multicellular immune response.

Antigen-stimulated delayed-type hypersensitivity response

An alternative method is the assessment of the delayed-type hypersensitivity (DTH) response. This method provides an indication of the *in vivo* cell-mediated immune response using novel (e.g. diphenylcyclopropenone, DPCP) or recall (e.g. tetanus and diphtheria toxoids, *Candida albicans*, streptococcus) antigens. Antigens are injected just under the skin, usually on the forearm, resulting in an inflammatory response of raised red swelling (oedema) at the point at which the antigen was applied. The diameter of the resulting oedema and the increase in redness (erythema) is usually recorded 24–48 hours later, with the greatest magnitude of oedema and erythema indicating the strongest *in vivo* cell-mediated immune response (see photograph). Novel antigens, such as DPCP, require prior sensitisation by skin exposure to elicit a primary allergic response; the strength of subsequent *in vivo* cell-mediated responses is later quantified with a dose series of the same antigen (Harper-Smith *et al.* 2011).

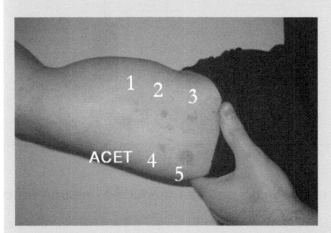

Skinfold thickening (oedema) response to a dose-series of DPCP (labelled 1–5) at 48 hours after topical application. Individuals had been sensitised to DPCP 1 month earlier. The dose series involved placing six 8-mm patches with DPCP on the inside of the upper arm for 6 hours. The patches were soaked in 10 µl of acetone (control, labelled ACET) and a range of low-dose DPCP concentrations from 0.0048% (patch 1) to 0.03125% (patch 5) made up in acetone design, after performing a two-hour treadmill run at 60% $\dot{V}O_2$ peak and a resting control trial, each separated by four weeks. It was found that exercise immediately before the antigen recall challenge elicited a lower recall response than when the same participants had been resting before the antigen recall challenge. Interestingly, compared with the corresponding control trial, the exercise-evoked impairment of the induction response to DPCP was greater (around 50% reduction) than the later recall response (around 20% reduction). This implies that the primary immune response to antigens is more susceptible to heavy exercise-evoked immune impairment than the later recall response (Figure 5.6).

Figure 5.6 The effects of a 2-hour run on a treadmill at 60% of peak oxygen uptake on the primary (induction) and secondary (recall) response to the novel antigen diphenylcyclopropenone (DPCP). The primary response was compared with that in a separate group who had been sensitised to DPCP after resting quietly. The recall response to the same antigen was determined in a group of participants who had been exposed to several monthly DPCP challenges before performing both an exercise test and a resting control trial. The impairment of the induction response to DPCP was greater (around 50% reduction) than the later recall response (around 20% reduction), implying that the primary response to antigens is more susceptible to immune impairment than the later memory response; con = controls, ex = exercise group (data from Harper Smith *et al.* 2011)

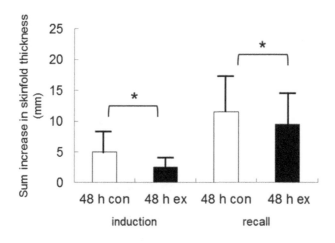

Summary of acute exercise and cell-mediated immune function

Acute exercise appears to stimulate changes in T-cell function that are, as with many other aspects of immune function, proportional to exercise intensity and duration. There is evidence that acute exercise stimulates T-cell activation, although it is not clear whether increases in activation are caused by an increase in the recruitment of activated cells into the circulation or an effect on the state of activation of individual cells themselves. Most likely it is a combination of both. Acute exercise is also associated with a decrease in T cell IL-2 and IFN-γ production immediately after exercise, although the importance of this in terms of any impairment of cell-mediated immunity is difficult to assess since total numbers of IL-2 and IFN-γ producing T cells had increased at this time. There are numerous reports in the literature detailing decreased mitogen-stimulated T-cell proliferation following acute exercise but interpretation of these findings may be confounded by the presence of NK cells and B cells in the cell cultures. Furthermore, it should be remembered that *in vitro* stimulation with mitogen does not necessarily reflect the more subtle responses of cells following a specific antigen encounter within the body. Moreover, exercise may alter T-cell function *in vitro* through an increase in the rate of cell death in cell culture rather than a decrease in T-cell division. Finally, while these impairments of specific T-cell functions in response to acute intensive exercise may be mathematically significant, it is important to recognise that in the absence of clinically normal reference ranges the biological importance of such findings is difficult to clarify.

ACUTE EXERCISE AND B-CELL FUNCTION

Upon stimulation, B cells proliferate and differentiate into memory cells and plasma cells, with plasma cells in the circulation or localised in lymph or mucosal tissue able to produce and secrete vast amounts of antigen-specific immunoglobulin (or antibody) that circulate in the body fluids. Compared with studies that have looked at the effect of exercise on T-cell responses, relatively few studies have concentrated on B-cell 'proliferation' itself. As described in the previous section, B cells also proliferate in response to certain mitogens; therefore, it is likely that some of the exercise-induced decline in T-cell proliferation from mitogen-stimulated lymphocyte cultures may be attributed changes in B-cell responses. However, any contribution is likely to be small given the relative size of the circulating B-cell population (B cells account for only 5–15% of all circulating lymphocytes). Therefore, to try to isolate B-cell functional capability, immunoglobulin levels have been more commonly assessed either *in vivo* or *in vitro* in response to mitogen-stimulated proliferation.

Circulating immunoglobulins

The predominant immunoglobulin in the blood is IgG (its normal serum concentration is around 12.0 g/L), with smaller amounts of IgA (around 1.8 g/L) and IgM (around 1.0 g/L). The amounts of IgD and IgE are negligible by comparison (less than 0.05 g/L). Therefore, it is not surprising that exercise-induced changes in serum IgA, IgG and IgM have received the most attention in the literature. On the whole, serum immunoglobulin concentrations appears to remain either unchanged or slightly increased in response to either brief or prolonged exercise. For example, modest increases in serum IgA, IgG and IgM were found following a maximal graded treadmill run in trained runners but these increases were similar to those found in a group of resting controls over the same duration. This suggests a possible diurnal effect and all changes were abolished when the data were adjusted for alterations in plasma volume (Nieman *et al.* 1989c). Serum concentrations of IgA, IgG and IgM were also unaffected by an acute bout of strenuous resistance exercise in both trained and untrained women (Potteiger *et al.* 2001). In contrast, a 45-minute walk at 60% was associated with small, yet significant, increases in serum IgA, IgG and IgM compared with rest over the same period of time (Nehlsen-Cannarella *et al.* 1991) suggesting that moderate exercise can lead to a transient rise in circulating antibody. Since there were no differences in plasma volume, the authors concluded that these increases might be due to exercise-induced influx of immunoglobulin into the blood from the lymph and extravascular pools.

In vitro immunoglobulin production

There are contrasting findings concerning *in vitro* immunoglobulin synthesis following mitogen-stimulation; these may depend upon the immunoglobulin being investigated. For example, Shek *et al.* (1995) found that, during a two hour treadmill run at 65% $\dot{V}O_2$max in trained males, IgM production by PWM-stimulated lymphocytes fell to 33% and 42% of pre-exercise values after 90 and 120 minutes of exercise, respectively, but IgA and IgG production did not appreciably change in response to exercise. Mackinnon *et al.* (1989) also report that a two-hour cycle bout at 90% of ventilatory threshold (70–80% $\dot{V}O_2$max) in trained cyclists had little effect on PWM-stimulated IgA and IgG production. In contrast, Tvede *et al.* (1989) observed a decline in the number of PWM-stimulated IgM, IgA and IgG producing B cells during and two hours after an intensive one-hour cycle bout in untrained individuals. These findings cannot be attributed to a redistribution of B cells, since circulating numbers did not change in response to the exercise. It is likely that differences in exercise duration and training status of the subjects involved in these studies account, at least in part, for these inconsistent findings. An alternative argument is that exercise-induced alterations in CD4+ cell numbers may have influenced these results because these studies used PWM to stimulate the lymphocytes. Pokeweed stimulates B cells via stimulation of CD4+ cell cytokine release. However, this cannot wholly account for the decreases in immunoglobulin synthesis reported: significant elevations in numbers of circulating CD4+ cells were observed at the same time as the decline in IgM production in the study of Shek *et al.* (1995) and the significant decreases in immunoglobulin synthesis at two hours post-exercise observed in the study of Tvede *et al.* (1989) occurred at a time when CD4+ cell numbers had returned to pre-exercise values.

In vivo immunoglobulin production

As explained earlier in this chapter, it should be remembered that *in vitro* measures of stimulated immunoglobulin production may not always accurately reflect an impairment of the *in vivo* response. The study by Bruunsgaard *et al.* (1997b), described earlier in this chapter, also assessed antibody responses to antigen-stimulation *in vivo*, by vaccinating trained triathletes 30 minutes after a half-Ironman event and comparing the responses in the group of non-exercised triathletes and a group of moderately trained controls. The vaccinations contained antigens that act on B cells via both T-cell dependent (tetanus and diphtheria toxoids) and T-cell independent (pneumococcal polysaccharide) pathways to assess any differential effects on cell function. Importantly, the antigens in these vaccines would have already been encountered by individuals (i.e. recall antigens) as part of general health vaccination programmes. No differences in the antibody response to any of the antigens were found between groups when assessed 14 days later, despite the lower *in vivo* cell-mediated immune responses observed in the exercising triathletes 48 hours after the event, as described in this chapter. These findings suggest that B-cell ability to generate antibody responses to recall antigens is not impaired following strenuous, high-intensity exercise.

The primary antibody response appears to be more susceptible to the effects of exercise. Injections with a novel antigen, such as keyhole limpet haemocyanin (KLH) will stimulate a primary antibody response in the form of B cell anti-KLH immunoglobulin production. KLH also has the advantage of being benign (i.e. it does not cause sickness). Although KLH is commonly used to stimulate primary antibody responses *in vivo* in both animals and humans, there are still relatively few studies that have used KLH to assess *in vivo* antibody responses to exercise. One study reports that progressive treadmill training in rats supresses anti-KLH IgM production compared with sedentary rats (Moraska *et al.* 2000). The effect of exercise on the primary antibody response may be intensity dependent; ten months of moderate aerobic exercise training in previously sedentary older adults resulted in greater anti-KLH IgM and IgG1 production than in a similar group who had undertaken flexibility training over the same time (Grant *et al.* 2008) (Figure 5.7).

Figure 5.7 Effects of a 10-month cardiovascular exercise (cardio) or flexibility/balance exercise (flex) intervention on the primary anti-KLH IgG1 response. Participants were vaccinated 8 months into the intervention. IgG1 responses were higher in the cardio group 2, 3 and 6 weeks after vaccination; * indicates a significant difference between cardio and flex groups at each time point post-vaccination ($P < 0.05$) (data from Grant *et al.* 2008)

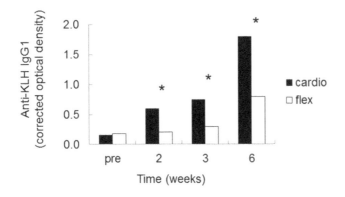

Effects of exercise training on acquired immune cell functions

In the true resting state (i.e. more than 24 hours after their last training session) circulating lymphocyte numbers and functions exhibit very few differences between athletes and non-athletes (Nieman 2000). Longitudinal studies in which previously sedentary people undertake weeks or months of exercise training have failed to show any marked changes in T and B cell functions, provided that blood samples are taken at least 24 hours after their last exercise bout. In contrast, T and B cell functions appear to be sensitive to increases in training load in well-trained athletes undertaking a period of intensified training, with decreases in circulating numbers of type-1 T cells, reduced T cell proliferative responses and falls in stimulated B cell immunoglobulin synthesis reported (Verde *et al.* 1992; Baj *et al.* 1994; Lancaster *et al.* 2004). This suggests that athletes engaging in longer periods of intensified training can exhibit decreases in T-cell functionality. The effects of intensified training on adaptive immune responses are discussed in more detail in Chapter 8.

KEY POINTS

- Acute exercise appears to result in changes in T-cell function that are proportional to exercise intensity and duration.
- A decrease in T-cell production of IL-2 and IFN-γ is reported immediately after acute, intensive exercise. The effect of this on type-1 T cell responses is unclear since it might be countered by a concomitant increase in the number of circulating IL-2 and IFN-γ producing T cells.
- Acute strenuous exercise decreases mitogen and antigen-stimulated T-cell proliferation but caution should be exercised when interpreting these findings because they may also reflect changes in the distribution of the circulating lymphocyte subpopulations and/or an increase in cells undergoing apoptosis.
- The ability of T cells to migrate towards to the chemical signals released by infected airway epithelial cells is reduced by prolonged, strenuous exercise.
- Serum immunoglobulin concentration appears to remain either unchanged or slightly increased in response to either brief or prolonged exercise.
- Mitogen-stimulated IgM concentration appears to increase in response to exercise independently of changes in T or B cell numbers. There are contrasting findings concerning any exercise effects on mitogen-stimulated IgA and IgG synthesis.
- *In vivo* assessments of both cell-mediated immune responses and antibody production suggest that the initial primary response is more affected by exercise than subsequent memory responses.
- Comparison of trained versus untrained individuals reveal little difference in measures of T and B cell functions, providing the blood samples are collected at least 24 hours after the last exercise bout.

FURTHER READING

Gleeson, M. (2007) Immune function in sport and exercise. *Journal of Applied Physiology* 103: 693–9.

Green, K. J. and Rowbottom, D. G. (2003) Exercise-induced changes to in vitro T-lymphocyte mitogen responses using CFSE. *Journal of Applied Physiology* 95: 57–63.

Green, K. J., Rowbottom, D. G. and Mackinnon, L. T. (2002) Exercise and T-lymphocyte function: a comparison of proliferation in PBMC and NK-cell depleted PMC culture. *Journal of Applied Physiology* 92: 2390–5.

Walsh, N. P., Gleeson, M., Shephard, R. J., Gleeson, M., Woods, J. A., Bishop, N. C., Fleshner, M., Green, C., Pedersen, B. K., Hoffman-Goetz, L., Rogers, C. J., Northoff, H., Abbasi, A. and Simon, P. (2011) Position statement. Part one: Immune function and exercise. Exercise Immunology Review 17: 6-63. Note: Information found on pages 21–4 relates specifically to acquired immunity and exercise and information found on pages 29–31 relates specifically to *in vivo* methods of assessing immune function.

6 Effects of exercise on mucosal immunity

Nicolette C. Bishop

LEARNING OBJECTIVES

After studying this chapter, you should be able to:

- understand the basic structure and effector mechanisms of immunoglobulin;
- identify the different antimicrobial proteins present in saliva;
- understand the effect of acute exercise and exercise training on levels of secretory immunoglobulins and other antimicrobial proteins;
- appreciate the potential mechanisms of mucosal immune system modulation by exercise;
- understand the relationship between levels of saliva secretory IgA and risk of upper respiratory tract infection.

INTRODUCTION

In Chapter 2, we looked at the different types of immune cells that make up our immune system and in Chapters 3, 4 and 5, we looked at the way in which exercise affects the circulating numbers and functions of these cells. However, important immune defence molecules called immunoglobulins are present in all bodily fluids, including blood plasma, lymph fluid, tears, sweat, mucous and breast milk. Immunoglobulin (Ig) is continuously secreted from terminally differentiated B cells known as plasma cells following antigen exposure. There are five classes of immunoglobulin: IgG, IgA, IgM, IgD and IgE. When secreted, immunoglobulin binds to antigen the immunoglobulin–antigen complex and is called an antibody.

IMMUNOGLOBULIN STRUCTURE AND ACTIONS

The main characteristics of the different types of immunoglobulin are summarised in Table 6.1. The structure of the IgG monomer is considered the basic characteristic Y-shaped structure of immunoglobulin (see Figure 2.9), with other classes existing as

Table 6.1 Concentrations and characteristics of the five classes of immunoglobulin (Ig)			
Ig CLASS	TYPICAL CONCENTRATION		CHARACTERISTICS AND MAIN ROLES
	SERUM (mg.ml^{-1})[a]	SALIVA (mg.l^{-1})[b]	
G	6.0–13.5	15–30	Most abundant in blood and tissue liquids (comprises 75–80% of all circulating Ig), lower amounts in saliva. Transfers across placenta. Binds to many types of pathogens. Monomeric, exists as 4 isotypes: IgG1, IgG2, IgG3, IgG4
M	0.5–3.0	5–10	'Natural antibody' found in serum without prior contact with antigen. Small amounts found in saliva. First antibody to appear after immunisation. Exists as a pentamer.
A	0.6–3.0	100–200	Major secretory antibody. Secreted across mucosal tract. Found in saliva, tears and breast milk. Exists as a monomer in serum and as a dimer in secretions. Has as two isotypes: IgA1 and IgA2
D	< 0.14	Not known	Exact role remains obscure. Recently found to be secreted in respiratory mucosa, where it binds bacteria and their products. Binds to circulating basophils stimulating release of antimicrobial and inflammatory proteins
E	< 0.0004	Not secreted	Binds strongly to receptors on basophils and mast cells, sensitising them for certain allergic reactions

Notes:
[a] Serum concentrations have been reported in mg.ml^{-1}, whereas those for saliva are in mg.l^{-1}; to compare the two directly, serum values should be multiplied by 1000
[b] Saliva values vary widely between individuals and will also depend on the method used for analysis

Sources: compiled using information from Engström *et al.* (1996), Pyne *et al.* (2000), Janeway *et al.* (2001), Chen and Cherutti (2011)

dimers (IgA) and pentamers (IgM). The arms of the Y are the fragment antigen (Fab) units containing antigen-binding sites where the molecule can bind to a wide variety of antigens. In this way, immunoglobulins act as opsonins, facilitating the recognition of the antigen–immunoglobulin complex by phagocytic cells. The tail of the Y contains the fragment crystallisable (Fc) unit; this is where the immunoglobulin binds to Fc receptors present on effector molecules and cells. Specific Fc receptors exist on neutrophils, monocytes/macrophages and natural killer (NK) cells for all types of antibody, although those for IgD and IgM are not so well characterised. It is important to remember that binding of antibody to a single Fc receptor on an effector cell is not enough to cause cellular activation on its own; rather, this requires the complex crosslinking of several Fc receptors bound to more than one immunoglobulin molecule. Following crosslinking, the receptors can activate several effector-cell actions, including activation of the complement pathway, phagocytosis, release of cytokines such as interferon gamma (IFN-γ) and other inflammatory mediators, and antibody-dependent cellular cytotoxicity, whereby NK cells actively lyse the target cell by release of cytotoxic molecules, such as granzyme and perforin, and also activate apoptosis (programmed cell death). Antigen-specific antibody can be detected in blood serum or plasma for decades after antigen encounter; the importance of this effect can be observed in the success of many global vaccination programmes.

THE COMMON MUCOSAL IMMUNE SYSTEM

To provide effective immune surveillance, antibody must be able to circulate readily throughout all bodily fluids. Unlike most other cells of the immune system, plasma cells are unable to migrate from tissue to tissue, so it is vital that these cells are located at vulnerable tissue sites or at sites where there is easy access to the circulation, such as the spleen, lymph and bone marrow. The mucosal surfaces of the body, such as those in the gut, nasal passages, respiratory passages, female reproductive tract and urinary tract, are examples of vulnerable sites which are exposed to a large number of different antigens. The 'common mucosal immune system' is a network of organised structures protecting these mucosal surfaces, including Peyer's patches and isolated lymphoid follicles in gut-associated lymphoid tissue, nasal-associated lymphoid tissue, bronchial/tracheal-associated lymphoid tissue and salivary glands. The sheer magnitude of these defences is easier to comprehend if you consider that the surface area of the human mucosae is around 400 m² – this is roughly equivalent to the size of a basketball court. In contrast, the surface area of another important defensive structure, the skin, is only 1.8 m².

SECRETORY IgA

The major effector function of the mucosal immune system is the production of IgA; it produces more IgA than its combined synthesis of the other four subclasses of immunoglobulin. This secretory IgA (SIgA) is considered to provide the 'first line of defence' against pathogens and antigens presented at mucosal surfaces and it does this with support from innate mucosal defences such as alpha-amylase (ptyalin), lactoferrin and lysozyme (Table 6.2). Salivary SIgA is the most commonly studied marker of mucosal immune system integrity, mainly because of the obvious advantage of being easy to collect in both field and laboratory situations. A high incidence of infections is reported in individuals with selective deficiency of IgA (Hanson *et al.* 1983) and low levels of SIgA are reported in children prone to respiratory infections (Lehtonen *et al.* 1987).

There are two isotypes of IgA: IgA1 and IgA2, with IgA1 forming about 90% of all IgA. Secretory IgA is a dimeric molecule, with the secreted IgA monomers joined 'tail-to tail' by a small polypeptide structure known as the J-chain. It also contains the epithelial-derived 'secretory component' (Figure 6.1), which is essentially a remnant of the receptor (known as the polymeric immunoglobulin receptor or pIgR) that binds IgA and allows its transport across the mucosal epithelium (Figure 6.2). The

PROTEIN	MAIN SOURCE	ACTION
α-amylase	Acinar cells in the secretory endpiece of salivary glands	Key digestive enzyme, breaking down starch into maltose; also inhibits the ability of bacteria to grow and attach to mucosal surfaces
Lysozyme	Acinar cells in the secretory endpiece of salivary glands	Destroys bacteria by breaking down the polysaccharide component of bacterial cell walls
Lactoferrin	Macrophages in the oral mucosa	Sequesters ferric iron to prevent bacterial growth; also acts against several viruses, including the respiratory viruses adenovirus and respiratory syncytial virus

Table 6.2 Characteristics of other antimicrobial proteins in saliva

Figure 6.1 Structure of dimeric secretory IgA. Two IgA monomers are joined tail-to-tail by the J chain. Secretory component is covalently bound to the IgA dimer providing resistance against degradation by proteases; Fab = fragment antigen unit; Fc = fragment crystallisable unit (adapted from Bishop and Gleeson 2009)

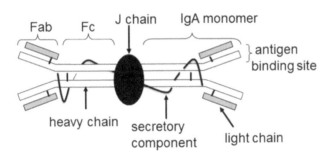

pIgR is synthesised by mucosal epithelial and glandular cells and expressed on the basolateral membrane, where it is perfectly placed to bind to IgA (and, to a far lesser extent, IgM) produced by local plasma cells. The receptor is proteolytically cleaved at the apical surface, leaving only the secretory component bound to the IgA dimer. However, the remaining secretory component is not just an artefact of previous cellular transport; rather, the covalent binding of secretory component makes secretory IgA more resistant to protease degradation in secretions such as saliva. The transport of IgA bound to pIgR across the mucosal epithelium essentially provides three aspects of protection by SIgA: (1) through prevention of pathogen adherence and penetration of the mucosal epithelium; (2) by neutralising viruses within the epithelial cells during transcytosis; and (3) by removal of locally formed immune complexes across mucosal epithelial cells to the luminal surface (Lamm 1998).

Figure 6.2 Transport of IgA across the mucosal epithelium. IgA monomers are secreted by terminally differentiated B cells (plasma cells) located in the basolateral surface. Dimeric IgA is formed when two IgA monomers are joined together by the J-chain. Dimeric IgA binds to the polymeric immunoglobulin receptor (pIgR) on the basolateral membrane of the epithelial cell and is transported to the apical surface where the pIgR is cleaved leaving only the secretory component bound to the secreted IgA. Secretory component acts to protect SIgA against breakdown by digestive enzymes (adapted from Bishop and Gleeson 2009)

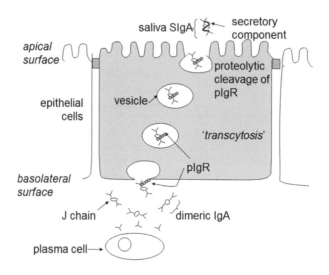

IMMUNE DEFENCES IN SALIVA

Humans produce around 1500 ml of saliva per day from three pairs of major salivary glands (the parotid, submandibular and sublingual glands), in addition to the around 600 smaller glands found in the submucosa under most soft tissue surfaces of the mouth (Figure 6.3). Although the parotid glands are the largest of the major salivary glands, they only contribute to around 25% of secreted saliva, with the submandibular glands accounting for 70% and the sublingual glands around 5%. Not only does the volume of saliva secreted vary between the pairs of major glands but the nature of the secretions also differs. Saliva secreted from the parotid glands tends to be watery ('serous'), whereas that from the sublingual glands is less watery but has a higher mucous content. The submandibular secretion is a mixture of the two.

Whereas IgA (and to a much lesser extent, IgM) is transported into saliva across salivary glandular epithelial cells as described above, the small amounts of IgG found in saliva are from the gingival crevicular fluid, a thin and watery fluid ('transudate') that is squeezed through the mucous membrane in the gingival crevice. Saliva alpha-amylase and lactoferrin are synthesised and secreted by acinar cells in the secretory endpiece of salivary glands. The main sources of lysozyme are macrophages in the oral mucosa, although there is some secretion of lysozyme from the basal cells of striated ducts in the parotid glands. Following secretion, both lysozyme and lactoferrin

Figure 6.3 Location of the main salivary glands

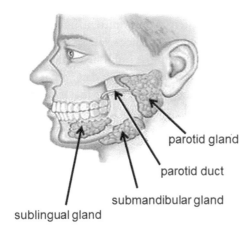

parotid gland

parotid duct

submandibular gland

sublingual gland

require pepsin digestion for conversion into an active form for their microbial activity (West *et al.* 2006). The fluid component of saliva is supplied by filtration of blood plasma in a dense network of blood vessels, via the interstitial space.

Control of saliva secretion

Saliva secretion is regulated by the autonomic nervous system. The salivary glands are innervated by branches of both the parasympathetic and sympathetic nervous systems that, unlike in many other physiological systems in the body, act synergistically rather than antagonistically. Parasympathetic stimulation produces a high volume of watery saliva that is low in protein content and this secretion is associated with a pronounced vasodilation of blood vessels supplying the gland, thought to be mediated by local release of vasoactive peptide. In contrast, saliva produced by sympathetic stimulation is relatively low in volume and high in protein, mainly owing to the increased exocytosis of salivary proteins from salivary gland or associated cells (Proctor and Carpenter 2007). The secretion of salivary SIgA can be increased by both parasympathetic and sympathetic nerve stimulation. Given that intensive exercise is associated with enhanced sympathetic nervous system activation it seems logical to assume that strenuous physical activity would modify secretion of saliva and its constituent proteins.

ACUTE EXERCISE AND MUCOSAL IMMUNITY

Following acute bouts of high-intensity exercise, many studies report a decrease in salivary SIgA concentration that recovers to resting levels within one hour of exercise completion. In contrast, other studies report either no change or even increases in SIgA concentration (Walsh *et al.* 2011a). The effects of exercise on salivary SIgA concentration and secretion rate appear to be largely dependent on overall exercise intensity and, to a lesser extent, exercise duration. Levels of salivary SIgA are generally unchanged, with moderate aerobic exercise lasting less than one hour (Bishop and Gleeson 2009), moderate and high-intensity intermittent/interval exercise protocols (Bishop *et al.* 1999, Davison 2011) and resistance-exercise sessions (Koch 2010).

A further reason for the inconsistency in the published literature is that there are several different methods used to express salivary SIgA data, often making it difficult to make direct comparisons between studies. One of the major sources of variation in salivary SIgA levels is an alteration in saliva flow rate (the volume of saliva secreted into the mouth per minute), which is not always accounted for. The literature is in general agreement that exercise of sufficient intensity (greater than 60% $\dot{V}O_2$ max) is associated with falls in rates of saliva flow (Walsh *et al.* 2011a). Therefore, even if the actual amount of salivary SIgA secreted across the epithelium remains constant, the concentration of salivary SIgA in that fluid would appear to increase because it is present in a smaller volume of saliva. This could give the artificial impression of enhanced mucosal defence. Similarly, stimulating saliva flow, for example by chewing, could result in a diluting effect on the concentration of SIgA in the saliva, giving the (perhaps misleading) notion of a decrease in salivary SIgA concentration. It is clear that researchers working in this area need a way of accounting for alterations in saliva flow.

A range of methods have been employed to overcome this problem. An early approach was to assess salivary SIgA concentration as a ratio to total saliva protein or albumin, with the assumption that total protein or albumin secretion rates into saliva do not change in response to exercise, allowing these proteins to act as a constant reference point. For example, in the first published study to look at the relationship between salivary SIgA and exercise, Tomasi *et al.* (1982) reported a 20% decrease in salivary SIgA concentration following two to three hours of competition in elite cross-country skiers that became a 40% decrease when expressed relative to saliva total protein concentration. However, it has been suggested that correcting for total protein is misleading, since protein secretion rate itself has been shown to increase during exercise (Blannin *et al.* 1998; Walsh *et al.* 1999). The expression of salivary SIgA as a secretion rate (concentration multiplied by saliva flow rate) is now generally viewed as a more appropriate indicator of mucosal protection because it takes any alterations in saliva volume directly into account. Furthermore, the mechanical washing effect that saliva production itself has on the oral mucosa is also important in host defence. A further method of expressing salivary SIgA data is relative to saliva osmolality, since osmolality rises in proportion to the fall in saliva flow rate and mainly reflects the inorganic electrolyte concentration, with protein accounting for less than one per cent of saliva osmolality.

Other influencing factors

Different methods of saliva collection are described in Technique box 6.1 and these may also contribute to the discrepancies in the literature (Bishop and Gleeson 2009). Cotton swabs are used to minimise the risk of gingival bleeding associated with the

Technique box 6.1

Saliva collection and analysis

There are several methods by which saliva samples can be collected but the most commonly used is cotton-swab collection or collection by passive dribble into a sterile plastic tube with a lid. It may be easier for some individuals (e.g. children) and in some situations (samples taken while exercise continues) for collections to be made using cotton swabs but there are some considerations with regard to volume collected that need to be taken into account, as outlined elsewhere in Chapter 6. Some collections are performed over a fixed time period (e.g. 2 minutes), others until a fixed volume (e.g. 1 or 2 ml) has been collected (these collections are usually into tubes with the target volume indicated on the side).

If you wish to report a secretion rate, you also need to determine saliva flow. To do this, make sure that you weigh the cotton swab and its tube or other collecting tube to the nearest 10 mg before and after collecting the sample, so that you are able to work out the saliva volume produced over the collection period. Assuming that saliva has a density of 1.0 g/ml, the difference in mass indicates the volume of saliva collected. This, divided by the collection time in minutes, gives you the volume of saliva produced each minute.

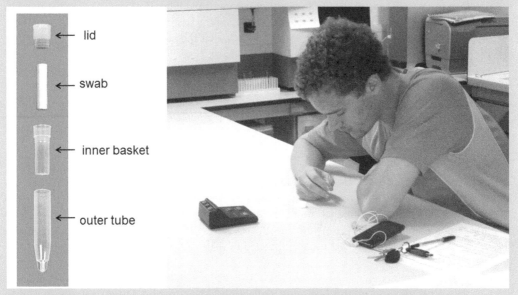

lid

swab

inner basket

outer tube

Collection of a saliva sample

Whichever method is being used, around 5 minutes before collection, provide the individual with a small (approximately 100 ml) drink of plain water to wash the mouth and remove any contaminants. Then, if using the swab method:

- give the individual an unopened swab tube and ask them to unscrew the tube lid and tip the swab out into their hand;
- ask the individual to swallow to empty the mouth and then ask them to place the swab under their tongue;

- ask the individual to sit quietly for the duration of the timed collection (normally 2 minutes but this may vary depending on the individual's saliva flow);
- at the end of the collection period, ask the individual to push the swab directly out of their mouths (without using their hands) into the plastic tube and replace the lid.

If using the passive dribble method:

- give the individual the unopened sterile screw-top tube and ask them to unscrew the lid;
- ask the individual to swallow to empty the mouth and then sit with their head tilted slightly forward;
- ask the individual to dribble the saliva as it collects under their tongue every 20 seconds for the duration of the timed collection (normally 2 minutes) or until the target volume has been reached, while making minimal facial movement and no talking (see photo).
- at the end of the collection period, ask the individual to replace the tube lid and pass the closed tube to you.

If using the passive dribble method, before analysis it is usual to aspirate the saliva into a fresh centrifuge tube and centrifuge at high speed (> 10,000 rpm) for two minutes to obtain a clear sample, with any contaminants (e.g. cells, mucous) collecting in the bottom of the tube. Cotton swabs are designed to be centrifuged in their outer tubes, with saliva collecting at the base of the outer tube via a small hole in the base of the inner basket. The supernatant (clear fluid) is then used for the analysis. Salivary IgA, lactoferrin and lysozyme concentrations are determined using specific enzyme linked immunosorbent assays (ELISA) as detailed in Chapter 2 (Technique box 2.1); whereby the target protein (e.g. IgA, lysozyme) is 'captured' by an initial antibody specific for that protein and detected by a second antibody that is also bound to an enzyme that can subsequently convert a substrate into a coloured product. The change in colour reflects the amount of the protein in the original sample and is compared with the change in a range of standard samples of known concentrations.

Alpha-amylase (α-amylase) activity is assessed by determining the activity of the enzyme in the saliva sample when a reagent is added containing a substrate (e.g. 2-chloro-p-nitrophenol linked to maltriose), which is broken down by α-amylase into a product that can be detected by the amount of light it absorbs (spectrophotometry). The amount of α-amylase activity present in the sample is directly proportional to the rate of increase in light absorbance after the reagent is added. For measurements of enzyme activity like this, it is important that the temperature of the reaction is recorded and remains constant. Values of enzyme activity (units/minute) are usually corrected to values at 37°C.

expectoration method of saliva collection. They are also easier to use with children than collections made by dribbling into a sterile collection pot. However, low (less than 0.2 ml) and high (over 2 ml) sample volumes may affect salivary SIgA concentrations obtained from cotton swabs. In addition, the placement of the cotton swab (e.g. under the tongue or against the inside of the cheek) could potentially affect the composition of the saliva collected, as this would preferentially collect saliva from and/or stimulate different saliva glands which, as outlined above, themselves differ in the composition of saliva that they produce. Another factor to consider when comparing studies, particularly those that have used swabs, is whether or not saliva flow has been stimulated by chewing. This tends to decrease the concentration of salivary SIgA, owing to a dilution effect of the increased saliva volume.

A further consideration when interpreting salivary SIgA data is its circadian variation: the salivary SIgA concentration decreases throughout the day from its highest value in the early morning to its lowest value in the evening. With this in mind, it is possible that reports of decreased SIgA after prolonged exercise performed in the morning may be at least partly reflecting usual diurnal variations in these markers.

Acute exercise effects on other antimicrobial proteins in saliva

Although the majority of studies investigating changes in mucosal immunity with exercise have focused on salivary SIgA, there is some evidence that concentrations of IgG in saliva are unchanged by acute bouts of exercise, whereas absolute concentrations of saliva IgM appear to parallel the decrease in SIgA levels and usually recover within 24 hours (Gleeson and Pyne 2000).

Increases in saliva alpha-amylase are stimulated by increased activity of the sympathetic nervous system, with most of this protein produced by the parotid gland. In accordance with this, several studies have found that exercise increases the alpha-amylase activity of saliva in a manner that is dependent on exercise intensity (Li and Gleeson 2004; Allgrove et al. 2008). Intense and exhaustive exercise of both shorter (around 20 minutes) and longer (around 3 hours) duration is associated with increases in saliva lysozyme secretion rate (Allgrove et al. 2008, West et al. 2010), although high-intensity intermittent exercise does not appear to affect saliva lysozyme concentrations (Davison 2011).

The effect of exercise on lactoferrin concentration and, particularly, salivary lactoferrin concentration, has received little attention to date. However, one study has shown a 50% increase in levels of salivary lactoferrin following a graded treadmill test to exhaustion in a cohort of elite rowers (West et al. 2010).

Potential mechanisms

The mechanisms by which acute exercise influences salivary responses have still not been fully determined. However, recent studies of salivary gland control and protein secretion in animal models have provided insights into several potential mechanisms which may be involved during exercise. Underlying these mechanisms are alterations in the stimulation of the autonomic nerves that innervate the salivary glands directly or the blood vessels that supply the glands.

Variations in the volume and/or source of secreted saliva will influence the resultant secretion rate of the constituent proteins. It has been suggested that stimulation of salivary glands by sympathetic nervous activity reduces saliva flow rate via vasoconstriction of the blood vessels supplying the salivary glands (Strazdins et al. 2005). While sympathetic stimulation is known to exert some control over glandular blood flow, it is important to note that this is not part of the reflex salivary response to stimuli such as anxiety, chewing, taste and sight of food. Under reflex conditions, it has been shown that vasoconstriction is not responsible for altered saliva volume because only sympathetic secretomotor nerve fibres and not vasoactive nerve fibres are stimulated (Proctor and Carpenter 2007). This suggests that the decrease in flow rate associated with exercise is more likely related to a removal of parasympathetic vasodilatory influences rather than sympathetically mediated vasoconstriction. This is further supported by the finding that 'dry mouth' sensations associated with psychological stress were related to parasympathetic withdrawal rather than sympathetic activation (Bosch *et al.* 2002) and that increased sympathetic activity through caffeine ingestion had no effect on saliva flow rate responses to intensive exercise (Bishop *et al.* 2006).

The rate of secretion of SIgA itself is depends on two factors: (1) the production of SIgA by the plasma cells; and (2) the rate of IgA transcytosis across the epithelial cell. It is unlikely that decreased production of SIgA by local plasma cells makes a major contribution to the alterations in salivary SIgA observed in response to acute exercise. This is because changes in salivary SIgA are evident relatively quickly (minutes) and B-cell ability to generate specific antibody secretory responses is not impaired even up to two weeks after strenuous, high-intensity exercise (Bruunsgaard *et al.* 1997b). Animal studies have demonstrated elevated IgA transcytosis from the glandular pool in response to acute stimulation of beta-adrenoreceptors, perhaps via increased availability of the pIgR (Proctor *et al.* 2003; Carpenter *et al.* 2004). Although such a mechanism has not yet been demonstrated in humans, the finding that increases in salivary SIgA secretion rate are associated with elevations in plasma adrenaline following caffeine ingestion lends some support to this suggestion (Bishop *et al.* 2006).

While enhanced IgA transcytosis may explain post-exercise elevations in salivary SIgA secretion, it does not account for contrasting findings of either no change or decreases in salivary SIgA secretion rate after acute exercise. Increased mobilisation of the pIgR only occurs above a certain threshold of frequency of stimulation (Proctor *et al.* 2003) and this could account for the finding of little change in salivary SIgA levels at more moderate intensities of exercise. However, the finding of decreased concentrations of IgA in response to exercise reported by some authors is harder to explain. The answer may lie in the findings of a study in rats, which reported decreases in SIgA concentration that were associated with a decline in pIgR mRNA expression following a treadmill run to exhaustion that lasted about one hour (Kimura *et al.* 2008). This may possibly imply that more intensive exercise (i.e. higher frequency of stimulation) exceeds a second critical threshold of stimulation above which pIgR expression becomes downregulated.

EXERCISE TRAINING AND MUCOSAL IMMUNITY

There is a consensus in the literature that falls in salivary SIgA concentration can occur during intensive periods of exercise training (Walsh *et al.* 2011a), with some studies also reporting a negative relationship between measurements of salivary SIgA and symptoms or incidence of upper respiratory tract illness (URTI). Several longitudinal studies have monitored immune function in high-level athletes over the course of a competitive season. For example, resting levels of salivary SIgA fell with each additional month of training in a cohort of elite Australian swimmers over a seven-month training season. Both the preseason and the mean pre-training SIgA concentrations were found to predict the number of infections in the swimmers (Gleeson *et al.* 1999a). In a study of American football players, the incidence of URTI was increased during periods of intense training and competition and this was associated with falls in SIgA concentration and secretion rate (Fahlman and Engels 2005). In this study, it was reported that the secretion rate of SIgA (which represents the amount of SIgA available on the mucosal surfaces for protection against pathogens) was significantly and inversely related to URTI incidence). Furthermore, a year-long study of America's Cup yachtsmen that collected saliva samples on a weekly basis found that levels of salivary SIgA were associated with rating of subjective fatigue and significant reductions in salivary SIgA occurred in the three weeks prior to clinically confirmed respiratory infection (Figure 6.4). Moreover, a salivary SIgA value of less than 40% of the individual's value when healthy indicated a 50% chance of contracting an infection within 3 weeks (Neville *et al.*, 2008).

Figure 6.4 Relative change in salivary secretory immunoglobulin A (SIgA) concentration in elite yachtsmen when compared with values when healthy in the weeks before and after clinically confirmed upper respiratory illness (URTI). A 40% decrease in IgA from an individual's healthy mean value was associated with a 1 in 2 chance of contracting URTI within 3 weeks; * URTI significantly different from −4 weeks, +1 week and +2 weeks ($P < 0.005$) (adapted from Neville *et al.* 2008)

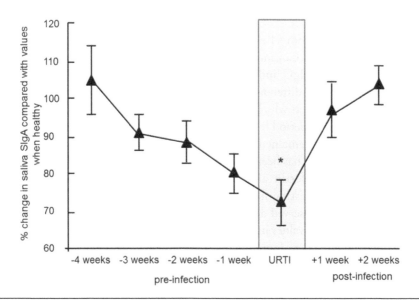

Short-term observations have not always been able to reproduce these outcomes, although this may be influenced by infrequent saliva collections. For example, saliva

Group activity 6.1

Discussion about the practicalities of collecting saliva for monitoring changes in immunoendocrine variables (e.g. SIgA, lysozyme, cortisol, testosterone) in athletes

The problem

Discuss the monitoring of saliva parameters in field settings (e.g. at a football training ground or swimming pool).

Points for discussion within your groups:

- What are the reasons for choosing saliva rather than blood for monitoring hormonal and immune status in athletes/teams?
- How should saliva be collected?
- How much saliva is needed?
- Is it better to use timed or fixed-volume collections?
- Which populations might provide the biggest problem in doing timed collections?
- What is the difference between stimulated and unstimulated samples?
- Does time of day matter?
- Should subjects be fed or fasted and does this matter?
- Where should you carry out the collection and are there any external influences that might affect saliva flow rate or composition?

samples taken from 41 elite Australian swimmers in the months of May and August before the 1998 Commonwealth Games found no differences in salivary concentrations of IgA, IgG and IgM between the two collection times (Pyne *et al.* 2000). Importantly, no differences in salivary immunoglobulin concentrations were found between swimmers who had experienced URTI (as confirmed by the team physician) in the six-week period leading up to and including the Commonwealth Games and those who had remained healthy.

To date, there has been little attention paid to the effect of training stress on saliva lysozyme, lactoferrin and alpha-amylase concentrations. With regard to saliva lysozyme, contrasting findings have been reported: lower saliva lysozyme concentrations were observed during periods of heavy training and competition compared with pre-season values in elite rugby players (Cunniffe *et al.* 2011), yet a five-month study of elite rowers found no difference in saliva lysozyme values between rowers and sedentary controls over the time-course of the study (West *et al.* 2010). Exercise training may have a clearer effect on saliva lactoferrin concentrations. Values were 60% lower in elite rowers than sedentary controls at baseline and mid-way through a five-month monitoring period (West *et al.* 2010) and periods of intense training and competition were associated with decreases in saliva lactoferrin concentration in National League basketball players (He *et al.* 2010). The effect of exercise training on alpha-amylase has received little attention in humans to date. However, a study in mice found no effect of 12 weeks free-running exercise on alpha-amylase levels (Yoshino *et al.* 2009).

Potential mechanisms

There is little research in either humans or animals to shed light on the potential mechanisms by which concentration and secretion rate of salivary SIgA decrease in response to long-term intensive training. Modification of IgA synthesis from local plasma cells could play a greater role in this chronic effect, particularly as this relationship is most consistently observed when salivary SIgA is monitored over periods of several months. In addition, it may be that repeated mobilisation of the pIgR could deplete the available formed IgA pool, leading to decreases in SIgA output. An inhibitory effect of cortisol exposure may also be involved here; increases in levels of salivary cortisol have been associated with decreased secretion rates of salivary SIgA, lysozyme and lactoferrin during the playing season in professional sportsmen (He *et al.* 2010; Cunniffe *et al.* 2011).

Clinical relevance

As we can see from the previous section, there is consensus that intensive training is associated with a decrease in salivary SIgA concentration and secretion rate. In many cases, particularly where monitoring has taken place over several months, falls in salivary SIgA levels have been related to either subsequent symptoms of, or confirmed, upper respiratory illness. However, this has not been shown unanimously and certainly observations over a shorter time period and/or with less frequent measurements have often not been able to replicate these findings.

Such observations highlight the challenge with which researchers find themselves presented when trying to identify relationships between SIgA levels and symptoms or incidence of URTI; individuals with lower levels of salivary SIgA will not necessarily present with URTI and those who present with URTI will not necessarily demonstrate low levels of salivary SIgA. There is no common threshold for salivary SIgA concentration or secretion rate below which all individuals are placed at increased risk for URTI. In addition, differences in collection methods and assay techniques mean that specific thresholds applied by particular research groups cannot necessarily be applied universally. Studies that have attempted to relate measures of salivary SIgA with symptoms or incidence of URTI have invariably used regression or correlation analyses, yet it is important to appreciate that the absence of a statistical relationship does not necessarily indicate the absence of a biological relationship. Measures of salivary SIgA vary widely between individuals and, with this in mind, it is probably more meaningful to monitor salivary SIgA responses on an individual basis, taking notice of any substantial deviations from the usual profile for that individual when healthy. The study in America's Cup yachtsmen mentioned in earlier in this chapter lends strong support for this approach: although a 40% deviation from an individual's healthy salivary SIgA concentration was associated with a one in two chance of contracting clinically confirmed URTI within three weeks, the authors failed to find any relationship between salivary IgA concentration (mg/L) and incidence of URTI (Neville *et al.* 2008).

KEY POINTS

- Immunoglobulin molecules are secreted by terminally differentiated B cells. There are five classes of Ig: IgG, IgM, IgA, IgD, and IgE.
- The common mucosal immune system is a structure protecting the mucosal surfaces of the gut, respiratory tract, nasal passages and female reproductive tract.
- The main effector function of the common mucosal immune system is secretion of IgA (known as secretory IgA, or SIgA). SIgA is a dimeric molecule (two immunoglobulin molecules joined together by a 'J-chain') and transported across the mucosal surfaces via the polymeric immunoglobulin receptor (pIgR).
- The SIgA response to acute exercise in inconsistent and is affected by several factors including exercise intensity, duration, method of collection, method of reporting and time of day. However, saliva flow rate is consistently reported to fall in response to exercise at moderate intensities and above.
- The changes in salivary SIgA with strenuous acute exercise may reflect altered mobilisation of the pIgR as a consequence of increase sympathetic nervous system activation. Decreases in saliva volume most likely reflect withdrawal of the inhibitory effects of the parasympathetic nervous system.
- Salivary SIgA concentrations and secretion rates tend to fall with longer-term, intensive exercise training. In many cases (but not all) this has been associated with increased risk of URTI.
- The mechanisms underlying the chronic effect of exercise are unclear but may reflect modified IgA synthesis from local plasma cells and/or depletion of the available pool of pIgR. An inhibitory effect of cortisol may be involved.
- Other antimicrobial proteins in saliva include alpha-amylase, lysozyme and lactoferrin. The effect of exercise on these has received far less attention than that of salivary SIgA and any changes tend to be less marked.
- Saliva can be collected easily in the field without the need for specialist equipment or training. In this way, monitoring salivary SIgA levels can be a useful tool for athletes and coaches to highlight athletes who may be at risk of URTI.
- Evaluation of salivary SIgA must be undertaken on an individual basis, with interpretation based on changes from the usual profile for that individual, rather than looking at overall changes within a group of athletes.

FURTHER READING

Allgrove, J. E., Gomes, E., Hough, J. and Gleeson, M. (2008) Effects of exercise intensity on salivary antimicrobial proteins and markers of stress in active men. *Journal of Sports Sciences* 26: 653–61.

Bishop, N. C. and Gleeson, M. (2009) Acute and chronic effects of exercise on markers of mucosal immunity. *Frontiers in Bioscience* 14: 4444–56.

Gleeson, M., Pyne, D. B. and Callister, R. (2004) The missing links in exercise effects on mucosal immunity. *Exercise Immunology Review* 10: 107–28.

Gleeson, M., McDonald, W. A., Pyne, D. B., Cripps, A. W., Francis, J. L., Fricker, P. A. and Clancy, R. L. (1999) Salivary IgA levels and infection risk in elite swimmers. *Medicine and Science in Sports and Exercise* 31: 67–73.

Neville, V., Gleeson, M. and Folland, J. P. (2008) Salivary IgA as a risk factor for upper respiratory infections in elite professional athletes. *Medicine and Science in Sports and Exercise* 40: 1228–36.

Walsh, N. P., Gleeson, M., Shephard, R. J., Gleeson, M., Woods, J. A., Bishop, N. C., Fleshner, M., Green, C., Pedersen, B. K., Hoffman-Goetz, L., Rogers, C. J., Northoff, H., Abbasi, A. and Simon, P. (2011) Position statement. Part one: Immune function and exercise. *Exercise Immunology Review* 17: 6–63. Note: the information found in pages 25–8 relates specifically to mucosal immunity and exercise.

7 Effect of extreme environments on immune responses to exercise

Neil P. Walsh and Samuel J. Oliver

LEARNING OBJECTIVES

After studying this chapter, you should be able to:

- describe research evidence from studies examining the effects of environmental extremes (e.g. heat, cold, high altitude, air pollution and spaceflight) on the immune response to exercise.
- demonstrate an understanding of the possible mechanisms by which environmental extremes have been hypothesised to alter the immune response to exercise.
- provide a case both for and against a possible role for immune dysregulation in exertional heat illness aetiology.
- critically discuss whether the commonly held belief that cold exposure increases the incidence of the common cold is credible and, if so, whether cold-induced depression of the immune function is responsible.
- demonstrate an understanding of the effects of high altitude on the incidence of infection and immune function.
- describe the effect of air pollution on immune function during exercise.
- describe the effect of space travel on infection and immune function.
- demonstrate an understanding of the strengths and weaknesses of laboratory and field studies investigating the effects of environmental extremes on the incidence of infection and immune function.

INTRODUCTION

Many factors have the potential to influence the immune response to exercise, including: age and sex (see Chapter 13); training status (see Chapter 8); nutrition (see Chapter 9); the psychological stress of training and competition and the quantity and quality of sleep (see Chapter 2) and the environmental conditions. Athletes, military personnel, fire fighters and mountaineers are often required to perform vigorous physical activity in adverse environmental conditions. These adverse environmental conditions may present themselves as extremes of heat and humidity, cold, high altitude, air pollution and, in a small number of cases, the hyper- and micro-gravity that accompanies spaceflight. Even in staged world sporting events, such as the Olympic Games, an athlete can be required to compete in adverse environmental conditions to which they are neither native nor resident, such as the altitude of Mexico City in 1968, the extreme heat and humidity of Athens in 2004 or the polluted air of Beijing in 2008. In spite of appropriate preparation, exercise in environmental extremes may induce a stereotyped stress hormone response over and above that seen during exercise in more favourable conditions (Shephard 1998).

Emergence of a new subdiscipline within exercise immunology

In the late 1990s, Dr Roy Shephard and his team at the University of Toronto presented the intriguing hypothesis that performing physical activity in stressful environments poses a greater threat than normal to immune function (Shephard 1998). Dr Shephard's pioneering work sparked a number of exercise immunologists to turn their attention to investigating the effects of environmental extremes on the immune response to exercise (Box 7.1).

Box 7.1 Dr Roy Shephard – a pioneer in exercise immunology

Dr Shephard is Professor Emeritus of Applied Physiology at the University of Toronto. He currently lives in Brackendale, British Columbia. He holds degrees from the University of London (BSc, MBBS, PhD and MD) and honorary doctorates from the Universities of Toronto, Ghent, Montréal and Québec, together with honour awards from the Canadian Society of Exercise Physiology, the American College of Sports Medicine and the North American Society for Pediatric Exercise Medicine. He is a former president of the Canadian Society of Exercise Physiology and the American College of Sports Medicine and has authored many books, including *Physical Activity, Training and the Immune Response* (1997), has published some 1,500 scientific papers and edited many journals. He was the founding editor of the journal, *Exercise Immunology Review* and is currently editor-in-chief of the *Year Book of Sports Medicine*.

Roy Shephard's research interests over a 63-year academic career in England, the United States, France and Canada have included many facets of fitness, exercise and environmental physiology. Retirement from the University of Toronto brought the opportunity for research at the Defence and Civil Institute of Environmental Medicine in a northern suburb of Toronto, where he found the opportunity to marry the emerging discipline of exercise immunology with personal experience in exercise physiology and the interests of the Institute in human survival under challenging environments. With a strong cadre of postgraduate fellows and graduate students, he authored a number of early reviews and research publications on these topics.

Considering the body's response to stressors such as exercise and environmental stress and the link with immune function (first described in Chapter 2 and summarised in Box 7.2), it is easy to understand why Dr Shephard hypothesised that exercise in adverse environmental conditions, with increased circulating stress hormone responses, would cause greater disruption to immune function and host defence. This chapter draws upon research evidence from studies investigating the effects of exercise in environmental extremes including heat, cold, high altitude, air pollution and spaceflight on immune responses and infection incidence to test this hypothesis.

Box 7.2 Neuroendocrine modulation of immune function – a coordinated response to stress

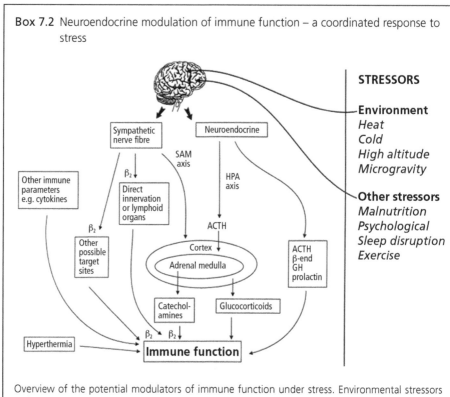

Overview of the potential modulators of immune function under stress. Environmental stressors such as heat, cold, high altitude or microgravity may indirectly influence immune function through the initiation of a stress-hormone response involving the hypothalamic-pituitary-adrenal axis and sympatheticoadrenal-medullary axis. Hyperthermia may have a direct effect on immune function (modified from Jonsdottir 2000)

Stressors such as exercise, heat or hypoxia are characteristically met by a series of coordinated hormonal responses controlled by the central nervous system (see Box 7.2) (Jonsdottir 2000). The central control station resides within the hypothalamus, with the hypothalamic-pituitary-adrenal (HPA) axis and sympatheticoadrenal–medullary (SAM) axis providing the effector limbs by which the brain influences the body's response to stress by controlling the production of adrenal hormones known to modulate immune function. The HPA axis regulates the production of cortisol by the adrenal cortex and the SAM axis regulates the production of catecholamines (adrenaline and noradrenaline) by the adrenal medulla. Aside from these dominant axes, anterior pituitary hormones with known immune regulatory effects, such as growth hormone and prolactin, may also be released during stressful situations. Evidence supports an interaction between neuroendocrine responses to exercise and immune responses to exercise (Hoffman-Goetz and Pedersen 1994). For example, sympathetic nerve innervation of organs of the immune system (e.g. primary lymphoid tissue) indicates an autonomic nervous system involvement in immune modulation under stress. The expression of β-adrenergic receptors on immune cells is well documented and, since these receptors are the targets for catecholamine signalling, it is generally considered that catecholamines have significant effects on immune cell function during stress. The immunosuppressive effects of cortisol are widely accepted.

HEAT STRESS AND IMMUNE FUNCTION

It is important to distinguish between the increase in body temperature that accompanies a fever (core temperature maintained at greater than 37.2°C) and the increase in body temperature that accompanies passive heat exposure (e.g. when taking a sauna or hot bath) or vigorous physical activity. An increase in endogenous pyrogens, such as IL-1, IL-6, IFN-γ and TNF-α, raise body temperature during a fever through an increase in the hypothalamic temperature set point. During passive heat exposure or vigorous physical activity, the hypothalamic temperature set point remains the same but problems with heat dissipation cause body temperature to rise. During vigorous exercise, particularly in warm weather, core body temperature frequently exceeds levels associated with fever and hyperthermia (over 39.5°C) (Pugh 1967; Byrne *et al.* 2006). Core body temperatures of 40–42°C have been reported in conscious runners and greater than 42°C in collapsed runners (Maron *et al.* 1977; Roberts 1989).

Passive heating and immune function

It has been known for some time that passive exposure to heat stress resulting in elevated core temperature evokes an increase in the circulating numbers of leukocytes. Inducing artificial fever (core temperature around 39.5°C) using whole-body immersion in warm water has been shown to increase circulating neutrophils, lymphocytes, NK cells and eosinophils and decrease monocyte numbers (Downing and Taylor 1987; Downing *et al.* 1988). The efficacy of inducing artificial fever as a potential therapy to increase immune function in cancer patients is reviewed in Box 7.3. The leukocytosis associated with hyperthermia may be partly accounted for by an increase in the demargination of leukocytes from the blood vessel walls as a result of the increase in cardiac output (increase in shear stress). Studies using hormonal blockade and hormone infusion do not support a role for catecholamines and β-endorphin in the circulating leukocyte response to hyperthermia but do support a role for growth hormone and cortisol as powerful mediators of neutrophil release into the circulation (Kappel *et al.* 1998).

Box 7.3 Does taking a regular sauna or hot bath reduce infection and improve immune function?

- It is a widely held belief that a hot bath or sauna can have therapeutic effects for many ailments. Is this why the Romans built so many spas?
- A small number of studies show that regular sauna bathing can decrease the symptoms of the common cold.
- Hot-water immersion has been shown to improve clinical outcomes for cancer patients, i.e. those with compromised immune function.
  - Whole-body hyperthermia (two degree Celsius rise in core temperature) in cancer patients increased circulating lymphocyte counts and mitogen-stimulated cytokine release in the hours after heating.
  - Whole-body hyperthermia in cancer patients using limb perfusion (heating the blood to 41.5°C) for up to six hours transiently raised neutrophil bactericidal capacity to healthy control levels.

Summary

Whole-body hyperthermia can be immunostimulatory in those with compromised immune function. However, it remains contentious whether taking a regular sauna or hot bath reduces respiratory tract infection incidence and improves immune function in otherwise healthy individuals.

With the exception of monocyte function, which does not appear to be affected by an increase in temperature within the range 37–39°C, an increase in *in vitro* or *in vivo* temperature of around 2°C is widely acknowledged to enhance neutrophil, lymphocyte and NK cell function (Walsh and Whitham 2006). The magnitude of the change in leukocyte function with passive heat stress appears to be dependent upon the magnitude of the temperature rise and also possibly the exposure duration. For example, leukocyte counts and function remained unaltered with a rise of around 0.7°C in core temperature but were enhanced with rise of around 2°C rise in core temperature (Kappel *et al.* 1991a; Severs *et al.* 1996). Furthermore, a brief increase in incubation temperature from 37°C to 39°C enhanced *in vitro* neutrophil migration but a similar increase in incubation temperature for a more prolonged period (72 hours) inhibited this important function (Nahas *et al.* 1971; Roberts and Sandberg 1979).

Exercise in the heat and immune function

Compared with exercise in thermoneutral conditions, exercise in hot conditions is associated with increased core temperature, higher heart rate (cardiovascular drift), increased circulating stress hormones and an increased reliance on carbohydrate as a fuel source (Galloway and Maughan 1997; Febbraio 2001). Unsurprisingly, compared with thermoneutral conditions, endurance performance in the heat is impaired (Galloway and Maughan 1997; Ely *et al.* 2010). Exercising in hot conditions in which core temperature rises by more than 1°C compared with thermoneutral conditions (where core temperature rise is less than 1°C) augments anticipated increases in circulating stress hormones, including catecholamines and cytokines, with associated elevations in circulating leukocyte counts (Cross *et al.* 1996; Rhind *et al.* 2004).

Using an elegant experimental model described as a 'thermal clamp' to assess the contribution of hyperthermia in the leukocytosis of exercise, two studies had subjects perform 40 minutes of cycling at 65% $\dot{V}O_2$ peak on one occasion with a rise in core temperature (cycling immersed to mid-chest in 39°C water) and on another occasion without a significant rise in core temperature – this thermal clamp condition involved cycling immersed to mid-chest in 18°C or 23°C water (Cross *et al.* 1996; Rhind *et al.* 1999). Exercising in the thermal clamp condition substantially reduced the rise in circulating leukocytes and neutrophils (Figure 7.1) and lymphocyte subsets (CD3+, CD4+ and CD8+) (Figure 7.2) and NK cell (CD16+CD56+) numbers but not the increase in circulating monocyte numbers. The thermal clamp reduced

Figure 7.1 Total leukocyte (A) and neutrophil (B) counts during and after 40 minutes of immersed cycling at 65% $\dot{V}O_2$ peak in hot and cold water. Values are mean ± SEM, n = 10 males. Significantly greater than resting: * $P < 0.05$ and ** $P < 0.001$. Significantly greater than cold: † $P < 0.05$ (modified from Rhind *et al.* 1999)

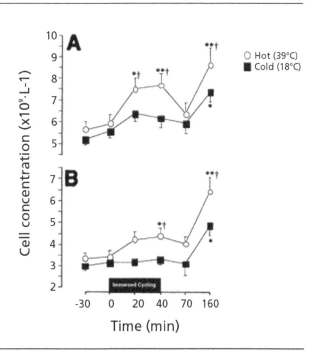

Figure 7.2 (A) T-lymphocyte (CD3+), (B) helper (CD4+) T-lymphocyte and (C) suppressor (CD8+) T-lymphocyte counts during and after 40 minutes of immersed cycling at 65% $\dot{V}O_2$ peak in hot and cold water. Values are mean ± SEM, n = 10 males. Significantly different from resting: * $P < 0.05$ and ** $P < 0.001$. Significant difference between trials: † P < 0.05 (modified from Rhind *et al.* 1999)

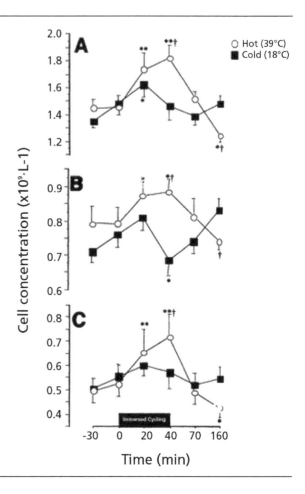

exercise-induced increments of plasma adrenaline, noradrenaline and growth hormone and abolished the increase in plasma cortisol concentration (Cross *et al.* 1996; Rhind *et al.* 1999) (Table 7.1). Multiple regression analysis showed that core temperature had no direct association with lymphocyte subsets but was significantly correlated with hormone levels. The authors stated that hyperthermia mediates exercise-induced leukocyte redistribution to the extent that it causes sympathoadrenal activation, with alterations in circulating adrenaline, noradrenaline and cortisol (Rhind *et al.* 1999).

These thermal clamp studies demonstrate a significant contribution of the rise in core temperature to the development of the leukocytosis and cytokinaemia of exercise (Cross *et al.* 1996; Rhind *et al.* 2004). However, with the exception of a reduction in stimulated lymphocyte responses after exercise in the heat (Severs *et al.* 1996), tightly controlled laboratory studies (see Group Activity 7.1) show a limited effect of exercise in the heat on: neutrophil function, monocyte function, NK cell cytotoxic activity (NKCA) and mucosal immunity (Walsh and Whitham 2006; Walsh *et al.* 2011a, 2011b).

Table 7.1 Plasma cortisol and catecholamine responses to 40 minutes of cycling at 65% $\dot{V}O_2$ peak in hot and cold water; values are mean ± SEM, $n = 10$ males

HORMONE	CONDITION	PRE-EXERCISE[a]	END OF EXERCISE[b]	RECOVERY[c]	LATER RECOVERY[d]
Cortisol (nmol/L)	Hot	470 ± 44	608 ± 60	768 ± 68[e]	373 ± 35
	Cold	535 ± 67	551 ± 63	384 ± 47[g]	295 ± 37
Adrenaline (nmol/L)	Hot	0.28 ± 0.03	1.78 ± 0.20[f]	1.07 ± 0.24[e]	0.47 ± 0.07
	Cold	0.24 ± 0.03	0.72 ± 0.13[e,g]	0.31 ± 0.05	0.26 ± 0.04
Noradrenaline (nmol/L)	Hot	2.53 ± 0.24	11.54 ± 1.72[f]	5.05 ± 2.46[e]	2.66 ± 0.26
	Cold	2.29 ± 0.20	4.49 ± 0.54[f,g]	3.68 ± 0.51[e]	2.82 ± 0.27

Notes:
[a]   0 minutes
[b]   40 minutes of cycling
[c]   30 minutes post-exercise
[d]   120 minutes post-exercise
[e]   Significantly different from resting pre-exercise values, $P < 0.05$
[f]   Significantly different from resting pre-exercise values, $P < 0.001$
[g]   Significant difference between trials, $P < 0.05$

Source: modified from Rhind *et al.* (1999)

Group activity 7.1

Discuss the strengths and weaknesses of the laboratory and field studies that investigate the effects of environmental stress on infection and immunity

The problem

Owing to the tight restrictions enforced by ethical committees, most laboratory studies that have examined immune responses to exercise in the heat have evoked only modest increases in core temperature (peak core temperature less than 39°C). Core temperature during exercise in the field often exceeds 40°C in athletes, military personnel and fire fighters undertaking vigorous physical activity in hot conditions.

Questions for group discussion

- What are the strengths and weaknesses of employing a laboratory design?
- What are the strengths and weaknesses of employing a field design?

These questions could equally form the basis of a group discussion about the strengths and weaknesses of the research in the other sections of this chapter dealing with cold stress, altitude, etc.

In summary, most of the available evidence does not support the contention that exercising in the heat poses a greater threat to immune function compared with thermoneutral conditions. It is worth noting that individuals exercising in the heat tend to fatigue sooner, compared with performing the same exercise in thermoneutral conditions, so their exposure to exercise stress in the heat tends to be self-limiting (Gonzalez-Alonso *et al.* 1999).

A controversial concept: a role for immune dysregulation in exertional heat illness

Without a doubt, the most compelling ongoing controversy in this subdiscipline of exercise immunology centres on whether the immune system is involved in the aetiology of exertional heat stroke (EHS). Unlike the more mild exertional heat illness (EHI), EHS is a life-threatening acute heat illness characterised by hyperthermia (core temperature above 40°C) and neurological abnormalities that can develop after exposure to high ambient temperature and humidity (Muldoon *et al.* 2004).

The possible involvement of immune dysregulation in the aetiology of EHS was first described in the exercise immunology literature by Dr Roy Shephard (see Box 7.1) and Dr Pang Shek (Shephard and Shek 1999b) and has been discussed more recently by others (Lim and Mackinnon 2006; Leon and Helwig 2010). During exercise heat stress, redistribution of blood flow can lead to gastrointestinal ischaemia which, in turn, can result in damage to the intestinal mucosa and the unwelcome leakage of lipopolysaccharide (LPS) into the portal circulation. The LPS is typically neutralised firstly by the liver and secondly by monocytes and macrophages. However, these defences may become overwhelmed, resulting in increased LPS in the peripheral circulation; the increase in circulating LPS may be exacerbated if immune function is impaired during heavy training (e.g. via decreased anti-LPS antibodies) (Bosenberg *et al.* 1988). In turn, a sequence of events ensues involving LPS binding to its binding protein, the transfer of LPS to its receptor complex, Toll-like receptor-4, with subsequent nuclear factor-kappa B activation and translation and production of inflammatory mediators including interleukins IL-1β, TNF-α, IL-6 and inducible nitric oxide synthase (Selkirk *et al.* 2008). These events can lead to the systemic inflammatory response syndrome (SIRS), intravascular coagulation and eventually to multi-organ failure. This is an attractive model (Figure 7.3), particularly for cases of EHS that are otherwise difficult to explain, because the pyrogenic cytokines (e.g. IL-1β and TNF-α) can alter thermoregulation (IL-1 induces fever) and cause cardiovascular instability resulting in collapse of the athlete or soldier. Arguments for and against a role for immune dysregulation in EHS aetiology are presented in Box 7.4.

Which came first, the chicken or the egg?

As Figure 7.3 shows, vascular damage and multi-organ failure induce cytokinaemia, so studies that report an increase in circulating cytokines in EHS casualties tells us very little, if anything, about a possible involvement of immune dysregulation in the aetiology of EHS. Prospective studies in humans are required to examine the extent of any immune dysregulation prior to collapse (Walsh and Whitham 2006).

Figure 7.3 Classical and immune pathways of exertional heat stroke; GI = gastrointestinal; LPS = lipopolysaccharide; RES = reticuloendothelial system; Ig = immunoglobulin; Mø = macrophage; LBP = lipopolysaccharide-binding protein; TLR-4 = Toll-like receptor-4; NF-κB = nuclear factor-kappa B; solid arrows indicate likely links in pathway; broken arrows indicate unsubstantiated in EHS aetiology from Walsh *et al.* 2011a, reproduced with kind permission)

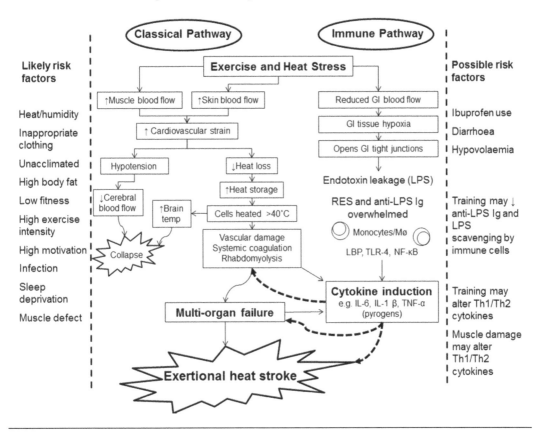

In summary, it is likely that the more traditional predisposing factors for EHS (Figure 7.3) such as high heat load and underlying illness (Rav-Acha *et al.* 2004), alongside a possible muscle defect causing excessive endogenous heat production (Rae *et al.* 2008), play a more prominent role in EHS aetiology than immune dysregulation. It remains to be seen whether immune dysregulation has a role to play in the aetiology of a small number of EHS cases that are otherwise difficult to explain by the more traditional predisposing factors. Emerging research will tell us more about the possible role for the immune system in recovery from heat stroke. For example, Lisa Leon and her colleagues at the United States Army Research Institute of Environmental Medicine in Natick have speculated that the cytokinaemia of heat stroke may be instrumental in the recovery process from this life-threatening event (Leon *et al.* 2006; Leon and Helwig 2010) and we must wait to see whether emerging research supports this exciting concept.

Box 7.4 Arguments for and against a role for immune dysregulation in EHS aetiology

Arguments for

Authors often cite support for an involvement of immune dysregulation in the aetiology of EHS from studies showing:

- Circulating LPS levels in ultramarathon runners similar to florid sepsis (Bosenberg *et al.* 1988);
- Improved heat tolerance in heat-stressed animals treated with corticosteroids and antibiotics to prevent increases in circulating LPS (Gathiram *et al.* 1987, 1988);
- Cytokinaemia in people with EHS (Bouchama *et al.* 1991);
- Symptoms of heat stroke in animals receiving IL-1β or TNF-α (Lin 1997);
- Enhanced survival in heat-stressed animals receiving IL-1 receptor antagonist (Chiu *et al.* 1996);
- Important roles for heat shock proteins (e.g. HSP72) in cellular acquired thermal tolerance (Kuennen *et al.* 2011);
- That experimentally induced inflammation compromises heat tolerance in rats (Lim *et al.* 2007).

Arguments against

There are many inconsistencies and gaps in knowledge that require elucidation. For example:

- There exists great variability in circulating LPS and cytokine levels in heat stroke and EHS casualties (Walsh *et al.* 2011a).
- There is no consensus about the level of circulating LPS associated with clinical manifestations of EHS, although one group (Moore *et al.* 1995) have suggested a threshold of 60 pg.ml^{-1};
- It seems unreasonable that one widely cited paper presents pre-exercise circulating LPS in ultra-distance triathletes of 81 pg.ml^{-1} (Bosenberg *et al.* 1988); surely, triathletes attend a race without initial clinical manifestations of heat illness?
- Circulating cytokine levels in heat stroke and people with EHS are more often than not below the magnitude seen during SIRS and sepsis (Bouchama *et al.* 1991).
- Lack of experimental control in field studies and delay in admitting patients to hospital for blood collection add to the confusing picture regarding cytokines and heat stroke pathology.

Acquired cellular thermal tolerance and heat acclimation – complementary or shared pathways of adaptation

Heat acclimation refers to the reduction in physiological strain that occurs after repeated days of heat exposures as a result of biological adaptations. For example, exercising heart rate and core temperature are decreased and sweating rate is increased at the same absolute work output during exercise in the heat after a period of heat acclimation – usually six days or more. Acquired thermal tolerance refers to cellular changes after repeated days of heat exposures that confer cytoprotection against subsequent, more extreme and potentially lethal heat exposure (Kregel 2002). These cellular changes, which include a blunting in the induction of heat shock proteins (e.g. HSP72) in mononuclear cells in response to heat shock, were thought to occur separately from the more traditional adaptations that accompany heat acclimation (i.e. those that reduce physiological strain during exercise-heat stress) (McClung *et al.* 2008; Leon and Helwig 2010). However, another study indicates that acquired thermal tolerance and heat acclimation may share a common mechanism (Kuennen *et al.* 2011). The authors showed that blocking the heat shock protein response (by daily supplementation of the polyphenol compound quercetin) prevented not only the cellular adaptations but also the normal thermoregulatory adaptations during a seven-day heat acclimation period – exercising core temperature was reduced by day seven in the placebo group but not in the group who received daily quercetin supplementation.

COLD STRESS AND IMMUNE FUNCTION

Cold stress and infection

Exercise immunologists have a keen interest in the effects of cold exposure on immune function and upper respiratory tract infection (URTI) incidence because athletes and soldiers regularly train and compete in cold ambient conditions (Castellani *et al.* 2006). Popular belief is that cold exposure increases susceptibility to URTI (see Box 7.5) but does exercising in a cold environment lead to immune function depression? This section examines the available evidence to answer this question.

Behavioural thermoregulation, e.g. adding extra clothes and finding shelter, maybe inadequate to prevent heat loss and maintain body temperature in a cold environment. In an attempt to defend core temperature, shivering thermogenesis and peripheral vasoconstriction begin (Figure 7.4). These responses are initiated by the SAM and HPA axis, which are also potent modulators of the immune system (Box 7.2). Alterations in thermoregulation may therefore also affect the immune system.

Research in athletes and soldiers shows that peak infection and illness typically occur at times of the year when ambient temperature is lowest; for example, a year-long study with elite cross-country skiers reported URTI incidence to be highest in the winter months (Berglund and Hemmingson 1990). Studies in soldiers also suggest an increase in incidence and severity of URTI during winter months or when deployed to colder regions (Whitham *et al.* 2006). From these epidemiological reports, it is not possible to establish that cold exposure was the cause of the URTI, as many other stressors were likely to have been present including arduous exercise (see Chapters 4–6), inadequate energy and fluid intake (see Chapter 9), psychological

---

Box 7.5 Does getting cold and wet increase your chances of developing a cold? It's called a 'cold' after all!

- It is a commonly held belief that getting a 'chill' causes acute viral respiratory infection (the 'common cold') but does the scientific evidence support this concept?
- Colds are most prevalent in winter months and when outside air temperature and humidity are low (Curwen 1997).
- Early studies that exposed people to the cold before or after a viral nasal inoculation reported no increases in URTI (Andrewes 1950).
- However, URTI symptoms were more than doubled in the four to five days after cold-water immersion of the feet for 20 minutes compared with non-chilled controls (Johnson and Eccles 2005).
- Furthermore, in a study of Finnish military conscripts, the onset of URTI, including the common cold, was preceded by three days of declining ambient temperature and humidity (Makinen *et al.* 2009).
- Acute peripheral cooling of the nose and upper airways has been suggested to inhibit the trafficking of immune cells. This creates a more suitable environment for viral replication that subsequently leads to the onset of common cold, by converting an asymptomatic sub-clinical infection into a symptomatic clinical infection (Figure 7.7) (Eccles 2002a).

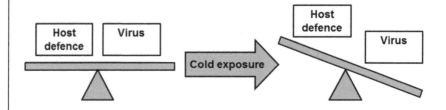

1. Infection but no symptoms (sub-clinical)   2. Infection with symptoms (clinically significant)

The hypothesised effect of cold exposure on infection

In summary, although not entirely conclusive, there is growing evidence to suggest that cold exposure often precedes, and is associated with increased incidence of, URTI including the 'common cold'.

---

stress and sleep disruption (see Chapter 2) and confined living. As discussed in the indicated chapters, these stressors are each purported to increase URTI. More compelling evidence for a link between low ambient temperature and increased URTI, including the common cold, has recently been provided from a two-year study in the Finnish military where ambient temperature and humidity were observed to decline in the three days before the onset of URTI (Makinen *et al.* 2009).

Figure 7.4 Potential mechanisms to explain increased infection in cold environments

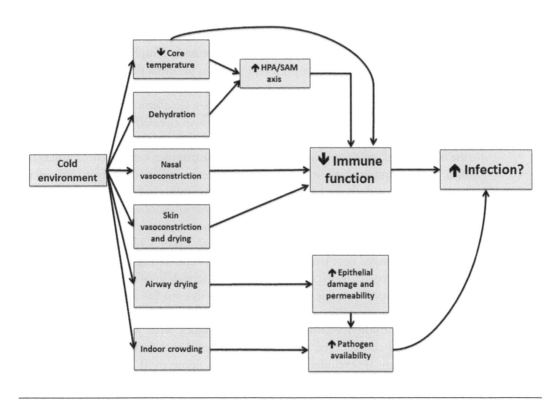

Decreased immune function with repeated cold exposure (Figure 7.4) is one mechanism of many that could explain the increase in infection reported by athletes and soldiers during the winter months. The following sections will focus on understanding this and other possible explanations.

Core body cooling and immune function

Hypothermia, defined as a core body temperature of less than 35°C, is uncommon in athletes because the heat produced as a by-product of exercise is normally adequate to offset heat loss. Nonetheless, hypothermia has been documented in some individuals exercising in cold water or in cold air intermittently for prolonged periods; for example, open-water swimmers and hill walkers (Pugh 1967). Indeed, many studies have identified hypothermia in open-water swimmers (Nuckton *et al.* 2000; Keatinge *et al.* 2001; Brannigan *et al.* 2009). Similarly, hypothermia is more common in some active occupational populations where cold air and water exposure is frequent during exercise or operations (e.g. naval and army personnel) (Beeley *et al.* 1993; Giesbrecht 2000).

A limited number of investigations have examined the effect of lowering core temperature on leukocyte cell trafficking and function in humans. Most studies have modestly lowered core temperature by 0.5–1°C, which causes a leukocytosis that typically remains for two hours after cooling: this leukocytosis is characterised by an increase in neutrophils and a simultaneous decrease in lymphocytes (Brenner *et al.* 1999; Costa *et al.* 2010). It has been reported that maximal shivering thermogenesis in adult humans can reach intensities equivalent to approximately 40% of $\dot{V}O_2$ max or approximately five times resting metabolic rate (Eyolfson *et al.* 2001), which is comparable with modest exercise. The modest rise in circulating leukocyte numbers associated with cold exposure may be attributed to demargination of leukocytes from the blood vessel walls as a result of increased cardiac output and catecholamines (Box 7.2). In these and in observational studies of patients undergoing surgery, where core temperature has decreased by 2°C to core temperatures of approximately 35°C, NKCA remained unaltered but saliva secretory immunoglobulin-A (SIgA) secretion rate, lymphocyte function and neutrophil function are reduced (Wenisch *et al.* 1996; Beilin *et al.* 1998; Brenner *et al.* 1999; Costa *et al.* 2010). Collectively, these studies suggest that lowered core temperature can disrupt circulating and mucosal immune function that may partly explain the increased infection in cold exposed athletes and soldiers. A limitation of this previous research is that studies in patients undergoing surgery have questionable relevance to healthy athletes because of anaesthesia and existing comorbidity. Furthermore, in the studies with healthy participants a thermoneutral control trial was not included and therefore an effect of diurnal variation cannot be excluded. More research is necessary if the effect of low core temperature on immune function is to be fully understood.

Exercise in cold conditions and immune function

Although decreases in core temperature are unusual, peripheral cold (low skin temperature) is common in outdoor enthusiasts and athletes because light clothing is often chosen for optimal athletic performance rather than thermal protection. Compared with steady-state exercise in thermoneutral conditions, exercise in cold air is associated with similar or slightly lower core and muscle temperature and cardiac output with increased respiratory heat loss, ventilation, oxygen uptake, carbohydrate oxidation and energy expenditure (Pugh 1967; Walsh *et al.* 2002). Because cold exposure causes an increased energy requirement, cold-induced diuresis and a blunted thirst response; as a consequence, negative energy balance and dehydration are more likely to affect those exercising and training in the cold (See Chapter 9 for effects of inadequate nutrition on immune function). Most of the small number of studies that have examined immune responses to exercise in cold conditions in humans have compared immune responses after short-duration exercise in cold with immune responses to exercise in hot, rather than thermoneutral conditions. For example, in one thermal clamp study healthy young men performed 40 minutes of cycling at 65% $\dot{V}O_2$ max immersed to mid-chest in cold (18–23°C) and hot (39°C) water where core temperature increased by around 0.5°C in cold and by around 2.0°C in hot conditions (Rhind *et al.* 1999). Exercising in cold water attenuated the leukocytosis observed after exercise in hot water with smaller increases in circulating neutrophils (Figure 7.1). The authors suggested that the significantly reduced plasma catecholamine and cortisol response to exercise in cold conditions was most likely responsible for the attenuated leukocytosis after exercising in the cold. Blunting plasma catecholamines and cortisol by exercising in cold water might therefore be favourable for immune function and host defence (Box 7.2). In another thermal clamp study, the same group had subjects perform a one-hour bout of cycling at 55% $\dot{V}O_2$ peak immersed in cold (18°C) and thermoneutral (35°C) water where a more modest (around 1°C) rise in core temperature occurred after exercise in thermoneutral water compared with around 0.2°C rise in core temperature after exercise in cold water (Brenner *et al.* 1999). Total and differential circulating leukocyte counts and NKCA were similar after exercise in cold and thermoneutral water. The previously noted blunting effect had therefore disappeared highlighting the importance of comparing exercise in cold conditions with thermoneutral rather than hot conditions.

Exercising in cold air conditions compared with thermoneutral conditions has been shown to have a limited effect on mucosal immunity. Compared with exercise in a thermoneutral environment, salivary SIgA secretion rate was similar immediately after and higher 30 minutes after a 30-minute exercise bout at 70% heart rate reserve in cold conditions (1°C) (Mylona *et al.* 2002). In line with this, immediately after prolonged cycling exercise (two hours at 70% $\dot{V}O_2$ max) salivary SIgA secretion rate was reduced similarly in cold (–6.4°C) and thermoneutral (19.8°C) conditions (Walsh *et al.* 2002). In summary, the limited evidence to date does not support the popular belief that exercising in cold compared with thermoneutral conditions decreases immune function, which might lead to greater infection. A limitation of studies to date is that they have focused predominantly on systemic circulating immune parameters assessed by *in vitro* immune tests. *In vitro* tests do not represent the whole-body and integrative function of the immune system. Peripheral blood samples only represent a small percentage of total leukocytes (around 5%) and therefore they can only poorly reflect a change in another part of the body that is important for the immune system (e.g. lymph nodes, bone, thymus). Circulating immune parameters are likely therefore to play a limited role in the drama of cold exposure, immune function and infection.

Alternative mechanisms to explain the increased URTI with cold exposure

Alternative mechanisms that might explain the increased URTI with cold exposure include decreased epithelial barrier function caused by upper airway drying from breathing cold air during exercise (Figure 7.4) (Giesbrecht 1995). Similarly, as the face is normally uncovered during exercise, cold exposure leads to decreases in nasal respiratory epithelium temperature and reduces mucociliary clearance of pathogens, which may impair immune cell trafficking and function, owing to peripheral vasoconstriction and decreased metabolism (Eccles 2002b). As more than half of body volume is less than three centimetres from the skin surface (Webb 1992), low skin temperature and subsequent cold induced peripheral vasoconstriction may impair whole body peripheral immune cell trafficking and function that may lead to greater infection, particularly if open wounds exist. This contention is supported by wound healing being slower and infection higher in surgical patients that become hypothermic (Kurz *et al.* 1996). Future research using *in vivo* skin measures, such as contact hypersensitivity (Harper Smith *et al.* 2011), are warranted to establish the effect of peripheral cooling on skin immune function (see Technique box 5.2 in Chapter 5). Additionally, although acute exercise in the cold has been shown to have a limited effect on mucosal immunity, future research should examine the chronic effects of breathing large volumes of cold air on mucosal and nasal immunity.

Owing to cold ambient temperature, poor weather and shorter daylight hours, athletes and soldiers spend a greater proportion of time living and training indoors during the winter months. Increased time spent in close contact with others can increase pathogen exposure and may therefore explain the increased URTI reported in the winter months. In the general population, indoor crowding has been suggested as a cause of increased infection for over 80 years (Hill and Clemen 1929). Whether crowding is really greater in winter compared with summer has been criticised, as it has been suggested that modern living means people lead a similarly crowded lifestyle all year round, e.g. share open-plan offices, factories and public transport. The idea that indoor crowding spreads infection is general accepted by scientists because few alternative explanations have been described (Eccles 2002a). As Figure 7.4 suggests, other possible explanations do exist for increased URTI incidence in athletes and other active populations during the winter months.

In summary, cold exposure is associated with a greater incidence of URTI in active populations. The mechanism(s) responsible for the increased URTI, however, remains elusive and may not be related to a reduced immune function. The limited evidence to date does not support that exercising in cold compared with thermoneutral conditions suppresses immune function.

ALTITUDE, IMMUNE FUNCTION AND INFECTION: INTO THE DEATH ZONE

Athletes must sometimes compete at modest altitudes up to 2,000 metres as numerous major sporting events are held at altitude (e.g. the 2010 South Africa Football World Cup). Moreover, altitude stress is common to athletes who complete training in altitude or hypoxia, with the aim of improving performance via hypoxia stimulated adaptations (e.g. increased red blood cell concentration and oxygen-carrying capacity). The two most used training paradigms are 'live high, train high', where athletes train and live at altitude, and 'live high, train low', where athletes are intermittently exposed to hypoxia by training at sea level but sleeping at natural or simulated altitude (Stray-Gundersen and Levine 2008). Simulated altitude is typically achieved in a chamber or tent with normobaric hypoxia (normal pressure but low

Figure 7.5 An athlete completes training in a hypoxic chamber at simulated altitude (normobaric hypoxia)

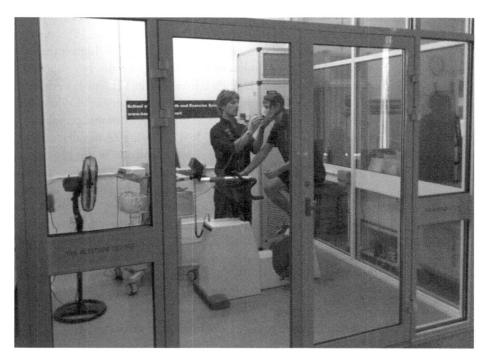

oxygen environment; Figure 7.5). Typically, these training periods are two to four weeks.

In contrast, trekkers, mountaineers and other active occupational groups (e.g. miners and soldiers) are exposed to high altitude for many weeks or months. Trekkers typically exceed 4,500 metres on trips to Himalayan or Andean mountain base camps, with mountaineers climbing into the death zone, greater than 8,000 metres, when attempting to scale the highest mountains in the world (Mount Everest 8,848 metres). In Nepal alone, over 130,000 foreigners visit each year to complete trekking and mountaineering activities. As more people become exposed to hypoxia, it is important to understand the effects of altitude and hypoxia *per se* on immune function and infection. This section describes what we know about this topic.

At high terrestrial locations, the reduced pressure (hypobaria) causes a reduction in the partial pressure of inspired oxygen in air that ultimately causes arterial hypoxaemia, a decrease in arterial oxygen content. To compensate, increases in ventilation, cardiac output and tissue vasodilation occur to improve blood oxygenation and delivery to tissues. Substrate selection also adapts to greater carbohydrate utilisation that ensures the most economical use of oxygen (Mazzeo 2005). As these adaptations are principally initiated by the SAM and HPA axes, it is plausible that adaptations for oxygen delivery may also affect the immune system (Box 7.2).

Altitude and infection

Reports suggest that elite athletes experience increased URTI symptoms during and immediately after altitude training camps (Bailey *et al.* 1998; Gore *et al.* 1998). Similarly, trekkers and mountaineers who travel to high altitude often report symptoms of URTI and studies indicate that upper-airway symptoms increase with increasing altitude (Murdoch 1995; Oliver *et al.* 2012). Further evidence that altitude exposure leads to greater infection comes from one large epidemiological study where soldiers stationed at 3,692 metres had greater pneumonia prevalence than those at lower altitudes (Singh *et al.* 1977). It is tempting to speculate that the increased incidence of URTI symptoms reported at altitude is the direct consequence of hypoxia-impaired immunity; however, limited evidence exists to support this notion (Walsh *et al.* 2011a). The increased infection incidence and URTI symptoms could be more simply explained by other factors common to high altitude (e.g. poor nutrition, cold exposure, ultraviolet radiation, personal hygiene and crowded living quarters). Moreover, diagnosing infection at altitude is difficult as there is a large degree of overlap in symptoms between URTI and acute mountain sickness (Bailey *et al.* 2003). Examining the effects of altitude and hypoxia on objective and clinically relevant measures of immune function is important to provide further confirmation as to whether depression of the immune system is responsible for the increased infection reported at altitude.

Altitude and immune function

Most human studies to examine immune function at altitude indicate that NKCA and humoral immunity are either unaffected or enhanced (Meehan *et al.* 1988; Biselli *et al.* 1991; Facco *et al.* 2005; Table 7.2). In contrast, T cell-mediated immune function has been shown to be impaired during altitude exposure (Pyne *et al.* 2000; Facco *et al.* 2005), which is likely related to the associated increases in circulating cortisol, adrenaline and noradrenaline reported at altitude (Mazzeo 2005).

Unfortunately, the few human studies to indicate an immunodepressive effect of high altitude have used *in vitro* techniques to assess cell-mediated immune function. The importance of using *in vivo* immune responses is that they reflect the coordinated, multi-cellular responses of the immune system and have an end result that is associated with clinical relevant endpoints, such as infection (Walsh *et al.* 2011a, 2011b). Although sparse, evidence does suggest that altitude exposure negatively affects clinically relevant immune function. For example, wound healing that is reliant on a well-orchestrated and functioning immune system (e.g. inflammation and phagocytosis) has been suggested in anecdotal reports by medical doctors of mountaineering expeditions to be impaired (Sarnquist 1983). Anecdotal reports of impaired wound healing in mountaineers at high altitude are supported by laboratory studies in animals showing that breathing hypoxic air (12% O_2 equivalent to 4,000 metres) impairs wound healing after intradermal injection with *Escherichia coli* (Knighton *et al.* 1984). Additionally, research using an *in vivo* immune measure also

Table 7.2 Immune function responses to acute exercise and periods of training in hypoxia or at altitude

	IMMUNE COMPONENT	IMMUNE RESPONSE COMPARED WITH SEA LEVEL[1]
Innate:		
Cellular	NK cell activity	Not different (Meehan *et al.* 1988; Klokker *et al.* 1995; Facco *et al.* 2005) or enhanced (Wang and Wu 2009)
	Neutrophil function	Increased (Hitomi *et al.* 2003; Wang and Chiu 2009) or not different (Chouker *et al.* 2005)
Soluble	Nasal lysozyme: protein	Not different (Meehan *et al.* 1988)
Adaptive:		
Cellular	T cell-mediated function	Decreased (Pyne *et al.* 2000; Facco *et al.* 2005; Zhang *et al.* 2007; Wang and Lin 2010)
Humoral	B cell-mediated function	Increased (Pyne *et al.* 2000) or not different (Biselli *et al.* 1991)
Soluble	Serum immunoglobulins	Not different (Biselli *et al.* 1991; Kleessen *et al.* 2005)
	Nasal and salivary SIgA	Not different (Meehan *et al.* 1988; Tiollier *et al.* 2005)

Note:
1 Where there are more studies to support a particular response the direction of effect is underlined

suggests that altitude exposure decreases T cell-mediated immune function (Oliver *et al.* 2011). Immune depression might therefore, at least in part, be responsible for the increased incidence of URTI reported at high altitude. The importance of using *in vivo*, rather than *in vitro*, immune measures has been highlighted because *in vivo* measures involve a whole-body integrated, multi-cellular response that is clinically relevant (Albers *et al.* 2005; Harper Smith *et al.* 2011). In the study by Oliver *et al.* (2011), the immune test involved the application of a novel antigen, diphenylcyclopropenone (DPCP), to the lower back of rested controls at sea level and mountaineers 28 hours after ascent to a cable car station at 3,777 metres. Four weeks after sensitisation, the strength of immune memory was quantified by measures of oedema (skinfold thickness) and redness (erythema) 48 hours after topical application of a low-dose series of DPCP. This test is described in Chapter 5 (Technique box 5.2). Compared with control responses, skinfold thickness and erythema were lower in the mountaineers (Figure 7.6). High-altitude exposure therefore impaired the induction of new immune memory as evidenced by the reduced immune response to the second exposure with the same antigen. Additionally, this study highlights the utility of this novel skin test as a feasible and sensitive *in vivo* immune function measure for field study use; therefore, overcoming many of the limitations with *in vitro* immune tests (e.g. the typical requirement for venepuncture, immediate sample processing, expensive laboratory facilities and highly-trained staff).

Altitude, exercise and immune function

As highlighted by the 1968 Mexico Olympics, where no records were set in endurance events, altitude greatly diminishes performance in aerobically demanding

Figure 7.6 Reduction in *in vivo* immune function at altitude (data from Oliver *et al.* 2011)

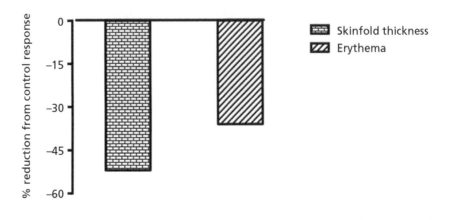

activities. This is primarily because $\dot{V}O_2$ max progressively declines at about 8% for every 1,000 metres of altitude gained after 700 metres (Grover *et al.* 1986). Consequently, submaximal performance is also affected at altitude, because an absolute workload completed at high altitude will require a greater relative oxygen uptake than at sea level (Lundby *et al.* 2007). Exercise at altitude is therefore associated with a number of responses that might further depress immune function that include increased circulating stress hormone concentrations. For example, when exercise workload is reduced to the same relative workload (same %$\dot{V}O_2$ max) plasma adrenaline is still found to be greater during exercise at 4,300 metres (Mazzeo and Reeves 2003). Further, during interval training sessions at 1,800 metres with well-trained runners, circulating noradrenaline and adrenaline were elevated more than during low-altitude training sessions, despite reducing running velocities by five per cent and the training sessions eliciting similar blood lactate responses (Niess *et al.* 2003). Given these additional stress responses and the widely acknowledged immune depression of exercise performed at sea level, we might expect a greater degree of immune suppression when exercise and training are performed at high altitude.

There are few tightly controlled studies that have assessed immune function responses to acute exercise and hypoxia stress (Table 7.2). In the most comprehensive examination, Wang and colleagues have shown that significant alterations in immune function tend to only occur when exercise is completed in severe hypoxia (12% inspired oxygen concentration, around 4,000 metres), when arterial hypoxaemia and catecholamines are greatest. As few immune alterations were noted at moderate hypoxia (15% inspired oxygen concentration, around 2,700 metres), this study suggests that immune function during exercise will only be altered above a particular hypoxic threshold. Compared with exercise at sea level, these studies suggest exercise under severe hypoxia is associated with increases in neutrophil function (i.e. phagocytic activity and oxidative burst; Wang and Chiu 2009), NK cell number and effector function potential (e.g. cytotoxic protein levels; Wang and Wu 2009) but unchanged NKCA (Wang and Wu 2009). Similar to studies of mountaineers and athletes training at altitude, Wang and colleagues also showed that lymphocyte function was impaired (decreased proliferation and increased apoptosis; Wang and Lin 2010). A notable feature of Wang and colleagues' study design is that participants completed the same absolute exercise workload, 30 minutes at 100 W, at sea level and in hypoxia and, therefore, it is presently unclear whether the immune modulation reported is an effect of hypoxia *per se* or because the same absolute workload completed at altitude requires a greater relative oxygen uptake than at sea level. Further studies are needed to demonstrate the effect of more realistic exercise workload and duration that are typically performed by athletes, trekkers, mountaineers and workers at altitude. This issue of exercise duration is key as one of the only studies to examine more prolonged exercise has shown that three to four hours of mountaineering from 1,780 to 3,198 metres suppressed neutrophil activation, a finding that was absent during ascent without exercise (Chouker *et al.* 2005). Chouker *et al.* (2005) speculated that downregulation of neutrophil function whilst climbing to high altitude may serve to limit exercise-induced inflammatory tissue damage which might otherwise be exacerbated by cytotoxic neutrophils. It remains unclear whether downregulation of neutrophil function whilst exercising at high altitude might alter host defence and risk of URTI. Furthermore, because athletes, trekkers and mountaineers typically select lower workloads with increasing altitude, future research where relative exercise intensities are comparable in normoxic and hypoxic environments is warranted to further understand the effects of hypoxia on the immune response to exercise.

In summary, high-altitude exposure has no negative effect on humoral immunity but has been shown to consistently suppress T cell-mediated immunity, which might at least partly account for the increased infection observed in those who travel to altitude.

AIR POLLUTION, EXERCISE AND IMMUNE FUNCTION

Pollution comes mainly from the burning of fossil fuels, which is why poor air quality is a characteristic of many cities that include former Olympic and World Cup hosts, including Los Angeles, Mexico City, Athens and Beijing (Florida-James *et al.* 2004). Air pollution is not, however, restricted to cities, as pollution can be blown into rural areas (Harrison 2006). The main air pollutants shown in well-controlled laboratory studies to reduce exercise capacity are carbon monoxide and ozone (Raven *et al.* 1974; Horvath *et al.* 1975; Schelegle and Adams 1986). In one dose-response study, ozone concentrations of 0, 120, 180 and 240 $\mu g/m^3$ caused 0%, 10%, 50% and 70% of participants to fail to complete a one-hour time trial (Schelegle and Adams 1986). Ozone levels exceeding even the upper dose in this study have been recorded on a frequent basis in many industrialised cities (Sivertsen 2006). Equally shocking is research that suggests that 30 minutes of jogging in a big city (New York) has been shown to raise circulating carboxyhaemoglobin concentration to a level associated with reduced exercise performance and similar to that found in a heavy smoker (Nicholson and Case 1983). Compared with a sedentary person, an athlete is more likely to suffer from the detrimental effects of air pollution, because greater breathing increases exposure to pollutants. During exercise, the exponential increase in ventilation causes a switch from predominantly nasal to predominantly mouth breathing, which means less pollutant is filtered by the nasal mucocilia and more pollutant travels deeper into the respiratory tract (Carlisle and Sharp 2001).

Air pollution and upper respiratory symptoms

Exercise performed in poor air quality is well established to increase URTI symptoms (e.g. cough and sore throat; Schelegle and Adams 1986; Brunekreef *et al.* 1994). Clearly, in well-controlled laboratory studies, it is easy to attribute these symptoms to inflammation and airway hyper-responsiveness that is caused by many pollutants (e.g. ozone, sulphur dioxide, nitrogen oxides and particulate matter). In practice, when an athlete presents with URTI symptoms, it is therefore important to consider the possible role of pollution in causing upper-respiratory symptoms. Interestingly, the immune system has a role to play irrespective of whether these URTI symptoms relate to infection or air pollution. The upper airways and lungs are very important in protecting us from illness and infection because the mouth and nose offer relatively easy access to our bodies for foreign material and pathogens. By virtue of the continuous exposure caused by breathing, which is increased during exercise and exacerbated further still at high altitude, they are also uniquely vulnerable to attack from these foreign materials. The important defence mechanisms include: (1) primary innate immune defence mechanisms such as the epithelial barrier, mucous secretions and mucociliary clearance that act as a physical barrier and contain neutralising agents (e.g. SIgA, lysozyme) that prevent inward passage of harmful foreign bodies and (2) secondary active immune components located in the epithelium, airway and alveoli include both innate and acquired immune cells (e.g. macrophages, neutrophils and lymphocytes; see Chapter 2 to learn more about these individual cell functions). These immune defences act in concert to neutralise and eradicate foreign matter (e.g. pollutants, bacteria, tumour cells) to the benefit of the host. Nonetheless, they are also implicated in debilitating airway hyper-responsiveness, inflammation and asthma (Holgate *et al.* 2009). Air pollution (e.g. ozone) and cold, dry air have been shown to damage these defences (Giesbrecht 1995; Al Hegelan *et al.* 2011), which help to explain, at least in part, why individuals exercising in extreme environments report increased upper-respiratory symptoms and infections.

Air pollution, exercise and immune function

Pollutants negatively affect the cardiorespiratory system and increase subjective sensations of effort, which likely reduce exercise capacity. Carbon monoxide reduces oxygen-carrying capacity because it competes with oxygen to bind with haemoglobin to form carboxyhaemoglobin. This consequently decreases $\dot{V}O_2$ max and exercise capacity (Raven *et al.* 1974; Horvath *et al.* 1975). High ozone has also been shown to reduce $\dot{V}O_2$ max (Brunekreef *et al.* 1994). As at altitude, any reduction in $\dot{V}O_2$ max will increase physiological stress for the same absolute workload and therefore it is tempting to speculate that immune function might be depressed in those that exercise in polluted air environments. However, as sensations of effort are higher during exercise in a polluted air environment, it is also plausible that exercise will be curtailed earlier or completed at a lower exercise intensity; as such, the immune response to exercise in a polluted air environment compared with a clean-air environment might be more similar than dissimilar.

Few studies have assessed the effect of air pollution on the immune response to exercise. Those that have suggest that even short-duration exercise (12–20 minutes) in polluted air (particulate matter and carbon monoxide) causes a greater increase in circulating leukocytes, specifically neutrophils (Jacobs *et al.* 2010; Kargarfard *et al.* 2011). A limitation of these studies is that immune measurements on blood samples are dissociated from the upper airways and lungs where the pollutants first meet the immune system. The leukocytosis indicates an increase in leukocyte trafficking that is most likely because neutrophils move toward the airways after exposure to pollutants (Seltzer *et al.* 1986; Vieira *et al.* 2012). Increases in neutrophils and other inflammatory factors (e.g. IL-6, IL-8 and prostaglandins) have been reported in bronchial lavage fluid and sputum following intermittent exercise in ozone levels that exceed air quality recommendations (Devlin *et al.* 1991, 1996; Hazucha *et al.* 1996; Holz *et al.* 1999). Ozone is suggested to cause inflammation from chemical reaction with the epithelial lining that generates free radicals and oxidative stress (Florida-James *et al.* 2004). Although the increased inflammation is part of an important process to clear foreign matter from the airways, it is also implicated in epithelial injury and increased permeability that may lead to future infection (Gomes *et al.* 2011). Limited studies have examined the effect of air pollution on immune function of regular exercisers. One longitudinal study in overweight women reported no alterations in lymphocyte proliferation but a decrease in NK cell cytotoxicity in those that regularly exercised within 150 metres of a major road (Williams *et al.* 2009). As it was detected at rest, the reduction in NK cell function is particularly striking and is suggestive of a chronic maladaptation. The effect of these changes on URTI incidence is unknown. This should be investigated in future studies that aim to better understand the effect of air pollution on immune function. In summary, the effect of air pollution on immune function during exercise is poorly understood.

SPACEFLIGHT, IMMUNE FUNCTION AND INFECTION: THE FINAL FRONTIER

Over the last 50 years, advancements in engineering have allowed humans to explore beyond the Earth's boundaries into the final frontier, space. The principal goal of space travel is planetary exploration with both the European Space Agency and the National Aeronautics and Space Administration having plans to send humans to the surface of Mars by 2040. Although robots are often used for space exploration, they have been shown in previous space missions to have limitations compared with humans (White and Averner 2001; Gueguinou *et al.* 2009). It is therefore likely that humans will be required for future planetary exploration. Unfortunately for the astronaut, space travel combines all the stressors of other extreme environments (extremes of temperature, changes in pressure, sleep deprivation, impaired nutrition and psychological stress), as well as some additional unique stressors that include hypergravity during take-off, and microgravity (weightlessness), confinement and radiation during space flight. The next section examines the effect of space travel on infection and immune function.

Space travel and infection

Medical reviews of both astronauts and cosmonauts have revealed a significant number of bacterial and viral infection episodes, which have included influenza, acute respiratory, conjunctivitis and dental infections (Hawkins and Ziegelschmid 1975). Indeed, 52% of crew members in early Apollo missions developed viral or bacterial infections during or one week after space flights (Hawkins and Ziegelschmid 1975). Living in close proximity to other crew greatly increases the likelihood of cross-transmission of infection and, without facilities to isolate crew members, a single infection may jeopardise the health and safety of an entire crew, as well as the success of any mission. Increased infection incidence during and immediately after space flight might be related to increased virulence of pathogenic microorganisms within microgravity (Taylor 1974; Nickerson *et al.* 2000; Wilson *et al.* 2007). For example, bacteria have been shown to proliferate more readily in space (Gueguinou *et al.* 2009) and bacteria from space-flight cultures when injected into mice decreased survival time (Wilson *et al.* 2007). An elevation of circulating stress hormones (e.g. catecholamines and cortisol) is, however, also a frequent observation in individuals returning from space and thus, as these hormones are potent modulators of the immune system (Box 7.2), it is possible that depressed immune function is responsible for the noted increase in infection.

Space travel and immune function

It is important to appreciate that the stress of space travel begins before launch day. Astronauts and space-station crew must complete intensive training and testing before flights and increases in plasma cortisol concentration have been reported two and ten days before launch (Stowe *et al.* 2000, 2011). Additionally in this period, astronaut neutrophil and monocyte function (phagocytosis and oxidative burst) is also lower than controls (Kaur *et al.* 2004, 2005). In combination, these studies suggest that astronauts and space-station crew may already be at a greater risk of infection before leaving Earth.

Owing to the practical difficulties of performing immune and neuroendocrine tests, very little is understood about immune function during space flight. For example, little is known about the innate immune response during space flight in humans. Despite the small numbers of astronauts and cosmonauts who have been studied, it has consistently been shown that humoral immunity remains intact during space flight, as serum immunoglobulins are typically unaltered (Voss 1984) or increased (Konstantinova *et al.* 1993). In contrast, cell-mediated immunity is suppressed during space flight of short or long duration (4–177 days; Taylor and Janney 1992; Gmunder *et al.* 1994). In these studies, astronaut cell-mediated immunity was assessed before and during space flight by their delayed-type hypersensitivity (DTH) response to an injection of seven common antigens (e.g. tetanus, diphtheria, streptococcus, candida). Whether assessed by the number of positive reactions or the sum of the diameters of all positive sites, the DTH response during space flight was approximately 30% lower than that assessed two months before flight (Figure. 7.7). Studies that have shown reactivation of latent viruses (Epstein-Barr, herpes, cytomegalovirus and varicella-zoster virus) also suggest that cell-mediated immunity is depressed during space flight (Mehta *et al.* 2000; Stowe *et al.* 2001; Pierson *et al.* 2005). Stress hormones measured during space flight suggest that short flights are associated with greater plasma cortisol (Stowe *et al.* 2001) but catecholamines and cortisol are within the normal range during longer flights (Kvetnansky *et al.* 1988). As only two astronauts were studied in each of these investigations, future research is required to substantiate these results and further examine neuroendocrine responses during space flight.

Reported increases in circulating stress hormones (cortisol and catecholamines) during the potentially lethal manoeuvres of re-entry and landing most likely account for the observed leukocytosis upon return to normal gravity (Stowe *et al.* 2003, 2011). The marked rise in circulating leukocyte numbers is most likely attributable

Figure 7.7 Suppressed *in vivo* cell-mediated immunity during space flight. Maximum possible number of reactions is 70 (*N* = 10) (data from Taylor and Janney 1992)

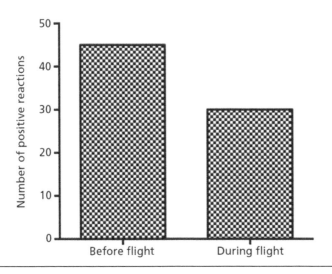

to a noradrenaline-mediated demargination of neutrophil cells (Taylor and Dardano 1983; Taylor *et al.* 1986; Stowe *et al.* 2003). Landing is, however, associated with suppressed phagocytosis and oxidative burst (Kaur *et al.* 2004). Additionally, monocyte number, phagocytosis, oxidative burst and degranulation have also been reported to decrease following space flight (Kaur *et al.* 2005). Additionally, monocytes stimulated by LPS have been shown to produce less IL-6, IL-10 and TNF-α but more IL-1β, which is characteristic of a shift from anti- to proinflammatory state and a shift from Th1 to Th2 (Crucian *et al.* 2011). Reductions in NK cell number and NKCA has also been reported after spaceflight (Konstantinova *et al.* 1993; Stowe *et al.* 2003). In general, cell-mediated immunity has been shown to decline after re-entry into the Earth's atmosphere, with changes including decreased *in vitro* mitogen-stimulated lymphocyte proliferation (IL-2 and IFN-γ production; Taylor and Dardano 1983; Taylor *et al.* 1986; Stowe *et al.* 2003). Similar to during space flight, serum immunoglobulin concentrations after exposure to microgravity have been shown to remain unchanged or increase after landing (Voss 1984; Konstantinova *et al.* 1993; Stowe *et al.* 2003).

In summary, space flight, including before launch, during flight and on return to Earth is associated with alterations in immune function that may increase susceptibility to infection. These immune alterations, alongside the increased microorganism virulence in microgravity, present considerable, as yet unresolved, challenges for future space travel to other planets.

KEY POINTS

- Since circulating stress hormones (e.g. cortisol and adrenaline) are known to be at least partly responsible for the immunosuppressive effects of exercise, larger increases in stress hormones after exercise in unfavourable conditions most likely accounts for the immune alterations compared with exercise in more favourable conditions.
- Passive heat stress that results in a core temperature greater than 39°C is associated with an increase in circulating total leukocyte and differential leukocyte number.
- An increase in *in vitro* or *in vivo* temperature of around 2°C is widely acknowledged to enhance neutrophil, lymphocyte and NK cell function.
- In comparison with prolonged exercise in thermoneutral conditions, prolonged exercise in hot conditions that evokes a larger increment in core temperature (greater than 1°C compared with thermoneutral conditions) is associated with larger numbers of circulating leukocytes during recovery.
- Studies that have clamped the rise in core temperature during exercise show that as much as half of the leukocytosis observed with exercise is attributable indirectly to the rise in core temperature through hyperthermia-induced sympathoadrenal activation.
- With the exception of PHA-stimulated lymphocyte proliferation, which decreased to a greater extent after prolonged exercise in the heat, studies show a limited

effect of prolonged exercise in the heat on neutrophil function, NKCA and salivary immunity.

- Hypothermia (core temperature less than 35°C) may lead to suppressed immune function and increase URTI incidence.
- Studies to date suggest that exercising in the cold does not depress immune function more so than exercising in thermoneutral conditions most probably because exercise prevents core cooling.
- Exposure to high altitude has been shown to increase URTI symptoms and decrease cell-mediated immunity but has a limited effect on other aspects of immunity (neutrophil and NK cell function, humoral and mucosal immunity).
- The effect of air pollution on immune function during exercise is presently unclear.
- Re-entry to normal gravity environment after microgravity exposure is associated with a leukocytosis, suppressed cell-mediated immunity and limited alterations in humoral immunity. Less is known about the effects of prolonged space flight on immune function but limited research also suggests cell-mediated immune function is impaired, which may explain the increased URTI incidence reported during and after space flight.

FURTHER READING

ACSM Position Stand (2006) Prevention of cold injuries during exercise. *Medicine and Science in Sports and Exercise* 38: 2012–29.

Armstrong, L. E. (2000) *Performing in Extreme Environments*. Champaign IL: Human Kinetics, chapters 2–6.

Gueguinou, N., Huin-Schohn, C., Bascove, M., Bueb, J. L., Tschirhart, E., Legrand-Frossi, C. and Frippiat, J. P. (2009) Could spaceflight-associated immune system weakening preclude the expansion of human presence beyond Earth's orbit? *Journal of Leukocyte Biology* 86: 1027–38.

Mazzeo, R. S. (2005) Altitude, exercise and immune function. *Exercise Immunology Review* 11: 6–16.

Walsh, N. P., Gleeson, M., Pyne, D. B., Nieman, D. C., Dhabhar, F. S., Shephard, R. J., Oliver, S. J., Bermon, S. and Kajeniene, A. (2011) Position statement. Part two: Maintaining immune health. *Exercise Immunology Review* 17: 64–103. [Information on pages 82–7 relates specifically to environmental extremes and the immune response to exercise.]

8 Immune responses to intensified periods of training

Michael Gleeson

LEARNING OBJECTIVES

After studying this chapter, you should be able to:

- summarise the effects of chronic exercise training on immune function;
- describe changes in innate, mucosal and acquired immune function that occur in response to short periods of intensified training in athletes;
- discuss associations between impaired immune function in athletes and increased incidence of infectious illness;
- describe the effects of overtraining syndrome on immune function and susceptibility to infection;
- discuss possible immune markers of impending overtraining.

INTRODUCTION

As discussed in Chapter 1, the relationship between exercise and susceptibility to infection has been modelled in the form of a J-shaped curve, as illustrated in Figure 1.1 (Nieman 1994a) and the relationship between exercise load and immune function is modelled as the inverse (mirror image of this curve). This model suggests that, while engaging in moderate activity may enhance immune function above sedentary levels, excessive amounts of prolonged high-intensity exercise induce detrimental effects on immune function. The literature provides strong evidence in support of the latter point (Nieman 1994a; Pyne 1994; Pedersen and Bruunsgaard 1995; Gleeson and Bishop 1999; Gleeson *et al.* 1999a; Mackinnon 1998; Shephard and Shek 1999a), although relatively little evidence is available to suggest that there is any clinically significant difference in immune function between sedentary and moderately active persons.

Retrospective and prospective longitudinal studies have identified that the majority of elite athletes experience symptoms of upper respiratory tract infection (URTI) at a rate similar to the general population (Cox *et al.* 2008; Fricker *et al.* 2000; Pyne and Gleeson 1998). However, the episodes of URTI in elite athletes do not follow the usual seasonal patterns of URTI observed in the general population (Matthews *et al.* 2002) but rather occur during or around competitions (Gleeson *et al.* 2002; Nieman *et al.* 2006; Peters and Bateman 1983; Spence *et al.* 2007; Walsh *et al.* 2011a). Symptoms occur more frequently during the high-intensity training and taper period before competitions in some sports, such as swimmers and kayakers (Fricker *et al.* 1999; Gleeson 2000b; Gleeson *et al.* 2000), while in other endurance sports, such as long distance runners, URTI symptoms appear more frequently after a competition (Cox *et al.* 2010c; Nieman *et al.* 2006; Peters and Bateman 1983). Illness-prone athletes may also be susceptible to URTI symptoms during regular training periods or following increases in training load (Fricker and Pyne 2005). The short-term duration of URTI symptoms (one to three days) reported in most studies suggests that, in most instances, a primary infection is unlikely and the symptoms may be due to viral reactivation (Gleeson *et al.* 2002; Reid *et al.* 2004) or other causes of exercise-induced inflammation.

RECAP OF THE EFFECTS OF EXERCISE TRAINING ON INNATE, MUCOSAL AND ACQUIRED IMMUNE FUNCTION

This section serves as a summary and reminder of the effects of exercise training on innate, mucosal and acquired immune function.

Exercise training effects on innate immune function

Regular exercise training does not appear to appreciably alter blood leukocyte counts, including those of neutrophils (Gleeson and Bishop 2005). However, there are a few reports that exercise training reduces blood neutrophil counts in those with chronic inflammatory conditions or neutrophils in sites of chronic inflammation (Michishita *et al.* 2010), raising the possibility that such exercise acts in an anti-inflammatory fashion in those with elevated inflammation. This effect could be beneficial or deleterious, depending upon the context. While there is little known about the influence of exercise training on neutrophil function, regular exercise, especially heavy, intense training, may attenuate neutrophil respiratory burst (Hack *et al.* 1994; Pyne *et al.* 1995). This could reflect a sustained effect of previous acute exercise, as attenuation of respiratory burst has been documented to last several days post-exercise (Suzuki *et al.* 1999). Both longitudinal exercise training and cross-sectional studies have shown that physically active persons exhibit reduced blood monocyte inflammatory responses to lipopolysaccharide, lower Toll-like receptor (TLR)-4 expression and a lower percentage of CD14+/CD16+ 'inflammatory' monocytes (Gleeson *et al.* 2011a). There are two reports from the same group demonstrating an effect of exercise training on rat dendritic cells. Liao *et al.* (2006) reported that dendritic cell numbers increased after training, with no difference in co-stimulatory molecule (CD80 or CD86) expression, while Chiang *et al.* (2007) found that major histocompatibility complex (MHC) II expression, mixed leukocyte reaction and interleukin

(IL)-12 production were increased in dendritic cells from exercise trained rats. Clearly, given the importance of dendritic cells in early immune regulation, this is an area ripe for further investigation.

Despite much research regarding the effects of exercise training on natural killer (NK) cell numbers and function, there appears to be much controversy regarding its effect. Early cross-sectional studies or interventions with limited subject numbers reported modest increases in NK cell cytolytic activity (NKCA) after moderate exercise training in previously sedentary subjects (McFarlin *et al.*, 2005; Nieman *et al.*, 1990, 1995; Peters *et al.*, 1994; Shephard and Shek, 1999; Woods *et al.*, 1999). In two of the larger trials, one study Fairey *et al.* (2005) found that 15 weeks of moderate exercise training increased NKCA compared with sedentary controls, while another 12-month trial found no change in NKCA in 115 post-menopausal women (Campbell *et al.* 2008). However, periods of very intensive training have been shown to alter NK-cell subsets and to reduce NKCA (Gleeson *et al.* 1995b; Suzui *et al.* 2004; Morgado *et al.* 2012).

Exercise training effects on mucosal immune function

The production of secretory immunoglobulin A (SIgA) is the major effector function of the mucosal immune system providing the 'first line of defence' against pathogens. To date, the majority of exercise studies have assessed salivary SIgA as a marker of mucosal immunity but, more recently, the importance of other antimicrobial proteins in saliva (e.g. α-amylase, lactoferrin and lysozyme) has gained greater recognition. Acute bouts of moderate exercise have little impact on mucosal immunity but prolonged exercise and intensified training can evoke decreases in salivary secretion of SIgA. Mechanisms underlying the alterations in mucosal immunity with acute exercise are probably largely related to the activation of the sympathetic nervous system and its associated effects on salivary protein exocytosis and IgA transcytosis. Depressed secretion of SIgA into saliva during periods of intensified training and chronic stress are probably linked to altered activity of the hypothalamic-pituitary-adrenal axis with inhibitory effects on IgA synthesis and/or transcytosis. Several studies support the hypothesis that reduced levels of salivary SIgA are associated with increased risk of URTI during heavy training. While study populations vary, the association of an increased risk of URTI with lower concentrations of salivary IgA and secretion rates has been consistent for high-performance endurance athletes undertaking intensive training regimens (Fahlman and Engels 2005; Gleeson *et al.* 1999a, 1999b, 2000b, 2002; Libicz *et al.* 2006; Neville *et al.* 2008; Nieman and Nelson-Cannarella 1992, 2002a, 2006; Pyne *et al.* 2000; Whitham *et al.* 2006). Similarly, the increases in salivary SIgA observed after moderate exercise training may contribute to the reduced susceptibility to URTI associated with regular moderate exercise (Akimoto *et al.* 2003; Klentrou *et al.* 2002).

A high incidence of infections is reported in individuals with selective deficiency of SIgA (Hanson *et al.* 1983) or very low saliva flow rates (Fox *et al.* 1985). Moreover, high levels of salivary SIgA are associated with low incidence of URTI (Rossen *et al.*

1970) and low levels of salivary SIgA in athletes (Fahlman and Engels 2005; Gleeson *et al.* 1999a, 2012b) or substantial transient falls in salivary SIgA (Neville *et al.* 2008) are associated with increased risk of URTI.

Levels of salivary SIgA vary widely between individuals and, although some early studies indicated that salivary SIgA concentrations are lower in endurance athletes compared with sedentary individuals (Tomasi *et al.* 1982), the majority of studies indicate that they are generally not different in athletes compared with non-athletes except when athletes are engaged in heavy training (Bishop and Gleeson 2009; Francis *et al.* 2005; Gleeson and Pyne 2000).

Exercise training effects on acquired immune function

In the true resting state (i.e. more than 24 hours after their last training session) circulating lymphocyte numbers and functions appear to be broadly similar in athletes compared with non-athletes (Nieman 2000). Longitudinal studies in which previously sedentary people undertake weeks or months of exercise training have failed to show any marked changes in T and B cell functions provided that blood samples are taken at least 24 hours after their last exercise bout. In contrast, T and B cell functions appear to be sensitive to increases in training load in well-trained athletes undertaking a period of intensified training, with decreases in circulating numbers of type-1 T cells, reduced T-cell proliferative responses and falls in stimulated B cell immunoglobulin synthesis reported (Baj *et al.* 1994; Lancaster *et al.* 2004; Verde *et al.* 1992). This suggests that athletes engaging in longer periods of intensified training can exhibit decreases in T-cell functionality. The cause of this depression in acquired immunity appears to be related to elevated circulating stress hormones, particularly cortisol, and alterations in the pro/anti-inflammatory cytokine balance in response to exercise. This appears to result in a temporary inhibition of type-1 T-cell cytokine production with a relative dampening of the type-1 (cell-mediated) response.

EFFECTS OF INTENSIFIED PERIODS OF EXERCISE TRAINING ON IMMUNE FUNCTION

The effects of intensified exercise training on immune function have been investigated in several athlete groups using relatively short-term (typically one to three weeks) longitudinal studies. There are a few longitudinal studies that have monitored immune function in athletes over the course of a competitive season lasting typically 4–10 months. There are also a handful of small cross-sectional studies that have compared immune function in athletes diagnosed as 'over-trained' with healthy athletes, as well as a few larger-scale studies that have compared 'illness-prone' with more healthy athletes.

Athletes commonly intensify their training for a few days or weeks at certain stages of the season. This may induce a state of overreaching, in which performance is temporarily reduced, but following a period of taper with only light training, results in super-compensation and an increase in performance. Several studies in recent years have investigated the effects of short periods of intensified training on resting immune function and on immunoendocrine responses to endurance exercise. These studies indicate that several indices of leukocyte function, including neutrophil and monocyte oxidative burst, T-lymphocyte CD4+/CD8+ ratios, mitogen-stimulated lymphocyte proliferation and antibody synthesis and NKCA are sensitive to increases in the training load in already well-trained athletes (Gleeson *et al.* 1995b; Lancaster *et al.* 2003, 2004; Robson *et al.* 1999b; Verde *et al.*, 1992). Even following relatively short periods (one to three weeks) of intensified training, marked reductions in neutrophil function, lymphocyte proliferation, SIgA and the circulating number of T-cells producing interferon-γ (IFN-γ) have been observed (Gleeson 2000b; Lancaster *et al.* 2003, 2004). For example, a two-week period of intensified training in already well-trained triathletes was associated with a 20% fall in the lipopolysac-charide-stimulated neutrophil degranulation response (Robson *et al.* 1999a; Table 8.1) and after only one week of intensified training in well-trained cyclists substantial falls in both neutrophil oxidative burst activity and lymphocyte proliferation responses were observed (Lancaster *et al.* 2003). Thus, with sustained periods of heavy training, several aspects of both innate and adaptive immunity are depressed but athletes are not clinically immune deficient. In other words, exercise-induced immune dysfunction does not put athletes in danger of serious illness but it could be sufficient to increase the risk of picking up common infections such as URTI or influenza should the dreaded outbreak occur.

Table 8.1 Effects of an acute increase in the training load on some immune variables in elite athletes

VARIABLE	TRAINING	
	NORMAL	INTENSIFIED
A		
Saliva IgA (mg/L)	115 ± 21	104 ± 25
Total leukocyte count ($\times 10^9$/L)	4.6 ± 0.2	5.1 ± 0.2
Neutrophil count ($\times 10^9$/L)	2.3 ± 0.2	2.7 ± 0.2
Neutrophil degranulation (fg/cell)[a]	166 ± 13	111 ± 7[b]
B		
T-cell CD4+/CD8+ ratio	2.91 ± 0.71	2.05 ± 0.32[b]
Mitogen-induced IgG synthesis (mg/L)	644 ± 207	537 ± 130[b]
Mitogen-induced IgM synthesis (mg/L)	730 ± 190	585 ± 445[b]

Notes:
A = Training was intensified over a 2-week period by the imposition of additional interval training sessions on top of the normal endurance training of eight male triathletes; data are mean ± SEM (data from Robson *et al.* 1998).
B = Weekly training distance was increased by 35% above the normal training for 3 weeks in ten male distance runners; data are mean (SEM) (data from Verde *et al.* 1992).
CD = clusters of differentiation; Ig = immunoglobulin.
[a] elastase release in response to stimulation with bacterial lipopolysaccharide.
[b] $P < 0.05$: significant effect of additional training.

Several longitudinal studies have monitored mucosal immune function in high-level athletes such as cyclists (Baj *et al.* 1994), swimmers (Gleeson 2000b; Gleeson *et al.* 1995b) and footballers (Bury *et al.* 1998; Fahlman and Engels 2005; Rebelo *et al.* 1998) over the course of a competitive season. In a study of American football players, the incidence of URTI was increased during intense training (Figure 8.1) and this was associated with falls in SIgA concentration and secretion rate. In that study, it was reported that the secretion rate of SIgA (which represents the amount

Figure 8.1 Incidence of upper respiratory tract infection (URTI) (A) and secretory immunoglobulin A (SIgA) concentrations (B) among male college American footballers ($N = 75$) and recreationally active male controls ($N = 25$) over a season of training and competition. The most intensive training and competition periods were in autumn (periods 2 and 3) and spring (periods 6 and 7)

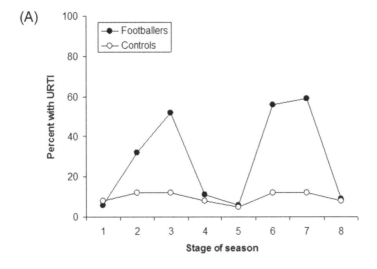

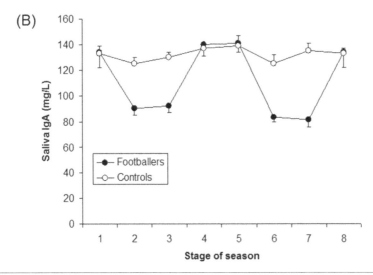

of SIgA available on the mucosal surfaces for protection against pathogens) was significantly and inversely related to URTI incidence (Fahlman and Engels 2005). In an earlier and much-cited study, the impact of long-term training on systemic and mucosal immunity was assessed prospectively in a cohort of elite Australian swimmers over a seven-month training season in preparation for the national championships (Gleeson *et al.* 1995b, 1999a). The results indicated significant depression of resting serum and salivary immunoglobulin concentrations in athletes, associated with long-term training at an intensive level. Furthermore, resting SIgA concentrations at the start of the training period showed significant correlations with infection rates (Figure 8.2) and the number of infections observed in the swimmers was predicted by the pre-season and mean pre-training SIgA levels (Figure 8.3). Among the markers of systemic immunity that were also measured, there were no significant changes in numbers or percentages of B- or T-cell subsets but there was a significant fall in NK cell numbers and percentages in the swimmers over the training season.

Figure 8.2 The relationship between resting salivary secretory immunoglobulin A (SIgA) concentration and incidence of infection among 26 elite swimmers during a 7-month training season. Resting SIgA fell during the 7-month training period on average by 4.1% per month of training and infection incidence was more frequent towards the end of the training period (data from Gleeson *et al.* 1995)

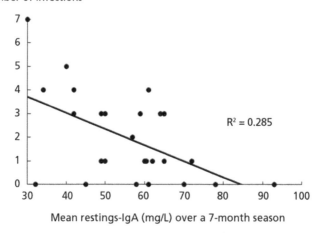

Number of infections

$R^2 = 0.285$

Mean restings-IgA (mg/L) over a 7-month season

Another study monitored elite yachtsmen over 50 weeks of training and competition and reported an inverse (i.e. negative) association between SIgA levels and training load as well as a significant inverse association between SIgA levels and URTI incidence (Neville *et al.* 2008). Furthermore, retrospective analysis of infection episodes and SIgA levels indicated that, before URTI episodes, SIgA levels fell in the preceding two to three weeks (see Figure 6.5).

These studies on mucosal immunity in athletes are representative of a very small number of studies that have established a relationship between some surrogate

Figure 8.3 Swimmers with resting salivary secretory immunoglobulin A (SIgA) concentrations below 30 mg/L had a higher incidence of upper respiratory tract infection (URTI; 4–7 episodes) than swimmers with higher secretory immunoglobulin A (SIgA) levels (0–3 episodes) during a 7-month training season (from Gleeson 2000)

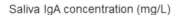
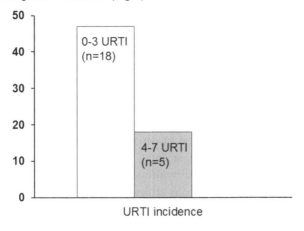

measure of immune function and infection incidence in athletes. A few studies of soldiers during intensive periods of military training have also reported a negative relationship between SIgA concentration and occurrence of URTI (Carins and Booth 2002, although others have not (Gomez-Merino et al. 2005; Tiollier et al. 2005a). SIgA was evaluated as a marker of the severity of stress during a 19-day Royal Australian Air Force survival course, during which the 29 participants experienced hunger, thirst, boredom, loneliness and extreme heat and cold, combined with demanding physical effort (Carins and Booth 2002). Dietary restriction, consumption of alcohol, body mass loss, occurrence of URTI and negative emotions were negatively associated with SIgA or the ratio of SIgA to albumin and the authors concluded that this ratio is a useful marker of the severity of stresses encountered during stressful training. Another study examined the impact of a three-week period of military training followed by an intensive five-day combat course in 21 French commandos on SIgA levels and incidence of URTI (Tiollier et al. 2005a). Saliva samples were collected at 8 a.m. before entry into the commando training, the morning following the three-week training period, after the five-day combat course and after one week of recovery. After the three-week training period, the SIgA concentration was not changed, although it was reduced by around 40% after the five-day course and returned to pre-training levels within a week of recovery. The incidence of URTI increased during the trial but was not related to SIgA. Among the 30 episodes of URTI reported, there were 12 rhinopharyngitis, six bronchitis, five tonsillitis, four sinusitis and three otitis. This study indicates that sustained stressful situations have an adverse effect on mucosal immunity and incidence of URTI, although a causal relationship between the two could not be established. However, in these military personnel studies, the training often involves not only strenuous physical activity but also dietary energy deficiency, sleep deprivation and psychological challenges. These multiple stressors are likely to induce a pattern of immunoendocrine responses that amplify the exercise-induced alterations.

In a study on competitive cyclists, the total number of leukocytes, T-lymphocyte subsets, mitogen-induced lymphocyte proliferation and IL-2 production, adherence capacity and oxidative burst activity of neutrophils were measured at rest at the beginning of a training season and after six months of intensive training and a racing season, cycling approximately 500 km a week (Baj *et al.* 1994). Baseline values of the tested immune parameters were within the range observed in non-trained healthy controls. At the end of the season, significant decreases in absolute numbers of CD3+ and CD4+ cells, diminished IL-2 production and reduced fMLP- and PMA-stimulated oxidative burst activity of neutrophils were noted. Surprisingly, a marked increase in lymphocyte proliferation induced by phytohaemagglutinin and anti-CD3 were also observed at rest after the training season.

In a study of 18 national level swimmers and 11 healthy non-athlete volunteers, blood samples were collected from athletes after 36 hours of resting recovery from exercise at four times during the training season and at similar times from the non-athlete controls (Morgado *et al.* 2012). The samples were incubated in the presence or the absence of LPS and IFN-γ and the frequency of cytokine producing neutrophils, monocytes and dendritic cells and the amount of each cytokine produced per cell were evaluated by flow cytometry. In addition, plasma cortisol levels were measured and upper respiratory symptoms recorded through daily logs. In the athletes, but not in the controls, a decrease in the number of monocytes, neutrophils and dendritic cell subsets and in the amount of IL-1β, IL-6, IL-12, TNF-α and MIP-1β produced by these cells in response to stimulation, was observed over the training season. The differences were most noticeable between the first (baseline values) and second blood collections, corresponding to the initial elevation of training volume. In the athletes, the plasma levels of cortisol partially correlated with training intensity and could, at least in part, explain the reduced response of cells to stimulation *in vitro*. The results from this study support the idea that long-term intensive training may affect the function of innate and antigen-presenting immune cells, reducing their capacity to respond to acute challenges, possibly contributing to an elevated risk of URTI.

There are only a few studies that have examined immunological changes in professional football players before, during and after a full season. Bury *et al.* (1998) reported that a competitive season in 15 Belgian professionals did not produce any change in the total number of leukocytes but increased neutrophil counts and decreased CD4+ T-lymphocyte counts. They also reported a slight decrease in T-cell proliferation and a significant decrease in neutrophil function. On the other hand, training and competitions did not induce significant changes in the number of NK cells nor NK cytotoxic activity. Rebelo *et al.* (1998) examined the effect of a soccer season on circulating leukocyte and lymphocyte subpopulations of 13 Portuguese players. At the end of the season, total leukocyte and neutrophil numbers and CD8+ cells were increased compared to pre-season values and the CD4/CD8 ratio was decreased.

Few studies have investigated the effects of intensified training on multiple markers of immune function. However, in one such study (Lancaster *et al.* 2003), seven healthy endurance-trained men completed three trials consisting of cycling exercise at a work rate equivalent to 74% $\dot{V}O_2$ max until volitional fatigue. The trials took place in the morning, before and after a six-day period of intensified training and after two weeks of light recovery training, as illustrated in Figure 8.4. Normal training consisted of around ten hours of cycling per week; during the intensive training phase, training load was increased on average by 73% (Figure 8.5). During recovery

Figure 8.4 Schematic representation of the experimental protocol used by Lancaster *et al.* (2003)

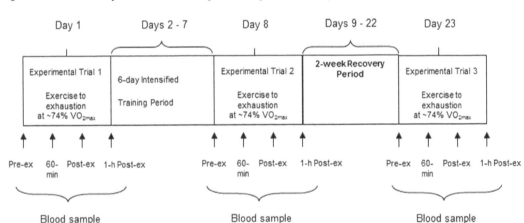

Figure 8.5 The weekly training load (hours : minutes) during the normal, intensified and recovery training periods in the study of Lancaster *et al.* (2003)

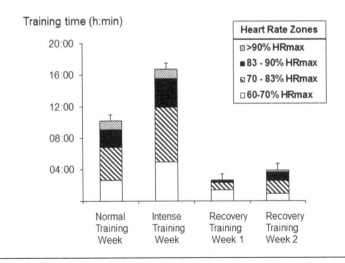

training, exercise was limited to no more than four hours per week for two weeks. Training intensity and duration were confirmed by the use of heart rate monitors. The percentage and number of T-cells producing IFN-γ was lower at rest following the intensified training period compared with normal training (Table 8.2). *Ex vivo* stimulated neutrophil oxidative burst activity (Figure 8.6) and lymphocyte proliferation (Figure 8.7) fell after acute exercise and were markedly depressed at rest after the intensified training period compared with normal training. *Ex vivo* stimulated monocyte oxidative burst activity was unchanged after acute exercise but was lower at rest following the intensified training period compared with normal training (Table 8.2). Following all acute exercise trials, the circulating number of IFN-γ+ T-cells and the amount of IFN-γ produced per cell was decreased (Figure 8.8). The six days of intensified training did not affect resting SIgA concentration but the latter was

Table 8.2 Monocyte oxidative burst activity (mean fluorescence intensity) and numbers of circulating interferon-γ+ (IFN-γ+) T-cells in blood taken at rest during normal, intensified and recovery training periods

| | CLASSIFICATION OF TRAINING PERIOD LOAD | | |
	NORMAL	INTENSIFIED	RECOVERY
Monocyte oxidative burst	178 ± 18	136 ± 24[a]	196 ± 21
IFN-γ+ T-cells ($\times$ 10^9 cells/L)	0.19 ± 0.02	0.12 ± 0.03[a]	0.20 ± 0.03

Note:
[a] $P < 0.05$ versus normal training

Source: data from Lancaster *et al.* (2003)

Figure 8.6 Effect of an exhaustive exercise bout performed during normal training (NT), intensified training (IT) and recovery training (RT) periods on neutrophil oxidative burst activity (mean fluorescence intensity, MFI). Analysis of variants revealed significant main effects of time and treatment (data from Lancaster *et al.* 2003)

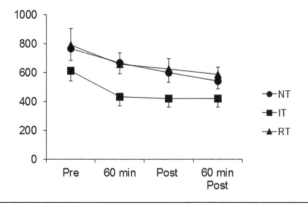

Figure 8.7 Effect of an exhaustive exercise bout performed during normal training (NT), intensified training (IT) and recovery training (RT) periods on mitogen-stimulated lymphocyte proliferation. Analysis of variants revealed significant main effects of time and treatment (data from Lancaster *et al.* 2003)

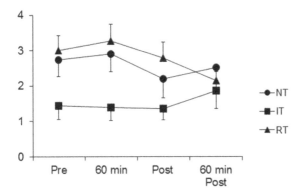

Lymphocyte proliferation (Stimulation Index)

Figure 8.8 Effect of an exhaustive exercise bout performed during normal training (NT), intensified training (IT) and recovery training (RT) periods on stimulated T lymphocyte interferon-γ (INF-γ) production (mean fluorescence intensity, MFI). Analysis of variants revealed significant main effect of time only (lower post-exercise compared with pre-exercise; $P < 0.05$) (data from Lancaster *et al.* 2003)

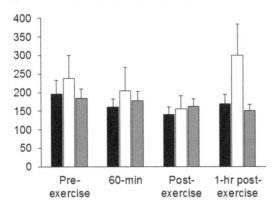

IFN-γ production by T lymphocytes (MFI)

significantly lower at the end of recovery training (SIgA values were 74.2 ± 13.1, 64.6 ± 12.5 and 49.0 ± 10.4 mg/L during normal training, intensified training and recovery training, respectively). Except for SIgA, all measured immune parameters were back to normal after two weeks of recovery training. These results indicate that: (1) acute exhaustive exercise causes a temporary fall in several aspects of immune cell function and a decrease in IFN-γ production by T cells; (2) resting immune function is decreased after only six days of intensified training and these effects are reversible with two weeks of relative rest; (3) in general, the immune response to an acute bout of exhaustive exercise is not affected by the weekly training load.

Although elite athletes are not clinically immune deficient, it is possible that the combined effects of small changes in several immune parameters may compromise resistance to common minor illnesses such as URTI. Protracted immune depression linked with prolonged intensive training may determine susceptibility to infection, particularly at times of major competitions.

COMPARISONS OF ILLNESS-PRONE ATHLETES WITH HEALTHY ATHLETES

Within the general healthy human population, there is a range of immunocompetency, owing to genetic differences, age, gender and lifestyle habits. Clearly, some individuals are more prone to illness than others (this is true for both the sedentary population and the athletic population) but it is not known which particular aspects of immune function (or dysfunction) are responsible for these differences in illness susceptibility. Biomarkers to predict infections could be of significant value among athletes and military personnel. As mentioned previously, several studies have reported associations between decreased SIgA concentration or secretion rate and URTI incidence in athletes (Gleeson *et al.* 1999a; Fahlman and Engels 2005; Neville *et al.* 2008) but these have been based on a relatively small number of subjects. Associations between URTI risk and blood immune parameters have not been extensively examined, though an impaired IFN-γ production in unstimulated whole-blood culture has been reported in fatigued and illness-prone endurance athletes (Clancy *et al.* 2006). However, the relevance of this measure of immune function to infection risk is unclear, as cytokine production in the unstimulated state is very low compared with the response to an infectious agent or antigen challenge.

One study attempted to examine immune factors (including the cytokine response to an antigen challenge) influencing susceptibility to URTI in men and women engaged in endurance-based physical activity during the winter months (Gleeson *et al.* 2012b). Eighty individuals provided resting blood and saliva samples for determination of markers of systemic immunity and each individual kept weekly training and illness logs for the following four months. Thirty of the subjects did not experience an URTI episode and 24 subjects experienced three or more weeks of URTI symptoms. Retrospective analysis revealed that these illness-prone subjects had higher training loads and had around 2.5-fold higher IL-4 and IL-10 production by multi-antigen-stimulated whole-blood culture than the illness-free subjects (Table 8.3). Illness-prone subjects also had significantly lower salivary SIgA secretion and saliva flow rate than the illness-free subjects. There were no differences in circulating numbers of leukocyte subtypes, lymphocyte subsets or plasma levels of IgA and IgG between the illness-prone and illness-free subjects. The production of IL-10 was positively correlated and the SIgA secretion rate was negatively correlated with the number of weeks with infection symptoms. The authors concluded that high IL-10 production in response to antigen challenge and low SIgA secretion are risk factors

Table 8.3 Differences between illness-prone and illness-free subjects

| | SUBJECTS | | P |
	ILLNESS-PRONE ($n = 24$)	ILLNESS-FREE ($n = 30$)	
URTI (weeks)	4.7 ± 2.2	0.0 ± 0.0	0.001
Training load (h/week)	10.7 ± 4.6	8.4 ± 4.4	0.046
Saliva flow rate (mL/min)	0.35 ± 0.19	0.53 ± 0.24	0.004
SIgA concentration (mg/L)	145 ± 79	155 ± 95	0.835
SIgA secretion rate (μg/min)	49 ± 36	80 ± 53	0.019
Plasma IgA (g/L)	1.38 ± 0.51	1.64 ± 0.80	0.183
Plasma IgG (g/L)	10.75 ± 1.83	11.31 ± 2.59	0.378
Leukocyte count ($\times\ 10^9$/L)	5.72 ± 1.88	5.78 ± 1.19	0.890
Neutrophil count ($\times\ 10^9$/L)	3.00 ± 1.46	2.94 ± 0.98	0.844
Monocyte count ($\times\ 10^9$/L)	0.48 ± 0.21	0.49 ± 0.13	0.831
Lymphocyte count ($\times\ 10^9$/L)	1.96 ± 0.56	2.13 ± 0.59	0.300
T cell count ($\times\ 10^9$/L)	1.21 ± 0.45	1.26 ± 0.42	0.688
B cell count ($\times\ 10^9$/L)	0.19 ± 0.08	0.23 ± 0.14	0.184
NK cell count ($\times\ 10^9$/L)	0.22 ± 0.11	0.25 ± 0.15	0.415
IL-1β production (pg/ml)	8.2 ± 7.1	8.5 ± 10.9	0.683
IL-2 production (pg/ml)	189 ± 258	76 ± 102	0.064
IL-4 production (pg/ml)	6.2 ± 9.6	2.3 ± 1.2	0.018
IL-6 production (pg/ml)	188 ± 137	126 ± 128	0.094
IL-8 production (pg/ml)	1119 ± 705	927 ± 717	0.264
IL-10 production (pg/ml)	6.8 ± 7.7	2.4 ± 2.5	0.008
IFN-γ production (pg/ml)	40 ± 62	26 ± 71	0.060
TNF-α production (pg/ml)	28 ± 32	26 ± 55	0.166

Note. Values are expressed as mean (± SD); cytokine levels are those observed after 24 hours *in vitro* incubation of whole blood with a multi-antigen vaccine

Source: data from Gleeson *et al.* (2012)

for development of URTI in physically active individuals. The significance of IL-10 may be its anti-inflammatory and immunosuppressive effects. Individuals that produce relatively large amounts of IL-10 during the early stages of an infection may not mount a sufficiently robust immune response to counter the pathogen and, consequently, may be more prone to developing the symptoms of infection. The results of this study also indicated that saliva flow rate is also an important factor in URTI risk. This might reflect the importance of other antimicrobial proteins in saliva, such as amylase, defensins, lysozyme and lactoferrin (West *et al.* 2009) in addition to SIgA. The multiple of the saliva flow rate and the saliva concentration of these antimicrobial proteins determines their secretion rates into the oral cavity.

A few other small-scale studies have attempted to determine if cytokine responses to exercise differ between healthy and illness-prone distance runners. One such study by Cox *et al.* (2007) classified runners as healthy (no more than two episodes of upper-respiratory symptoms per year; N = 10) or illness-prone (four or more episodes per year; N = 8) and reported that the resting plasma IL-8, IL-10 and IL-1ra concentrations were 19–38% lower in illness-prone runners. After a standardised bout of treadmill running, post-exercise plasma IL-10 and IL-1ra concentrations were 10–20% lower, whereas IL-6 elevations were 84–185% higher in illness-prone subjects, suggesting that cytokine responses to exercise differ between healthy and illness-prone athletes. This might reflect impaired inflammatory regulation in the hours after exercise that may account for the greater frequency of upper-respiratory symptoms experienced. Such differences in cytokine production in response to exercise or infection may be, at least in part, due to differences in cytokine gene polymorphisms (Cox *et al.* 2010a) but more work is needed to establish whether this is an important factor influencing illness risk among athletes or other populations.

EFFECTS OF OVERTRAINING ON IMMUNITY

As athletes strive to produce improved performances, they are under pressure to increase their training load; this is epitomised by the Olympic motto '*citius, altius, fortius*' (faster, higher, stronger). Paradoxically, there is much anecdotal evidence cited in the literature that links excessive exercise with a chronic decrease in athletic performance. This is highlighted by elite athletes failing to improve on the previous year's performances, despite undergoing ever more intensive training programmes, or athletes reporting an inability to regain previous form following a tough competition.

An athlete must undergo significant stress during training to provide sufficient stimulus for physiological adaptation and the subsequent improvement in performance. To ensure that the athlete adapts favourably to the training load, imposed adequate rest is a crucial part of any training programme. If rest is not sufficient and the exercise stress alone or combined with other stressors (physical, nutritional, environmental or psychological) is too great, the athlete may fail to adapt (maladapt) and become overreached. If insufficient rest continues when overreached and the athlete is exposed to further stressors, then a state of chronic fatigue, non-recovery and, in some instances, immunodepression may occur; this is classified as overtraining syndrome (OTS). For an up-to-date review on the diagnosis, treatment and prevention of OTS see Meeusen *et al.* (2013).

Redefinition of overtraining syndrome

To date, the aetiology of OTS remains elusive but the recent redefinition of the syndrome may help to resolve this conundrum. The term 'overtraining syndrome' is, in fact, a misnomer, since it implies that exercise is the sole causative factor of the syndrome, whereas the aetiology of OTS appears to be multifactorial. This has been a major limiting factor in identifying the cause of OTS. Therefore, the syndrome has been redefined as unexplained underperformance syndrome (UPS; Budgett *et al.* 2000); hence, for the purposes of clarity, the syndrome will be referred to as UPS for much of this chapter.

Unexplained UPS has been defined as a persistent decrement in athletic performance capacity despite two weeks of relative rest, which is acknowledged by both the coach and the athlete (Budgett *et al.* 2000). UPS should not be confused with overreaching, which causes a temporary deterioration in performance but, with sufficient rest and recovery, the overreached athlete recovers fully and, in many instances, their athletic performance is improved.

Symptoms of unexplained UPS

The most prominent symptom of UPS is general/local fatigue and heightened sense of effort during training. Other commonly reported symptoms include general malaise/flu-like symptoms, sleep and mood disturbances, unexplained or unusually heavy, stiff and/or sore muscles, loss of appetite, gastrointestinal disturbances and slow wound healing.

Anecdotal reports from athletes and coaches of an increased infection rate with UPS have also been supported by several empirical studies. In a cohort study of highly trained athletes before the Olympic Games, over 50% of the athletes who reported symptoms of UPS presented with infection compared with none of the athletes in the overreached group (Kingsbury *et al.* 1998). It appears, therefore, that suppression of immune system function as a consequence of excessive physical and/or psychological stress can clinically manifest as an increased susceptibility to infectious illness. The most commonly reported infection and most acutely disabling for elite athletes is that of the upper respiratory tract.

Hypotheses to explain immunodepression in UPS

There are several possible causes of the diminution of immune function associated with periods of heavy training. Although, at present, there is no encompassing theory to explain the altered immune competence experienced by athletes with UPS, several hypotheses have been proposed.

Glutamine hypothesis

The most frequently cited theory is the glutamine hypothesis of overtraining which was first proposed by Eric Newsholme (Newsholme 1994). Glutamine is an amino acid essential for the optimal functioning of lymphocytes and *in vitro* studies by Newsholme and his colleagues have demonstrated that, in the absence of glutamine, lymphocytes are unable to proliferate (see Box 8.2). Since many athletes with UPS and those undergoing intense exercising training present with low plasma glutamine concentrations (Keast *et al.* 1995, Kingsbury *et al.* 1998; Rowbottom *et al.* 1995), it is hypothesised that the fall in plasma glutamine levels causes lymphocyte function to become depressed, thus rendering the athlete more susceptible to infections. However,

Box 8.2 Dr Eric A. Newsholme, PhD

The late Professor Eric Newsholme read natural science at Cambridge and this was followed by a PhD in biochemistry. In 1964, he moved to Oxford University to work with Sir Hans Krebs: he became a Fellow of Merton College and a Lecturer at the Department of Biochemistry in 1973. Eric was a rare example of a talented researcher who was also an outstanding teacher. He could make even drab topics in biochemistry sound exciting and he had many original ideas and hypotheses that have informed exercise biochemistry and immunology over several decades. More than 50 PhD students and a similar number of postdoctoral scientists received research training in Eric's laboratory. Eric published over 300 research papers and reviews. His textbooks (*Regulation in Metabolism* by Newsholme and Start, 1973, and *Biochemistry for the Medical Sciences* by Newsholme and Leech, 1983) provided many biochemists with much knowledge of intermediary metabolism and metabolic control. Eric recently updated his 1983 textbook to become *Functional Biochemistry in Health and Disease* with Tony Leech (2010).

Eric took up marathon running in his mid-30s and successfully completed around 40 marathons. This gave him a considerable appreciation of energy metabolism in exercise. Work in the late 1970s and early 1980s with a DPhil student, M. S. M. Ardawi, resulted in the discovery (among others) that the amino acid, glutamine, was used as a fuel at a surprisingly high level in resting, unstimulated lymphocytes. *In vitro* work in Eric's laboratory by another student, Mark Parry Billings, demonstrated that, despite the presence of all other essential nutritional components in cell culture medium, only when glutamine was decreased did a decrease in the proliferative ability of lymphocytes occur. Philip Newsholme (Eric's son) and, later, Philip Calder (also students) showed that glutamine was essential for macrophage function.

On becoming aware of a decrease in some key immune cell numbers and functions after prolonged, exhaustive exercise, Eric hypothesised that a lack of glutamine might be responsible. Glutamine is a metabolic fuel for many cells and a nitrogen donor for purine and pyrimidine nucleotide synthesis and, thus, for DNA synthesis. There is an extensive literature on the role of glutamine in clinical situations, to which Eric's group has contributed, showing that burns and major trauma are associated with very low glutamine levels in the blood. Several field studies confirmed that the plasma concentration of glutamine was indeed low (by 20–25%) in endurance runners after an event, as well as in overtrained athletes at rest (Parry-Billings *et al.* 1992). Subsequent studies on more than 150 marathon runners showed that the provision of glutamine within the recovery period reduced self-reported illness (mostly URTI) by around 43% compared with placebo.

The other major aspect of Eric's input into exercise immunology concerns fatty acids and the immune system. This work was carried out largely with his former student, Philip Calder (now a professor at Southampton University). Eric's key contributions almost certainly emanated from his desire to provide quantitative descriptions of complex metabolic pathways and to consider whole-body metabolism, not just the cell or tissue in which the study was conducted. Another principle which he liked to instil in his students was: 'you can never prove or disprove a hypothesis: you can only add to the evidence for or against it'. Bear that in mind when you read this book!

a weakness in this theory concerns the *in vitro* studies. When lymphocytes are cultured with identical glutamine concentrations to the lowest plasma glutamine concentrations reported in athletes following intense exercise or with UPS (300–400 µM), lymphocyte proliferation and lymphokine-activated killing cell activity are identical to when they are cultured in normal resting glutamine levels (600 µM). Furthermore, Kingsbury *et al.* (1998) found no differences in the plasma glutamine concentrations of athletes with UPS, either with or without infections. Although plasma glutamine does not appear to be involved with exercise-induced immunodepression, it may still provide a useful marker of excessive exercise and impending UPS.

Open window theory

An alternative theory is the 'open window' theory, as detailed in previous chapters. The period of post-exercise suppression of some aspects of the immune system has been identified as a potential window of opportunity for infections. This window can remain open for 3–72 hours (although in most cases, 3–24 hours is probably the norm) following exercise, during which an infectious agent may be able to gain a foothold on the host and increase the risk of an opportunistic infection (Pedersen and Ullum 1994). It is feasible that the combination of stressors that lead to the onset of UPS in athletes may cause the post-exercise 'window of vulnerability to infection' to be open for a longer period, consequently rendering the athlete with UPS more susceptible to infection.

Tissue injury or cytokine theory

The most recent theory, which holds much promise, is the 'tissue injury theory' of immunodepression in UPS proposed by Smith (2003, 2004). Over the first decade of the twenty-first century, it has been established that T-helper lymphocytes (Th), an integral part of immune function, comprise two functional subsets, namely Th1 and Th2, which are associated with cell-mediated immunity and humoral immunity, respectively (as described in Chapter 2). When Th-precursor cells are activated, one subset is upregulated in favour of the other subset, such that either the Th1 or the Th2 lymphocytes are activated, depending on the nature of the stimulus. The upregulation of one subset over the other is determined by the predominant circulating cytokine pattern. The tissue injury theory proposes that the exercise-induced immunodepression in UPS is due to excessive tissue trauma (i.e. muscle fibre damage) induced by intense exercise with insufficient rest, which produces a pattern of cytokines that drive the Th2 lymphocyte profile. The upregulation of the Th2 lymphocytes is further augmented by the elevation of circulating glucocorticoids, catecholamines and prostaglandin E_2 following prolonged exercise. The Th2 proliferation results in a suppression of the Th1 lymphocyte profile, thereby suppressing cell-mediated immunity. It has been suggested that this may be an important mechanism in exercise-induced depression of immune cell functions (Northoff *et al.* 1998) and in increasing susceptibility to viral infections (Smith, 2003).

The observed tissue trauma and cytokine pattern following prolonged exercise lends some credence to this hypothesis, although whether this is a causal factor in the incidence of post-exercise infection remains unknown. The theory concludes that the increased incidence of infection in some athletes with UPS is not due to a global immunosuppression but rather to an altered aspect of immune function resulting in a down-regulation of cell-mediated immunity. This theory may provide insight into the increased incidence of viral infections in some athletes with UPS, since cell-mediated immunity predominantly protects against intracellular viral infections. However, this theory cannot account for the bacterial infections of the upper respiratory tract (e.g. streptococcal and staphylococcal infections), which are associated with depression of non-specific immunity and are commonly reported in athletes with UPS.

It is also possible that chronic elevation of stress hormones, particularly glucocorticoids such as cortisol, resulting from repeated bouts of intense exercise with insufficient recovery, could cause temporary immunodepression, even in the absence of tissue trauma. It is known that both acute glucocorticosteroid administration (Moynihan et al. 1998) and exercise cause a temporary inhibition of IFN-γ production by T-lymphocytes and a shift in the Th1/Th2 cytokine profile towards one that favours a Th2 (humoral) response with a relative dampening of the Th1 (cell-mediated) response.

Whilst the theories discussed above describe the possible causes of compromised immune function in UPS, the universal and most debilitating symptom in UPS is the persistent fatigue reported by athletes. This may also be attributable to elevated levels of cytokines in the blood causing 'sickness behaviour'. Cytokines communicate with the central nervous system and induce a set of behaviours referred to as 'sickness behaviour', characterised by mood changes, a disinclination to exercise and fatigue, until the inflammatory response is resolved. This is thought to be a protective mechanism as it dampens the individual's desire to expend energy in times of excessive physical and psychological stress. This theory has received some support from a study that reported elevated levels of cytokines (e.g. IL-6) in the circulation at rest, at the same time as markers of muscle damage were evident in well-trained triathletes undergoing periods of intensified training (Robson-Ansley et al. 2007) and a study that reported positive associations between elevated levels of plasma cytokines and mood disturbance (including increased sensations of fatigue) during intensified periods of training in elite rowers (Main et al. 2010).

The cytokine theory has been further refined into the 'IL-6 hypothesis of UPS' (Robson 2003). This theory proposes that factors aside from exercise-induced tissue trauma trigger a dysregulated inflammatory response in UPS, causing either increased levels of circulating cytokines or an increased sensitivity to cytokines. The theory is primarily focused on the fatigue-inducing properties of the cytokine, IL-6, which increases sensations of fatigue as its circulating concentration rises during prolonged exercise (Robson-Ansley et al. 2004). Studies investigating the effect of IL-6 on resting healthy individuals showed that low doses of recombinant human IL-6 (rhIL-6, a synthesised form of IL-6) induce an increased sensation of fatigue, depressed mood state, as well as elevated heart rate and disrupted sleep pattern, which are strikingly similar symptoms to those reported by athletes with UPS, although the symptoms of IL-6 administration are relatively short-term in healthy individuals compared with the chronic fatigue associated with UPS. The IL-6 link in the association of chronic fatigue with UPS is further advanced by a study that showed a heightened sensitivity to rhIL-6 administration in patients with chronic fatigue syndrome (CFS) compared with normal control subjects (Arnold *et al.* 2002). The CFS group experienced an immediate increase in flu-like symptoms following rhIL-6 administration, whereas the control group did not experience any symptoms until six hours post-administration. Furthermore, the feelings of fatigue and malaise remained up to 24 hours after the rhIL-6 administration in the CFS group. This suggests that an athlete with UPS undergoing physical and/or psychological stress resulting in elevated IL-6 concentrations could experience an exacerbated sensation of fatigue during exercise. Of significant interest is the finding that IL-6 administration in healthy individuals induces temporary symptoms that are akin to those experienced during influenza infection. This may explain why some athletes with UPS complain of flu-like symptoms in the absence of clinically confirmed infection and suggests a cytokine-mediated sickness behaviour.

KEY POINTS

- Resting immune function is not very different in athletes compared with non-athletes.
- Periods of intensified training (overreaching) in already well trained athletes can result in a depression of immunity in the resting state.
- Illness-prone athletes appear to have an altered cytokine response to antigen stimulation and exercise. Having low levels of salivary IgA secretion makes athletes more susceptible to URTI.
- Overtraining is associated with recurrent infections and immunodepression is common but immune functions do not seem to be reliable markers of impending overtraining.
- There are several possible causes of the diminution of immune function associated with periods of heavy training. One mechanism may simply be the cumulative effects of repeated bouts of intense exercise (with or without tissue damage) with the consequent elevation of stress hormones, particularly glucocorticoids such as cortisol, causing temporary inhibition of Th1 cytokines with a relative dampening of the cell-mediated response. When exercise is repeated frequently there may not be sufficient time for the immune system to recover fully.
- The IL-6 hypothesis of UPS postulates that a heightened sensitivity to IL-6 or a dysregulated production of IL-6 during exposure to physical and/or psychological stress are possible mechanisms for the development of UPS in athletes. Furthermore, the absence of clinical confirmation of infection despite the flu-like symptoms reported by some athletes following excessive exercise suggests a cytokine-mediated sickness behaviour response to physical stress.

FURTHER READING

Bishop, N. C. and Gleeson, M. (2009) Acute and chronic effects of exercise on markers of mucosal immunity. *Frontiers in Bioscience* 14: 4444–56.

Fahlman, M. M. and Engels, H. J. (2005) Mucosal IgA and URTI in American college football players: A year longitudinal study. *Medicine and Science in Sports and Exercise* 37: 374–80.

Gleeson, M., McDonald, W. A., Cripps, A. W., Pyne, D. B., Clancy, R. L. and Fricker, P. A. (1995) The effect on immunity of long-term intensive training in elite swimmers. *Clinical and Experimental Immunology* 102: 210–16.

Meeusen, R. , Duclos, M., Foster, C., Fry, A., Gleeson, M., Nieman, D., Raglin, J., Rietjens, G., Steinacker, J. and Urhausen, A. (2013) Prevention, diagnosis and treatment of the Overtraining Syndrome. Joint consensus statement of the European College of Sport Science (ECSS) and the American College of Sports Medicine (ACSM). *European Journal of Sport Science* 13: 1–24.

Morgado, J. M., Rama, L., Matos, A., Silva I., Inacio M. J., Henriques A., Laranjeira, P., Rosado, F., Alves, F., Gleeson, M., Pais, M. L., Paiva, A. and Teixeira, A. M. (2012) Cytokine production by monocytes, neutrophils and dendritic cells is hampered by long term intensive training in elite swimmers. *European Journal of Applied Physiology* 112: 471–82.

Smith, L. L. (2003) Overtraining, excessive exercise, and altered immunity. Is this a T helper-1 versus T helper-2 lymphocyte response? *Sports Medicine* 33: 347–64.

9 Exercise, nutrition and immune function

Neil P. Walsh and Michael Gleeson

LEARNING OBJECTIVES

After studying this chapter, you should be able to:

- describe the mechanisms by which nutrient availability may alter the immune response to heavy exercise and training;
- describe how poor dietary practices during training and competition may be involved in the aetiology of exercise-induced immune depression;
- provide examples of research findings from studies investigating the effects of macronutrient and micronutrient availability on the immune response to heavy exercise and training;
- critically evaluate the evidence that diet and nutritional supplements can modify immune responses and reduce infection incidence, severity and duration during heavy training and competition.

INTRODUCTION

Athletes engaged in heavy training programmes, particularly those involved in endurance events, appear to be more susceptible to upper respiratory tract infections (URTI) as discussed in Chapter 1. Laboratory and field-based investigations have implicated immune depression, particularly in the hour after heavy exercise ('open window hypothesis'), as being at least partly responsible for the increased incidence of URTI in athletes (discussed in Chapters 4–6). It is noteworthy, though, that evidence showing a causal relationship between immune depression and increased incidence of URTI in athletes is currently lacking (Walsh *et al.* 2011b). Many factors are known to influence the immune response to exercise; these include nutrition (discussed in this chapter), environmental conditions (discussed in Chapter 7) and the psychological stress of training and competition (briefly discussed in Chapter 2).

Nutritional deficiencies are widely acknowledged to impair immune function and there exists a large body of evidence showing that the incidence and/or severity of many infections is increased by specific nutritional deficiencies. Insufficient energy, macronutrient and micronutrient intake have all been shown to impair immune function. This chapter firstly highlights the probable mechanisms by which nutrient availability influences the immune response to heavy exercise and training. A summary of the research evidence investigating the effects of the day-to-day training diet and competition diet on immune function and susceptibility to infection follows. Where available, recommendations for macronutrient and micronutrient intake are included to help athletes to counter some of the negative effects of heavy exercise and training on immune function. The remainder of this chapter focuses on the controversial question: do nutritional supplements augment immune function and reduce illness in athletes?

NUTRIENT AVAILABILITY AND IMMUNE FUNCTION: MECHANISMS OF ACTION

Nutrient availability has the potential to affect almost all aspects of the immune system because macronutrients are involved in immune cell metabolism and protein synthesis and micronutrients are involved in immune cell replication and antioxidant defences (Gleeson 2006a). Inadequate nutrient availability is known to cause alterations in immune function including depressed cell-mediated immunity, T-lymphocyte proliferation, complement formation, phagocyte function, humoral and secretory antibody production and altered cytokine production. Deficiencies or excesses of specific nutrients may alter the immune response by 'direct' and/or 'indirect' mechanisms (Figure 9.1). A nutritional deficiency is said to have a 'direct effect' when the nutritional factor being considered has primary activity within the lymphoid system (e.g. as a fuel source) and an 'indirect effect' when the primary activity affects all cellular material or another organ system that acts as an immune regulator. A reduction in the availability of carbohydrate (e.g. decreased blood glucose concentration during prolonged exercise) might decrease immune cell energy metabolism and protein synthesis (e.g. cytokine, antibody and acute phase protein production); this would be described as a 'direct effect' (Figure 9.1). Alternatively, decreased blood glucose availability might have an 'indirect effect' on immune function through its stimulatory effect on the secretion of stress hormones. The immunosuppressive effects of the stress hormones (e.g. cortisol and adrenaline) are widely acknowledged to explain much of the exercise-induced immune depression ('indirect effect'; Figure 9.1) (Walsh et al. 2011b). The duration and severity of a nutrient deficiency also have a potentiating influence on the magnitude of immune impairment; although, even a mild deficiency of a single nutrient can result in an altered immune response (Gleeson 2006a). Studies in animals and humans have shown that adding the deficient nutrient back to the diet can restore immune function and resistance to infection (Calder and Kew 2002). Diets that are excessively high in some nutrients (e.g. omega-3 polyunsaturated fatty acids and zinc) also have the potential to cause detrimental effects on immune function (Bishop et al. 1999). Athletes often consume diets that are excessively high in carbohydrate, to maintain

Figure 9.1 Nutrient availability and immune function: direct and indirect mechanisms. Deficiencies in macro/micronutrients may modify immune responses directly by altering the availability of energy and nutrients required for cell proliferation and protein synthesis and indirectly by influencing circulating levels of stress hormones known to have immunoregulatory effects. Evidence is lacking to show that inadequate nutrition and associated immune impairment translates into the increased susceptibility to URTI observed in athletes undergoing heavy training. Solid arrows (⇨) = Research evidence mostly supports link; dotted arrow = limited research evidence to support link in athletes; CHO = carbohydrate; ACTH = adrenocorticotrophic hormone; URTI = upper respiratory tract infection

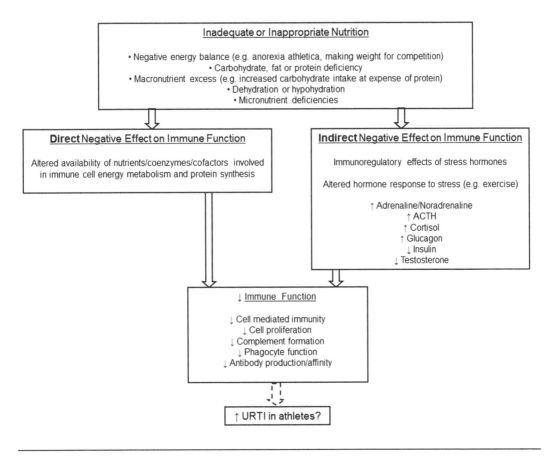

muscle glycogen stores, at the expense of protein which might be detrimental as protein is an important nutrient for immune function.

It is important to understand that decreased nutrient availability during prolonged high-intensity exercise, and poor dietary practices that limit nutrient availability in athletes and soldiers during training, may be involved in the aetiology of exercise-induced immune depression. For example, carbohydrate beverage ingestion during prolonged exercise is purported to prevent some of the observed immune depression by blunting changes in circulating blood glucose and stress-hormone concentrations (Henson *et al.* 1998). This indicates a more than likely involvement of nutrient availability in the aetiology of exercise-induced immune depression. Whether the immune depression associated with nutrient deficiencies during heavy training translates into the increased reports of URTI observed in athletes remains unclear (Walsh *et al.* 2011a).

THE TRAINING AND COMPETITION DIET AND IMMUNE FUNCTION

Energy and body water deficits and immune function

Relatively little is known about the effects of dietary energy restriction, hypohydration (body water deficit) and dehydration (dynamic loss of body water, e.g. through sweat losses) on immune responses at rest or after exercise. Both cellular and humoral immunity have been shown to be depressed in soldiers surviving for 12 days on ration packs providing only half of their daily energy requirements (around 7.5 MJ or around 1,800 kcal) compared with a control group who consumed sufficient energy to maintain energy balance (Booth *et al.* 2003). Another study has shown that soldiers undertaking an eight-week training programme with a modest daily energy deficit (around 2.2 MJ or around 500 kcal) experienced decreases in circulating lymphocyte and monocyte counts that were prevented with additional feeding to offset the energy deficit (Figure 9.2; Diment *et al.* 2012). A particularly novel finding in this study was that nutritional supplementation to offset the energy deficit increased the salivary secretory immunoglobulin A (SIgA) secretion rate during the eight-week training programme (Figure 9.2). This finding can be considered favourable for host defence (see Chapter 6).

A 36-hour fast has been shown to decrease both neutrophil chemotaxis and oxidative burst activity, although this was reversed with re-feeding in only four hours (Walrand *et al.* 2001). Another study in humans has shown that a seven-day fast lowered total T and helper T-lymphocyte numbers, together with lymphocyte interleukin (IL)-2 release in response to bacterial stimulation (Savendahl and Underwood 1997). The authors noted that, during prolonged starvation, large reductions in lymphocyte IL-2 production might impair immune function; indeed, IL-2 is known to enhance a number of immune functions, including lymphocyte cytotoxicity by both natural killer (NK) cells and cytotoxic T cells. Starvation in anorexia nervosa has also been associated with a reduction in memory T cells (CD45RO+) although, once again, normalisation occurred rapidly after re-feeding (Mustafa *et al.* 1997). The authors speculated that elevated circulating cortisol during starvation in people with anorexia nervosa may have had differential effects on T lymphocyte populations, resulting in the decrease in memory T cells. One might argue that the results from studies involving prolonged fasting (e.g. for periods up to seven days) have little relevance for competitive athletes but it is worth noting that many athletes adopt very low energy diets and periods of fasting in sports where leanness or low body weight are thought to confer an advantage (e.g. gymnastics, dance) or to make weight for competition (e.g. boxing, martial arts, rowing). In one

Figure 9.2 Circulating lymphocyte count (A) and salivary secretory immunoglobulin A (SIgA) secretion rate response (B) to an 8-week military training programme where soldiers consumed either a habitual diet alone (CON – open circle) or a habitual diet plus a daily mixed nutritional supplement (SUP – solid circle); baseline (week 0), pre-field exercise (week 6) and after an arduous 2-week field exercise (week 8); data are mean (SEM); * $P < 0.05$ and ** $P < 0.01$ vs. baseline; ## $P < 0.01$ vs. CON (from Diment et al. 2012)

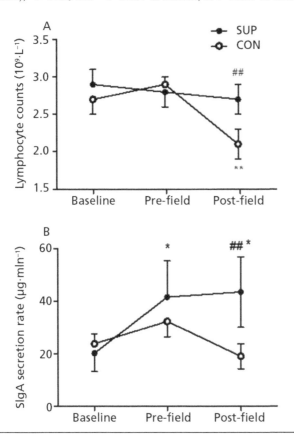

study, circulating lymphocyte counts, total T and helper T lymphocyte counts were lowered after only 24 hours of energy restriction (90% restriction) in an experimental protocol that resembled an athlete making weight for competition (Laing et al. 2008). In addition, the subclinical disorder 'anorexia athletica' has been associated with an increased susceptibility to infection (Beals and Manore 1994). As such, when feasible, athletes are advised to consume sufficient energy during training, competition and recovery to limit the potential detrimental effects of an energy deficit on immune function. Performing standardised measurements of nude body mass at weekly intervals and, if possible, body composition (e.g. using a bioelectrical impedance device), will provide the athlete with valuable information in this regard (i.e. whether they are in energy balance, gain or deficit). As described in the next paragraph, day-to-day changes in nude body mass on rising in the morning probably reflect changes in hydration status rather than energy balance.

Elevated plasma cortisol has been observed during dehydration in ruminants (Parker *et al.* 2003) and during prolonged exercise with restricted fluid intake compared with exercise performed with sufficient fluid intake to offset sweat losses (Bishop *et al.* 2004). Given that the immunosuppressive effects of cortisol are widely acknowledged, we might expect these observations of increased plasma cortisol with fluid deficits to be associated with depressed immune function. Indeed, one elegant study demonstrated that intravenous endotoxin injection in dehydrated rats caused a fever that was absent when the endotoxin was injected into euhydrated rats (Morimoto *et al.* 1986). Until recently, very little was known about the effects of hydration status on the immune response to heavy exercise and training. As fluid intake sufficient to offset fluid losses during prolonged exercise can prevent the decrease in saliva flow rate (Walsh *et al.* 2004), one would expect this to maintain the secretion rate of several saliva proteins known to have important antimicrobial properties (e.g. SIgA, lysozyme and α-amylase) (Bishop and Gleeson 2009). Very recent evidence provides some support for this notion as modest dehydration (three per cent body mass loss evoked by exercise-heat stress without fluid intake) decreased saliva secretion rates of lysozyme and α-amylase; albeit, the secretion rate of salivary SIgA remained unchanged (Figure 9.3; Fortes *et al.* 2012). Fluid deficits during heavy exercise and training (particularly in hot environments) might therefore play a role in the observed immune impairment. It is quite possible that combining a modest fluid deficit and a modest energy deficit has additive or, in some cases, even synergistic effects on immune function. For example, a 48-hour period of either fluid restriction alone (75% restriction, 2.9 litres per day deficit) or energy restriction alone (90% restriction, 11 MJ or around 2,600 kcal per day deficit) did not significantly affect the salivary SIgA secretion rate but combining these fluid and energy restrictions significantly decreased the response (Figure 9.4; Oliver *et al.* 2007). With the available information in mind, athletes are advised to consume sufficient fluids during training, competition and recovery to limit the potential detrimental effects of fluid deficits on immune function. By weighing themselves nude before and after exercise, athletes can estimate sweat losses and determine the appropriate amount of fluid that should be replaced (where one kilogram of body mass loss = around one litre of sweat loss). Coaches and support staff should also consider monitoring changes in their athletes' hydration status, particularly whilst training and competing in hot environments. The simplest method of monitoring hydration is to assess daily nude body mass changes on rising in the morning but support staff should also consider using urinary indices (e.g. colour, osmolality and specific gravity) salivary indices (e.g. osmolality) and possibly even ocular indices of hydration (e.g. tear fluid osmolality) (Walsh *et al.* 2004; Armstrong *et al.* 2010; Fortes *et al.* 2011).

From a critical standpoint, studies in athletes and soldiers that investigate the effects of energy and fluid deficits on clinically relevant *in vivo* immune measures and clinical outcomes, such as infection or wound healing, are currently lacking and are sorely needed.

Figure 9.3 Salivary antimicrobial protein responses to progressive exercise-heat induced dehydration to 1%, 2% and 3% body mass loss (BML), subsequent overnight fluid restriction (8 a.m.) and rehydration (11 a.m.) during fluid restriction (DEH – solid circle) and with fluid intake to offset fluid losses (CON – open circle). Shown are salivary secretory immunoglobulin A (SIgA) secretion rate (A), α-amylase secretion rate (B) and lysozyme secretion rate (C). Values are means (SEM); * $P < 0.05$, ** $P < 0.01$ vs. 0% BML; # $P < 0.05$, ## $P < 0.01$ indicate differences between trials (© 2008 Canadian Science Publishing or its licensors; reproduced with permission from Fortes *et al.* 2012)

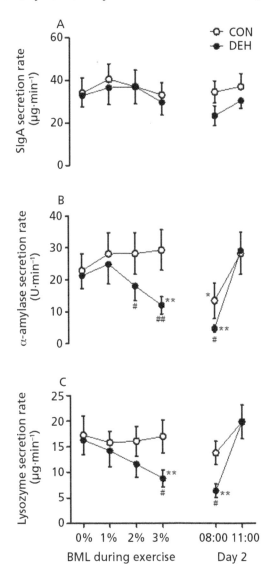

Figure 9.4 Percentage change (Δ) in salivary secretory immunoglobulin A (SIgA) secretion rate after a 48-hour period of fluid restriction (FR), energy restriction (ER) and combined fluid and energy restriction (F+ER); ** *P* < 0.01 indicates that SIgA secretion rate (μg·min⁻¹) was lower than baseline (from Oliver *et al.* 2007)

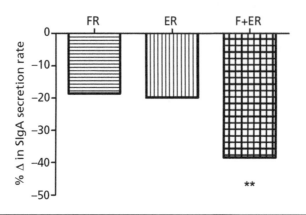

Dietary carbohydrate, exercise and immune function

The importance of adequate carbohydrate availability for maintenance of heavy training schedules and successful athletic performance has long been recognised. During periods of heavy training, athletes should consume sufficient carbohydrate to cover about 60% of their energy costs. The recommended daily carbohydrate intake is 6–10 g/kg body mass for athletes who train for one to three hours each day and 8–12 g/kg body mass for athletes training more than four hours each day (Burke *et al.* 2011). These recommendations are principally aimed at restoring muscle and liver glycogen stores to ensure sufficient carbohydrate availability for skeletal muscle contraction for training on successive days and to avoid the development of hypoglycaemia during long training sessions without carbohydrate ingestion.

Since many aspects of exercise-induced immune function impairment seem to be caused by elevated levels of stress hormones (Figure 9.1), nutritional strategies that effectively reduce the stress-hormone response to exercise would be expected to limit the degree of exercise-induced immune dysfunction. The size of the glycogen stores in muscle and liver at the onset of exercise influences the hormonal and immune response to exercise. The amount of glycogen stored in the body is rather limited (usually less than 500 grams) and is affected by recent physical activity and dietary carbohydrate intake. When individuals perform prolonged exercise following several days on very low carbohydrate diets (typically less than ten per cent of dietary energy intake from carbohydrate), the magnitude of the circulating stress hormone response (e.g. adrenaline and cortisol) and cytokine response (e.g. IL-6, IL-10 and IL-1ra) is markedly higher than on normal or high carbohydrate diets (Figure 9.5; Mitchell *et al.* 1998; Bishop *et al.* 2001b). Nevertheless, with the exception of a modest depression in circulating lymphocyte counts (Mitchell *et al.* 1998), there is limited

Figure 9.5 Changes in the concentrations of (A) plasma cortisol, (B) plasma interleukin-6 (IL-6) and (C) plasma interleukin-1 receptor antagonist (IL-1ra) after 1 hour of cycling at 60% $\dot{V}O_2$ max immediately followed by a 30-minute time trial (work rate around 80% $\dot{V}O_2$ max). For the three days prior to the exercise trial, participants consumed either a high-carbohydrate (CHO) diet where > 70% of total dietary energy from CHO (open circle) or a low-CHO diet where < 10% of total dietary energy from CHO (solid circle); data are presented as mean (SEM); significantly different from Low-CHO, # $P < 0.05$, ## $P < 0.01$ (from Bishop *et al.* 2001b)

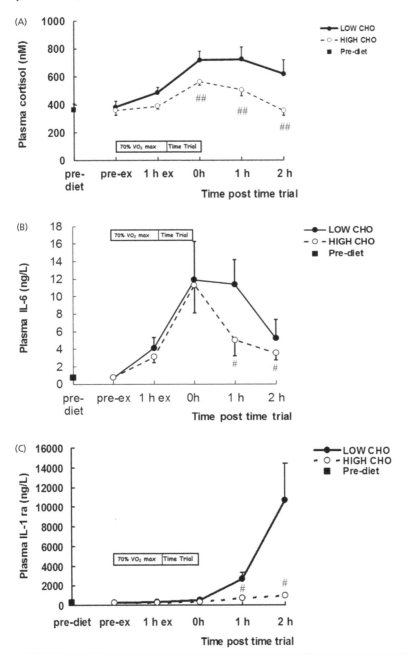

evidence showing that immune indices are depressed to a much greater extent after prolonged exercise in participants on a very low carbohydrate compared with a high carbohydrate diet. Given, though, that the cortisol response to prolonged exercise is greater in participants on a very low carbohydrate diet, athletes with carbohydrate intake well below the recommended intake will not only jeopardise athletic performance, by limiting muscle and liver glycogen availability but may also place themselves at risk from the known immunosuppressive effects of cortisol.

Dietary fats, exercise and immune function

Fat is an essential substrate in the diet, not only because of the important contribution of fat metabolism to energy production but also because lipids are important constituents of cell membranes. In contrast to the small carbohydrate stores within the body, those of lipids are, from a practical standpoint, unlimited. The UK Department of Health recommends that total fat intake should contribute no more than 35% of daily energy intake in sedentary individuals; of which, saturated fats should contribute no more than 10% of total daily energy intake, with the remainder of fat intake provided by monosaturated fatty acids (15%), polyunsaturated fatty acids (PUFAs; 6%), linoleic acid (1%), linolenic acid (0.2%) and trans-fatty acids (less than 2%). The American College of Sports Medicine recommends that athletes consume a diet where 20–35% of daily energy intake should come from fat (Rodriguez *et al.* 2009). Relatively little is known about the potential contribution of dietary fatty acids to the regulation of exercise-induced modification of immune function. Two groups of PUFAs are essential to the body: the omega-6 (*n*–6) series, derived from linoleic acid and the omega-3 (*n*–3) series, derived from α-linolenic acid. These PUFAs cannot be synthesised in the body and so must be derived from the diet. Fatty acids may influence immune function either by acting as a fuel for immune cells ('direct effect'), in their important role as membrane constituents in immune cells ('direct effect') or by regulating eicosanoid (particularly prostaglandin) formation ('indirect effect'; Figure 9.1). Prostaglandins are known to have immunomodulatory effects. There are reports that diets rich in omega-6 and omega-3 PUFAs improve the conditions of patients suffering from diseases characterised by an overactive immune system, such as rheumatoid arthritis; that is to say, they have anti-inflammatory effects (Calder 2011). Whether increasing dietary intake of PUFAs in healthy athletes alters immune function remains an ongoing topic of debate.

Immune function is often compromised on a high-fat diet (Pedersen *et al.* 2000) and so a diet high in fats would not be recommended to athletes for optimal immune functioning. For example, resting NK cell activity decreased during a seven-week endurance training programme in previously untrained men who consumed a fat-rich diet (62% daily energy intake as fat) but increased in men who consumed a carbohydrate-rich diet (65% daily energy intake as carbohydrate) (Pedersen *et al.* 2000). It is difficult to clarify whether the negative effect of the fat-rich diet on NK cell activity was caused by a lack of dietary carbohydrate or an excess of a specific dietary fat component. Although low fat diets (less than 15% daily energy intake as fat) have been shown to enhance some aspects of immune function (Pedersen *et al.* 2000), exercise performance may be decreased on a low-fat diet and micronutrient intake (e.g. vitamin E, iron, calcium and zinc) will probably be below the recommended level on a low-fat diet. Given that these micronutrients are essential to immune function (e.g. vitamin E is an important lipid-soluble antioxidant), when athletes consume a low-fat diet, they may be more susceptible to oxidative stress. On the basis that exercise performance may be decreased and the immune response to exercise may be impaired, athletes are not recommended to consume low-fat diets (less than 15% daily energy intake as fat).

Dietary protein, exercise and immune function

The World Health Organization advises that a minimum protein intake of 0.8 g/kg body mass per day is adequate for the needs of sedentary individuals. During certain circumstances, such as heavy endurance exercise or an intense strength training programme, protein turnover substantially increases, which, in turn, increases the individual's daily protein requirement. The American College of Sports Medicine recommends a daily protein intake of 1.2–1.4 g/kg body mass per day to maintain nitrogen balance for endurance athletes and 1.2–1.7 g/kg body mass per day to support muscle growth for strength athletes (Rodriguez *et al.* 2009). There is little evidence to show that either endurance- or resistance-trained athletes are protein deficient. As long as athletes consume sufficient energy from food to maintain energy balance and their diet is well-balanced, the increased requirement for protein will likely be met. Consequently, those athletes most at risk of protein deficiency would be those undertaking a programme of food restriction to lose weight, vegetarians, and athletes consuming unbalanced diets (e.g. with excess carbohydrate intake at the expense of protein). Inadequate protein intake is widely acknowledged to impair immune function and increase the incidence of opportunistic infections (Li *et al.* 2007). The effects of dietary protein deficiency on the immune system include atrophy of lymphoid tissue, decreased mature T-lymphocyte numbers and T-lymphocyte proliferation response to mitogens, decreased T-lymphocyte helper/suppressor ratio (CD4+/CD8+) and decreased macrophage phagocytic activity and IL-1 production. As expected, the severity of the protein deficiency tends to dictate the magnitude of immune impairment, although even moderate protein deficiency has long been known to impair immune function (Daly *et al.* 1990).

DIETARY SUPPLEMENTS AND IMMUNE FUNCTION IN ATHLETES

This section critically reviews the research evidence on dietary supplements and immune function. You should find Table 9.1 useful, as it provides a rating of the strength of the supporting evidence for the chosen supplement to improve immunity and/or reduce infection risk in athletes.

Table 9.1 Dietary supplements and immune function in athletes: proposed mechanism of action and evidence for efficacy

SUPPLEMENT	PROPOSED MECHANISM OF ACTION	EVIDENCE FOR EFFICACY	EVIDENCE RATING[1]
Carbohydrate	Maintains blood glucose during exercise, lowers stress hormones and thus counters immune dysfunction.	Ingestion of carbohydrate (30–60 g/hour) attenuates stress hormones and some, but not all, immune perturbations during exercise. Only very limited evidence that this modifies infection risk in human athletes.	●●●○○
N-3 polyunsaturated fatty acid	Found in fish oil. May influence immune function by acting as a fuel, in their role as membrane constituents or by regulating eicosanoid formation e.g. prostaglandin. Prostaglandin is immunosuppressive. Exert anti-inflammatory effects post-exercise.	Some evidence of limiting inflammation after muscle damaging eccentric exercise in humans but no evidence of reducing infection risk in athletes.	●○○○○
Glutamine	Non-essential amino acid that is an important energy substrate for immune cells, particularly lymphocytes. Circulating glutamine is lowered after prolonged exercise and very heavy training.	Supplementation before and after exercise does not alter immune perturbations despite maintenance of circulating glutamine.	●○○○○
Caffeine	Stimulant found in a variety of foods and drinks (e.g. coffee and sports drinks). Caffeine is an adenosine receptor antagonist and immune cells express adenosine receptors. Caffeine elevates blood adrenaline at rest and in response to exercise.	Some evidence that caffeine supplementation activates lymphocytes and attenuates the fall in neutrophil function after exercise. Efficacy for altering URTI incidence in athletes remains unknown.	●○○○○
Vitamin C	An essential water-soluble antioxidant vitamin that quenches ROS and augments immunity. Reduces interleukin-6 and cortisol responses to exercise in humans.	Relatively small effects on cortisol compared with carbohydrate; immune measures no different from placebo. Patchy evidence of efficacy in reducing URTI symptoms after ultra-marathon events.	●●○○○
Vitamin E	An essential fat-soluble antioxidant vitamin that quenches exercise-induced ROS and augments immunity. Good evidence for some immune enhancing effects in the frail elderly.	No evidence of benefit for younger healthy humans or athletes. High doses may even be pro-oxidative.	●○○○○

Table 9.1 continued

SUPPLEMENT	PROPOSED MECHANISM OF ACTION	EVIDENCE FOR EFFICACY	EVIDENCE RATING[1]
Vitamin D	An essential fat-soluble vitamin known to influence several aspects of immunity, particularly innate immunity (e.g. expression of antimicrobial proteins). Skin exposure to sunlight accounts for 90% of the source of vitamin D.	Some evidence for deficiency in athletes and soldiers, particularly in northerly latitudes and in the winter months (decreased skin sunlight exposure). Deficiency has been associated with increased URTI in soldiers. More evidence supporting the efficacy of supplementation is required.	●●●○○
Zinc	An essential mineral that is claimed to reduce incidence and duration of colds. Zinc is required for DNA synthesis and as an enzyme cofactor for immune cells. Zinc deficiency results in impaired immunity (e.g. lymphoid atrophy) and zinc deficiency is not uncommon in athletes.	No evidence for reduced infection incidence with zinc supplementation in humans. Some, but not all, human studies suggest a reduction in duration of cold symptoms if zinc gluconate lozenges are administered within 24 hours of onset of cold symptoms. Unlikely to be of any real benefit to athletes unless they are zinc deficient. High doses of zinc supplementation can decrease lymphocyte function.	●●○○○
Echinacea	Herbal extract claimed to enhance immunity via stimulatory effects on macrophages. There is some *in vitro* evidence for this.	Early human studies indicated possible beneficial effects but more recent, larger-scale and better-controlled studies indicate no effect of Echinacea on infection incidence or severity of cold symptoms.	●○○○○
Quercetin	A plant flavonoid. *In vitro* studies show strong anti-inflammatory, anti-oxidant and anti-pathogenic effects. Animal data indicate an increase in mitochondrial biogenesis and endurance performance.	Human studies show some reduction in illness rates during short periods of intensified training and mild stimulation of mitochondrial biogenesis and endurance performance in untrained subjects.	●●○○○
β-glucans	Polysaccharides derived from the cell walls of yeast, fungi, algae and oats that stimulate innate immunity.	Effective in mice inoculated with influenza virus but human studies with athletes showed no benefits.	●○○○○
Probiotics	Live microorganisms that, when administered orally for several weeks, can increase the numbers of beneficial bacteria in the gut. This has been associated with a range of potential benefits to gut health, as well as modulation of immune function.	Some, but not all, human studies show improvements in aspects of acquired immunity and reduced incidence of URTI and gastrointestinal problems.	●●●○○

Table 9.1 continued

SUPPLEMENT	PROPOSED MECHANISM OF ACTION	EVIDENCE FOR EFFICACY	EVIDENCE RATING[1]
Bovine colostrum	First milk of the cow that contains antibodies, growth factors and cytokines. Claimed to improve mucosal immunity and increase resistance to infection.	One study suggests an effect in elevating salivary SIgA in human endurance runners but evidence is not forthcoming that this modifies infection risk.	●○○○○

Notes:
[1] Scientific evidence is rated on a continuum where: ○○○○○ indicates no supporting evidence; ●●●○○ indicates modest supporting evidence and ●●●●● indicates very strong supporting evidence.
URTI = upper respiratory tract infection; ROS = reactive oxygen species; SIgA = secretory immunoglobulin A

Carbohydrate

Dr David Nieman (Box 9.1) and his team have shown that consumption of carbohydrate during prolonged exercise attenuates the rise in plasma adrenaline, cortisol, and cytokines (Nehlsen-Cannarella *et al.* 1997); attenuates the trafficking of most leukocyte and lymphocyte subsets (Nieman *et al.* 1993b, 1994, 1998a); prevents the exercise-induced fall in neutrophil function and reduces the diminution of mitogen-stimulated T lymphocyte proliferation (on a per-cell basis) after prolonged exercise (Henson *et al.* 1998). Consuming 30–60 grams of carbohydrate per hour during 2.5 hours of strenuous cycling prevented both the decrease in the number and percentage of interferon-gamma (IFN-γ) positive T lymphocytes and the suppression of IFN-γ production from stimulated T lymphocytes observed with a placebo treatment (Lancaster *et al.* 2005a). IFN-γ production is critical to antiviral defence and it has been suggested that the suppression of IFN-γ production may be an important mechanism leading to an increased risk of infection after prolonged exercise bouts (Northoff *et al.* 1998). Carbohydrate ingestion during prolonged exercise has also recently been shown to attenuate the post-exercise fall in T-lymphocyte migration into human rhinovirus-infected airway epithelial tissue (Figure 9.6; Bishop *et al.* 2009).

Box 9.1 David C. Nieman, DrPH, FACSM

Dr David Nieman is a professor in the College of Health Sciences at Appalachian State University, and Director of the Human Performance Laboratory at the North Carolina Research Campus in Kannapolis, North Carolina (www.nrcresearchcampus.net). Dr Nieman has been a pioneer in exercise immunology and his team has devoted great energy to better understanding the influence of dietary supplements on immune health in athletes. His work has helped to establish that: (1) regular moderate exercise lowers upper respiratory tract infection rates while improving immunosurveillance (Nieman *et al.* 2011a); (2) heavy exertion increases infection rates (Nieman *et al.* 1989a, 1990a) while causing transient changes in immune function (Nieman *et al.*, 1993b, 1994, 1998a); and (3) that carbohydrate (Nieman *et al.*, 2004) and flavonoid (Nieman *et al.* 2007, 2009a) ingestion by athletes attenuates exercise-induced immune depression. Dr Nieman's current work is centred on investigating unique nutritional products as countermeasures to exercise- and obesity-induced immune dysfunction, inflammation, illness and oxidative stress (www.ncrc.appstate.edu). Dr Nieman has received US$6 million in research grants and published more than 280 peer-reviewed publications in journals and books, and sits on ten journal editorial boards, including the *Journal of Applied Physiology* and *Medicine and Science in Sports and Exercise*. He is the author of nine books on health, exercise science and nutrition, *including Exercise Testing and Prescription: A Health-Related Approach* (New York: McGraw-Hill, 2011, now in its 7th edition). Dr Nieman served as Vice-president of the American College of Sports Medicine and two terms as President of the International Society of Exercise and Immunology. He was an acrobatic gymnast and coach for ten years and has run 58 marathons (personal best 2 hours 37 minutes) and ultra-marathons.

Figure 9.6 Influence of heavy exercise and carbohydrate intake on T-lymphocyte migration towards human rhinovirus-infected cell line. A shows migration of T-helper cells (CD4+); B shows migration of naïve T-helper cells (CD4+CD45RA+); # $P < 0.05$ higher on CHO than PLA; ** $P < 0.01$ vs. resting value (reproduced with permission from Bishop *et al.* 2009)

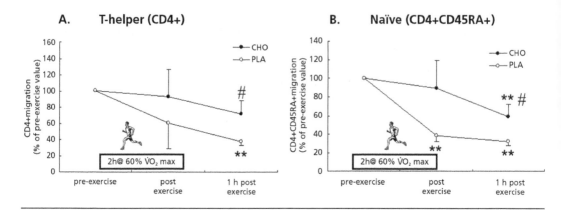

Although carbohydrate feeding during exercise appears to be effective in minimising some of the immune perturbations associated with prolonged strenuous exercise, it does not prevent the falls in NK cell function or salivary SIgA secretion and seems less effective at minimising the more modest immune alterations during exercise, which includes regular rest intervals; in for example, football (Bishop *et al.* 1999a) or resistance exercise (Nieman *et al.*, 2004). Furthermore, carbohydrate feeding during exercise is not as effective in reducing immune-cell trafficking and functional depression when exercise is performed to the point of fatigue (Bishop *et al.* 2001a). Findings show that carbohydrate/protein feeding immediately after but not one hour after prolonged, heavy exercise can prevent the post-exercise decrease in bacterially stimulated neutrophil degranulation (Costa *et al.* 2009). In line with the work where carbohydrate was fed during exercise, this immediate post-exercise feeding strategy had little influence on salivary antimicrobial proteins during recovery (Costa *et al.* 2012). Thus, carbohydrate is seen as only a partial countermeasure against exercise-induced immune impairment and evidence that the beneficial effect of feeding carbohydrate on immune responses to exercise actually translates into a reduced incidence of URTI after prolonged exercise, such as marathon races is currently lacking. Although a trend for a beneficial effect of carbohydrate ingestion on post-race URTI was reported in a study of 98 marathon runners, this did not achieve statistical significance and larger scale studies are needed to investigate this possibility (Nieman *et al.* 2002a). A current paradox, described in more detail in Box 9.2, is that the train-low strategy (i.e. with low carbohydrate availability) adopted by many endurance athletes to maximise training adaptations might pose a greater threat to the immune system (compared with training high) via increases in circulating immunosuppressive stress hormones (e.g. cortisol).

Box 9.2 The carbohydrate training adaptation–immune maintenance paradox

Train low and compete high – a new perspective on dietary carbohydrate to maximise training adaptations

- *What is train low and compete high?*
  This relatively new concept is where the athlete trains with low carbohydrate availability to promote a greater training response, before switching to high carbohydrate availability to optimise competitive performance.

- *How might an athlete train low?*
  - By training twice-a-day an athlete commences half of their training sessions with a low muscle glycogen concentration.
  - By training after an overnight fast.
  - By consuming only water during longer training sessions.
  - By withholding carbohydrate in the hours after exercise.

- *What evidence supports the concept that training low increases training adaptations?*
  Commencing training with low muscle glycogen (vs. high muscle glycogen) has been shown to enhance metabolic adaptations by inducing a greater transcriptional activation of muscle enzymes involved in carbohydrate metabolism; including, AMP-activated protein kinase (AMPK), GLUT4, hexokinase and pyruvate dehydrogenase (PDH) complex. Training low has also been shown to enhance adaptive responses favouring fat metabolism (for a comprehensive review see Burke *et al.* 2011).

- *Does train low and compete high improve athletic performance?*
  Although training low can improve metabolic adaptations, this has not, as yet, been shown to translate into better athletic performance compared with more conventional diet and training practices.

- *What are the disadvantages of training low?*
  One obvious disadvantage is that an athlete would not be able to train as hard when training low.
  The athlete and support staff would need to carefully consider the scheduling of train-low sessions within the periodised training programme to avoid the potentially deleterious effects of overreaching and chronic maladaptation (coined the 'overtraining syndrome').

- *What is meant by the carbohydrate training adaptation–immune maintenance paradox?*
  By training low to maximise metabolic adaptations (e.g. training twice a day), the athlete may be penalised with decreased immune function and an increased risk of infection. It is widely accepted that training with low carbohydrate availability increases the immunosuppressive stress hormones. Indeed, it has long been known that the second of two daily training bouts causes greater immune perturbations than the first (Ronsen *et al.* 2001b).

n-3 polyunsaturated fatty acid

As described in Table 9.1, n-3 PUFAs are found in fish oils and can modulate immune function by acting as a fuel source for immune cells, in their role as membrane constituents or by regulating eicosanoid formation (e.g. leukotrienes and prostaglandins); indeed, prostaglandins are known for their anti-inflammatory effects. One study in untrained men reported that the inflammatory response to eccentric exercise-induced muscle damage, evaluated by increases in circulating IL-6 and C-reactive protein, was attenuated by 14 days of daily supplementation with docosahexaenoic acid (an n-3 PUFA: 800 mg), tocopherols (300 mg) and flavonoids (100 mg hesperetin and 200 mg quercetin) (Phillips *et al.* 2003). However, it has been suggested that high intakes of PUFA may exert an undesirable influence on inflammation and immune function during and after exercise (Konig *et al.* 1997) and some human studies have shown that dietary supplements with n-3 PUFA (e.g. eicosapentaenoic acid) decrease NK-cell activity in healthy humans (Thies *et al.* 2001). Another study, however, indicated that supplementation with a combination of n-3 PUFA (eicosapentaenoic acid and docosahexaenoic acid) in 2.4 g/day of fish oils for six weeks had no effect on selected immune responses to prolonged exercise, although in this study NK-cell activity was not measured (Nieman *et al.* 2009b). A follow-up study by the same group has generated some concern after reporting an increase in the oxidative stress marker, F2-isoprostane in plasma after exercise when trained cyclists were supplemented daily with the same n-3 PUFA combination (McAnulty *et al.* 2010). More research is needed on the effects of altering essential fatty acid intake on immune function after exercise and during periods of heavy training.

Glutamine and branched-chain amino acids

Glutamine is the most abundant free amino acid in human muscle and plasma and is utilised at very high rates by leukocytes to provide energy and optimal conditions for nucleotide biosynthesis. Indeed, glutamine is important, if not essential, to lymphocytes and other rapidly dividing cells, including the gut mucosa and bone marrow stem cells. Glutamine is also required for optimal macrophage phagocytic activity. Prolonged bouts of exercise (Rennie *et al.* 1981), periods of heavy training (MacKinnon and Hooper 1996) and maladaptation to training (coined the 'overtraining syndrome') (Parry-Billings *et al.* 1992) have all been associated with a fall in the blood plasma concentration of glutamine. This decrease was hypothesised to explain the exercise-induced immune impairment (Parry-Billings *et al.* 1990). The glutamine hypothesis is discussed in more detail in Box 9.3.

Caffeine

Caffeine is the most widely consumed drug in Europe and America. It has long been used by athletes because of the convincing evidence that even modest doses of caffeine (e.g. 3 mg/kg body mass) improve endurance performance (Bridge and Jones 2006).

Box 9.3 The glutamine hypothesis

The late Professor Eric Newsholme aroused early interest with his hypothesis that the exercise-induced suppression of immune function was due to a decrease in plasma glutamine availability (Parry-Billings *et al*. 1992). Glutamine is certainly needed for leukocyte metabolism. Studies from his Oxford University laboratory found a 20% fall of plasma glutamine following a marathon run. A controlled trial showed a reduced risk of immunosuppression after endurance races in those who consumed two drinks each containing 5 g glutamine, (19% compared with 51% reported infections in those given a maltodextrin placebo; Castell *et al*. 1996; Castell and Newsholme 1998). A severe lack of glutamine can undoubtedly impair immune function in malnourished populations but glutamine lack seems less plausible in athletes who are eating a high-protein diet. Subsequent research has generally failed to support any benefit of glutamine supplements for reducing immune impairments after exercise (Rohde *et al*. 1995, 1998; Walsh *et al*. 2000).

   Several scientists have suggested that exogenous provision of glutamine supplements may be beneficial by preventing the impairment of immune function after prolonged exercise. However, the evidence that oral glutamine supplements reduce the incidence of URTI after endurance events is limited (Castell *et al*. 1996). Several studies that have investigated the effect of oral glutamine supplementation during and after exercise on various indices of immune function have failed to find any beneficial effect. A glutamine solution (0.1 g/kg body mass) given during exercise, immediately post-exercise and 30 minutes after prolonged bouts of cycling at 75% $\dot{V}O_2$ max prevented the fall in the plasma glutamine concentration but did not prevent the fall in mitogen-induced lymphocyte proliferation and lymphokine-activated NK-cell activity (Rohde *et al*. 1998). Similarly, maintaining the plasma glutamine concentration by consuming glutamine in drinks taken both during and after two hours of cycling at 60% $\dot{V}O_2$ max did not affect leukocyte subset trafficking or prevent the exercise-induced fall in neutrophil function (Walsh *et al*. 2000). Unlike the feeding of carbohydrate during exercise, glutamine supplements do not seem to affect immune function perturbations (Table 9.1) and review articles (Walsh *et al*. 1998b; Hiscock and Pedersen 2002) conclude that falls in plasma glutamine are not responsible for exercise-induced immunodepression.

   Bassit and colleagues reported that supplementation (6 g/day for 15 days) with branched-chain amino acids (BCAAs) before a triathlon or a 30-km run prevented the approximately 40% decline in mitogen-stimulated lymphocyte proliferation observed in the placebo control group after exercise (Bassit *et al*. 2002). BCAAs (valine, isoleucine and leucine) are precursors for glutamine, and BCAA supplementation prevented the post-exercise fall in plasma glutamine concentration and was also associated with increased IL-2 and IFN production. However, these findings need to be viewed with caution as there were flaws in the experimental design and statistical analysis; as such, these results need to be confirmed in more controlled studies. In summary, the evidence to date does not support a role for decreased plasma glutamine in the aetiology of exercise-induced immune depression (the 'glutamine hypothesis') and there is little data to support the contention that athletes should supplement glutamine to maintain immune function.

In 2004, caffeine was removed from the list of banned substances by the International Olympic Committee. Caffeine originates naturally in 63 species of plants as several types of methylated xanthines. Caffeine and caffeine-like substances can be found in a variety of foods and drinks (now including several sports drinks and energy drinks) but the main sources for these substances are coffee beans, tea leaves, cocoa beans, and cola nuts. Although consumption varies greatly, typical caffeine consumption in the UK and USA is 200 mg/day (around 3 mg/kg body mass) but this may be as high as 400 mg/day in parts of Scandinavia, where habitual caffeine intake is high (around 6 mg/kg body mass). Coffee accounts for 75% of all caffeine consumption (typically there is 40–180 mg of caffeine per cup). Caffeine is an adenosine-receptor antagonist and several immune cell types, including neutrophils and lymphocytes express adenosine receptors. Furthermore, caffeine ingestion results in elevated circulating adrenaline concentration both at rest and during exercise and so could conceivably affect immune cell functions 'indirectly' (Figure 9.1) via actions on adrenoreceptors. At present, there is little information on the effects of caffeine on immune function at rest. The addition of pharmacological doses of caffeine to cell culture media has been associated with a dose-dependent suppression of mitogen-stimulated proliferative responses of human lymphocytes (Rosenthal *et al.* 1992). However, *in vivo* administration of 18 mg/kg/day of caffeine in rats was associated with a significant increase in mitogen-stimulated T-cell proliferation (Kantamala *et al.* 1990). In the same study, B-cell proliferative responses to mitogen were significantly decreased following administration of a more physiologically relevant caffeine dose of 6 mg/kg/day.

Exercise studies have demonstrated that caffeine ingestion (6 mg/kg body mass) one hour before a bout of intensive endurance exercise was associated with greater perturbations in numbers of circulating lymphocytes, CD4+ and CD8+ cells compared with placebo. Moreover, caffeine ingestion was associated with an increased percentage of CD4+ and CD8+ cells expressing the early activation marker CD69 *in vivo* before and after exercise (Bishop *et al.* 2005a). Other findings from a series of studies by Dr Bishop's group show that caffeine ingestion (6 mg/kg body mass) increased salivary SIgA responses during prolonged exercise (Bishop *et al.* 2006), attenuated the post-exercise fall in stimulated neutrophil oxidative burst (Walker *et al.* 2006) and, more recently, increased NK-cell recruitment to the circulation and NK-cell activation one hour after prolonged, high-intensity exercise (Fletcher and Bishop 2011). From a critical standpoint, 6 mg/kg body mass is a relatively high dose of caffeine, so a particular strength of the latter study is that a 2 mg/kg body mass 'low dose' of caffeine was also shown to increase NK-cell activation during recovery from prolonged, high-intensity exercise. It is thought that at least some of these effects may be mediated through caffeine's action as an adenosine receptor antagonist. More work is needed to determine the efficacy of caffeine supplementation to maintain immune health in athletes; for example, the influence of caffeine supplementation on *in vivo* immune function and infection incidence in athletes remains unknown.

Megadoses of antioxidant vitamins

Vitamins with antioxidant properties, including vitamins C, E, and β-carotene (provitamin A), may be required in increased quantities in athletes to inactivate the products of exercise-induced lipid peroxidation. Oxygen free-radical formation that accompanies the dramatic increase in oxidative metabolism during exercise could potentially inhibit immune responses. Sustained endurance training appears to be associated with an adaptive upregulation of the antioxidant defence system; however, such adaptations may be insufficient to protect athletes who train extensively (Powers *et al.* 2004).

Vitamin C (ascorbic acid) occurs in high concentration in leukocytes and is implicated in a variety of anti-infective functions, including promotion of T-lymphocyte proliferation, prevention of corticosteroid-induced suppression of neutrophil activity, production of IFN and inhibition of virus replication. It is also a major water-soluble antioxidant that is effective as a scavenger of ROS in both intracellular and extracellular fluids. It can act as an antioxidant both directly (e.g. in the prevention of auto-oxidative dysfunction of neutrophil bactericidal activity) and indirectly via its regeneration of reduced vitamin E. Good sources of vitamin C, include fruit and vegetables and the recommended daily amount (RDA) is 40 mg in the UK.

In a study by Peters and colleagues, using a double-blind placebo research design, it was determined that daily supplementation of 600 mg of vitamin C (15 times the RDA) for three weeks before a 90-km ultra-marathon reduced the incidence of URTI symptoms (incidence was 33% compared with 68% in age- and sex-matched control runners) in the two-week post-race period (Peters *et al.* 1993). Caution is needed when interpreting the results for URTI from self-report logs as it is unlikely that 68% of the athletes in the placebo group were suffering from an infection in the two-week post-race period. The limitations with using self-report to record URTI are discussed in detail in Chapter 1. A follow-up study also showed that the supplementation of additional dietary antioxidants (vitamin E and β-carotene) did not confer any additional beneficial effect (Peters *et al.* 1996). The doses of vitamin C used in these studies (600–1,000 mg/day) are considerably higher than the daily dosage of 200 mg that is needed to saturate body tissues with vitamin C. In a more recent randomised, double blinded, placebo-controlled study, 1,500 mg/day vitamin C for seven days before an ultra-marathon race with consumption of vitamin C in a carbohydrate beverage during the race (athletes in the placebo group consumed the same carbohydrate beverage without added vitamin C) did not affect oxidative stress, cytokine or immune function measures during and after the race (Nieman *et al.* 2002b). In contrast, it has been reported (Fischer *et al.* 2004) that four weeks of combined supplementation with vitamin C (500 mg/day) and vitamin E (400 iu/day equivalent to around 270 mg which is around 27 times the RDA of 10 mg) before a three-hour knee-extension exercise protocol reduced muscle IL-6 release and reduced the systemic rise in both circulating IL-6 and cortisol. Some degree of blunting of the plasma cortisol response to exercise and better maintained neutrophil function after exercise was reported in a placebo-controlled study that used the same dose of daily vitamin C and E supplements and examined immunoendocrine responses to 2.5 hours of cycling after four weeks of supplementation (Davison *et al.* 2007). Furthermore, administration of the antioxidant N-acetyl-L-cysteine (a precursor of glutathione) to mice prevented the exercise-induced reduction in intracellular glutathione concentration and markedly reduced post-exercise apoptosis in intestinal lymphocytes (Quadrilatero and Hoffman-Goetz 2004). Thus, although there are some inconsistencies in the literature regarding antioxidant supplementation and immune responses to exercise, there is at least a sound scientific basis for believing that such supplementation could have beneficial effects in alleviating exercise-induced immunodepression via the mechanisms summarised in Figure 9.7 and Table 9.1.

The most recent Cochrane meta-analysis examined the evidence that daily doses of more than 200 mg vitamin C were more effective in preventing or treating the common cold than placebo (Douglas *et al.* 2007) Twenty-nine trial comparisons involving 11,077 study participants contributed to this meta-analysis of the relative risk (RR) of developing a cold while taking prophylactic vitamin C. The pooled RR was 0.96 (95% confidence interval [CI] 0.92 to 1.00). A subgroup of six trials that involved physically active participants (a total of 642 marathon runners, skiers and soldiers on sub-Arctic exercises) reported a pooled RR of 0.50 (95% CI 0.38 to 0.66). Thirty comparisons involving 9,676 respiratory episodes contributed to the meta-analysis on the duration of the common cold during vitamin C or placebo

Figure 9.7 Possible mechanisms by which dietary antioxidant supplementation reduces stress-induced or exercise-induced immunodepression. Also shown is the effect of carbohydrate ingestion during prolonged exercise (reproduced, with permission, from Gleeson 2006a)

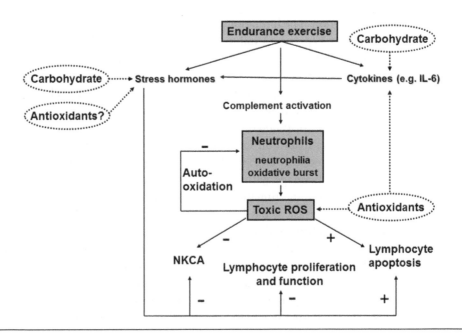

supplementation. A consistent benefit of vitamin C was observed, representing a reduction in cold duration of 8% (95% CI 3% to 13%) for adult participants and 14% (95% CI 5% to 21%) for child participants. Fifteen trial comparisons that involved 7,045 respiratory episodes contributed to the meta-analysis of severity of episodes experienced while on prophylaxis and the results revealed a benefit of vitamin C when days confined to home and off work or school were taken as a measure of severity. A limited number of trials had examined cold duration and severity during therapy with vitamin C that was initiated after the onset of cold symptoms and no significant differences from placebo were found. The authors concluded that the failure of vitamin C supplementation to reduce the incidence of colds in the normal population indicates that routine mega-dose prophylaxis is not generally justified but that individuals subjected to brief periods of severe physical exercise and/or cold environments may gain some benefit. However, even if some protective effects of high-dose antioxidant supplementation on infection risk is indeed a reality, athletes need to consider the risks, which may include the blunting of some of the adaptations to training with a high intake of antioxidants (Ristow *et al.* 2009), although whether or not this is likely to affect adaptations in already well-trained athletes performing intensive training has been questioned (Yfanti *et al.* 2010).

Vitamin D

Vitamin D is not actually a vitamin but a secosteroid hormone produced in the skin from 7-dehydrocholesterol after exposure to sunlight ultraviolet-B radiation. The classical role of vitamin D in bone mineralisation is very well known but much less is known about a putative role for vitamin D in maintaining immune function. New insights indicate that sufficient vitamin D is required for the production of antimicrobial proteins (e.g. cathelicidin and defensins) following Toll-like receptor stimulation; as such, vitamin D is purported to play a central role in the antibacterial defences that characterise the innate immune response (Table 9.1; Laaksi 2012). Under most circumstances, the major source of vitamin D (around 90%) comes from exposure of the skin to sunlight, thus dietary vitamin D (e.g. from oily fish, eggs and fortified cereals) typically accounts for a small component (around 10%). However, diet becomes a very important source of vitamin D in northerly latitudes during the wintertime because the limited sunlight exposure is known to be inadequate for inducing endogenous vitamin D production (Laaksi *et al.* 2010). Adequate exposure of the skin to sunlight to avoid vitamin D deficiency is 5–30 minutes in the middle of the day several times each week (Powers *et al.* 2011). The Institute of Medicine in the USA has recommended that daily vitamin D intake should be 15 µg (600 iu/day) for skeletal outcomes but the vitamin D requirements for extraskeletal outcomes, such as maintaining immune function remain poorly understood (Ross *et al.* 2011). Vitamin D status is determined by measuring the serum concentration of the major circulating form of the hormone, 25-hydroxyvitamin D (25(OH)D) which is formed in the liver. Vitamin D deficiency (serum

25(OH)D less than 40 nmol/l) is not uncommon and reaches epidemic levels among adults with limited sunlight exposure. Such was the level of concern about vitamin D deficiency in Finland that in 2003 the Ministry of Social Affairs and Health instigated the fortification of milk (0.5 µg/dl) and margarines (10 µg/100 g) with vitamin D; this fortification has substantially improved vitamin D status in Finland (Laaksi 2012).

Emerging evidence indicates that some athletes also experience vitamin D deficiency. Particularly susceptible appear to be athletes who:

- live in the northern hemisphere during the winter months
- have darker skin (owing to the relationship of skin pigmentation to vitamin D synthesis)
- train indoors; and finally
- wear protective clothing that covers the skin (Powers *et al.* 2011).

Vitamin D deficiency has been associated with increased infection in a small number of studies. In one study in 756 conscripts serving on a military base in Finland, those with serum 25(OH)D less than 40 nmol/l (N = 24, 3.6%) experienced significantly more days of absence from duty owing to respiratory infection than those with serum 25(OH)D greater than 40 nmol/l (Laaksi *et al.* 2007). A follow-up study in 164 military conscripts, by the same group in Finland, showed that supplementation with 10 µg/day vitamin D for six months prevented the typical wintertime fall in serum 25(OH)D (data for N = 58) but did not alter the number of days absent, owing to respiratory tract infection. Although, a positive finding was that the proportion of men remaining healthy throughout the six-month period was greater in the intervention group (51%) than in the placebo group (36%; Laaksi *et al.* 2010). Clearly, there is a pressing need for studies to determine the efficacy of vitamin D supplementation to improve immunity in athletes (Table 9.1).

Zinc

Zinc is essential for the development of the immune system and more than 100 metalloenzymes are dependent on it, including those involved in the transcription of DNA and synthesis of proteins. Zinc also functions as an intracellular signal molecule for immune cells (Prasad 2009). The effects of zinc deficiency on immune function include lymphoid atrophy, decreased delayed-hypersensitivity cutaneous responses, decreased IL-2 production, impaired mitogen-stimulated lymphocyte proliferative responses and decreased NK-cell cytolytic activity (Overbeck *et al.* 2008; Prasad 2009).

Vegetarian athletes are at risk for zinc deficiency because meat and seafood are the richest zinc sources and, although nuts, legumes, and whole grains are good sources of zinc, the high levels of fibre in these foods can decrease zinc absorption. Zinc deficiency can also be a problem for athletes in sports where a low body mass confers a performance advantage. Very-low-energy or starvation-type diets may induce significant zinc losses. Because zinc is lost from the body mainly in sweat and urine and these losses are increased by exercise, a heavy schedule of exercise training (particularly in the heat) could conceivably induce a zinc deficiency in athletes.

Studies concerning the relationship between immune function, exercise and zinc status in athletes are lacking. However, megadoses of zinc (the RDA is 10 mg and 12 mg for females and males, respectively) can actually have detrimental effects on immune function. The administration of zinc (150 mg twice a day) to 11 healthy males for six weeks was associated with reduced T-lymphocyte proliferative responses to mitogen stimulation and impaired neutrophil phagocytic activity (Chandra 1984). A study of male runners found that six days of zinc supplementation (25 mg of zinc and 1.5 mg of copper, twice a day) exaggerated the exercise-induced suppression of T-lymphocyte proliferation in response to mitogens; although this did not reach statistical significance (Singh et al. 1994). These two studies should be viewed with some caution, as the work of R. K. Chandra has since been brought into question (Smith 2005) and the Singh study tested only five male runners, and thus was underpowered to determine statistical significance. Potential problems with zinc supplements of more than 30 mg per day include nausea, bad taste reactions, lowering of high-density lipoprotein cholesterol, depression of some immune cell functions and interference with the absorption of copper. Hence, large doses of zinc are not recommended. Instead, athletes should be encouraged to consume some zinc-rich foods in their training and competition diet (e.g. poultry, meat, fish and dairy produce). Vegetarians might consider a 10–20 mg supplement of zinc daily but, in view of the above findings, supplements at the lower end of this range may be more suitable for vegetarian athletes.

The efficacy of zinc supplementation as a treatment for the common cold has been investigated in at least a dozen studies published since 1984. Unfortunately, the findings have largely been equivocal and are often presented in obscure rather than mainstream nutrition journals. Several reviews of this topic conclude that zinc supplementation may be of benefit in the treatment of some diseases such as pneumonia and acute lower respiratory infection but that the results for the common cold are not conclusive (Macknin 1999; Marshall 2000; Roxas and Jurenka 2007; Overbeck et al. 2008; Prasad 2009). Although only limited evidence suggests that taking zinc supplements reduces the incidence of URTI (McElroy and Miller 2002; Veverka et al. 2009), in the studies that have reported a beneficial effect of zinc lozenges in treating the common cold (i.e. reduction of symptom duration, severity or both) zinc lozenges (greater than 75 mg/day) had to be taken within 24 hours of the onset of symptoms to be of any benefit (Hemila 2011).

Echinacea

Several herbal preparations are reputed to have immunostimulatory effects and consumption of products containing *Echinacea purpurea* is widespread among athletes. In a double-blind, placebo-controlled study, the effect of a daily oral pre-treatment for 28 days with pressed juice of *E. purpurea* was investigated in 42 triathletes before and after a sprint triathlon (Berg *et al.* 1998). A subgroup of athletes was also treated with magnesium as a reference for supplementation with a micronutrient important for optimal muscular function. During the 28-day pre-treatment period, none of the athletes in the Echinacea group became ill, compared with three athletes in the magnesium group and four athletes in the placebo group.

Numerous experiments have shown that *E. purpurea* extracts exert significant immunomodulatory effects *in vitro*. Among the many pharmacological properties reported, activation of macrophages, polymorphonuclear leukocytes and NK cells has been reasonably well demonstrated (Barrett 2003). Changes in the numbers and activities of T-cell and B-cell leukocytes have been reported but are less certain. Despite this cellular evidence of *in vitro* immunostimulation, pathways leading to enhanced resistance to infectious disease have not been adequately described. Several dozen human experiments, including a number of blind, randomised trials report health benefits. The most robust data come from trials testing *E. purpurea* extracts in the treatment of acute URTI. Although suggesting a modest benefit, these trials are limited both in size and in methodological quality. In a randomised, double-blind, placebo-controlled trial, administering unrefined Echinacea at the onset of symptoms of URTI in 148 college students did not provide any detectable benefit or harm compared with placebo (Table 9.1) (Barrett *et al.*, 2002).

In a meta-analysis of trials on Echinacea (Linde *et al.*, 2006) that included 22 well-controlled trials, three trials investigated prevention of colds and 19 trials tested treatment of colds. A variety of different Echinacea preparations were used. None of the three comparisons in the prevention trials showed an effect of Echinacea over placebo. Comparing an Echinacea preparation with placebo as a treatment for colds, a significant beneficial effect was reported in nine comparisons, a trend in one and no difference in six. The authors' main conclusions were that Echinacea preparations tested in clinical trials differ greatly but that there is some evidence that preparations based on the aerial parts of the Echinacea plant might be effective for the early treatment of colds in adults but results are not fully consistent. Beneficial effects in preventing colds have not been shown in independently replicated, rigorous randomised trials. Hence, although a great deal of moderately good-quality scientific data regarding Echinacea has been gathered, its effectiveness in treating illness or in enhancing human health has not yet been proved beyond a reasonable doubt.

Quercetin

The physiological effects of dietary plant polyphenols including the flavonol quercetin are of great current interest, owing to their antioxidant, anti-inflammatory, anti-pathogenic, cardioprotective, and anti-carcinogenic actions. The richest food sources of quercetin are apples, blueberries, broccoli, curly kale, hot peppers, onions and tea. Total daily flavonol intake (with quercetin representing about 75%) varies from 13 mg to 64 mg, depending on the study sample and the population studied. Humans can absorb significant amounts of quercetin from food or supplements, and elimination is quite slow, with a reported half-life ranging from 11–28 hours. Animal studies indicate that seven days of quercetin feeding improves survival from influenza virus inoculation (Davis *et al.* 2008).

A few human trials have now been conducted and a double-blind, placebo-controlled study with 40 cyclists showed that 1,000 mg/day quercetin for three weeks significantly increased plasma quercetin levels and reduced URTI incidence during the two-week period following three successive days of exhaustive exercise (Nieman *et al.* 2007). A surprisingly high proportion (45%) of participants in the placebo group reported URTI symptoms in the two-week post-training period. Once again, you are recommended to familiarise yourself with the limitations of using self-report for recording URTI as discussed in Chapter 1. In this study, markers of immune dysfunction, inflammation and oxidative stress were not different from the quercetin treated group, suggesting that quercetin exerted direct anti-viral effects, at least within the context of the study design. There is some support for co-ingestion of quercetin with other flavonoids and food components to improve and extend quercetin's bioavailability and bioactive effects. These include the flavonoid epigallocatechin 3-gallate (EGCG) from tea, isoquercetin, which is the glycosylated form of quercetin in onions and other foods, n-3 PUFA, such as eicosapentaenoic acid (EPA) and docosahexaenoic acid (DHA), vitamin C and folate. In a study with 39 trained cyclists, a quercetin supplement combined with EGCG, isoquercetin and n-3 PUFA was more effective than quercetin alone in partially countering exercise-induced inflammation and oxidative stress (Nieman *et al.* 2009a). It remains a matter of contention whether blunting inflammation and oxidative stress during training with supplement cocktails (e.g. quercetin with EGCG and n-3 PUFA) attenuates some of the important metabolic adaptations that occur during training.

Beta-glucans

Beta-glucans are not only present as major structural components of the cell walls of yeast, fungi and some bacteria but are also present in the diet as part of the endosperm cell wall in cereals, such as barley and oat. Beta-glucans are carbohydrates consisting of linked glucose molecules and differ in macromolecular structure depending on the source; β-glucans from bacteria are unbranched 1,3 β-linked glycopyranosyl residues. The cell wall β-glucans of yeast and fungi consists of 1,3 β-linked glycopyranosyl residues with small numbers of 1,6 β-linked branches, whereas oat and barley cell walls contain unbranched β-glucans with 1,3 and 1,4 β-linked glycopyranosyl residues. The specific characteristics of the various β-glucans may influence their immune modulating effects. For example, it has been suggested that high molecular weight and/or particulate β-glucans from fungi directly activate leukocytes, whilst low molecular weight β-glucans from fungi only modulate the response of immune cells when they are stimulated (e.g. with cytokines) (Brown and Gordon 2003). This implies that the addition of β-glucans to the diet may be used to modulate immune function and so might improve the resistance against invading pathogens in humans.

To date, there is limited evidence for immune-promoting effects of orally administered oat β-glucans in animals and humans. Intragastric administration of oat β-glucans in mice enhanced resistance to bacterial and parasitic infections (reviewed by Volman *et al.* 2008). Furthermore, another study demonstrated that daily ingestion of oat β-glucan counteracted the decrease in macrophage antiviral resistance induced by exercise stress in mice (Davis *et al.* 2004). Results from *in vitro* studies in animals treated with β-glucans suggest that β-glucans enhance the immune response in leukocytes and epithelial cells. In the *in vivo* situation, there is now substantial evidence in animals that these effects ultimately translate into an enhanced survival after infection with pathogens (Volman *et al.* 2008). In this respect, effects are observed irrespective of the β-glucan source and/or route of administration. It has been suggested that the protective effects of orally administered 1,3 β-glucans are mediated through receptor-mediated interactions with microfold cells – specialised epithelial cells for the transport of macromolecules in the Peyer's patches – which lead to increased cytokine production and enhanced resistance to infection. Therefore, it might be possible to modulate human immune function by increasing the dietary β-glucan intake, for example, by developing functional foods. This may have benefits for specific, immunocompromised target populations like, for example, the elderly or people with type II diabetes but possibly also for athletes involved in heavy training; all of these populations are characterised by some degree of suppression of the (Th1) immune response (Gleeson 2006b). However, one trial in humans found no effect of three weeks of β-glucan supplementation (5.6 g/day) on immune responses to exercise or infection incidence during the two-week period following three successive days of exhaustive exercise (Nieman *et al.* 2008).

Probiotics

Probiotics are food supplements that contain live microorganisms which when administered in adequate amounts confer a health benefit on the host. There is now a reasonable body of evidence that regular consumption of probiotics can modify the population of the gut dwelling bacteria (microbiota) and influence immune function (Matsuzaki 1998; Mengheri 2008; Borchers *et al.*, 2009; Minocha 2009), although it should be noted that such effects are strain specific. Probiotics survive gut transit and modify the intestinal microbiota such that the numbers of beneficial bacteria increase and, usually, numbers of species considered harmful are decreased, which has been associated with a range of potential benefits to the health and functioning of the digestive system, as well as modulation of immune function. Probiotics have many mechanisms of action. By their growth and metabolism, they help to inhibit the growth and to reduce any harmful effects of other bacteria, antigens, toxins and carcinogens in the gut but, in addition, probiotics are known to interact with the gut-associated lymphoid tissue, leading to positive effects on the innate and even the acquired immune system. This is possible because the gut, as the largest surface area of the body, has a significant role to play in immunity, as every day it has to deal with three different immune challenges. Firstly, it must differentiate and tolerate the large commensal microbiota otherwise inflammation will occur and, secondly, it must also tolerate the food antigens. On the other hand, the gut must be able to mount a defence against any potential pathogens when required. This explains why 85% of the body's lymph nodes are located in the gut and why probiotics, as functional foods that target the gut, have the potential to affect the health of the whole body including parts of the body distant from the gut.

Studies have shown that probiotic intake can improve rates of recovery from rotavirus diarrhoea, increase resistance to enteric pathogens, and promote anti-tumour activity. Some evidence even suggests that probiotics may be effective in alleviating some allergic and respiratory disorders in young children (Kopp-Hoolihan 2001). Although, to date, there are few published studies of the effectiveness of probiotic use in athletes, interest is beginning to grow, mostly in examining their potential in helping to maintain overall general health, enhancing immune function or reducing URTI incidence and symptom severity or duration (West *et al.* 2009).

In a double-blind, placebo-controlled, crossover trial in which healthy elite distance runners received the probiotic *Lactobacillus fermentum* or placebo daily for 28 days, with a 28-day washout period between the initial and the second treatment, athletes (n = 20) suffered fewer days of respiratory illness and lower severity of respiratory illness symptoms when taking the daily probiotic (Cox *et al.* 2010c; Figure 9.8). There was also a significant change in the whole blood culture IFN-γ production, with the probiotic treatment eliciting a two-fold greater change in whole-blood culture IFN-γ production compared with placebo, which may be one mechanism underpinning the positive clinical outcomes. In another study in athletes presenting with fatigue and impaired performance and who had a deficit in blood CD4+ (T-helper) cell IFN-γ production compared with healthy control athletes, this apparent T cell impairment was reversed following a one-month course of daily probiotic (*L. acidophilus*) ingestion (Clancy *et al.* 2006).

Another probiotic supplement was investigated in 119 marathon runners who completed a randomised, double-blind intervention study in which they received

Figure 9.8 Number of days of respiratory tract illness (RTI) symptoms for 20 endurance athletes during 1 month of supplementation with a probiotic or placebo. Also shown is the mean severity of RTI symptoms on the probiotic and placebo treatments (data from Cox *et al.* 2010)

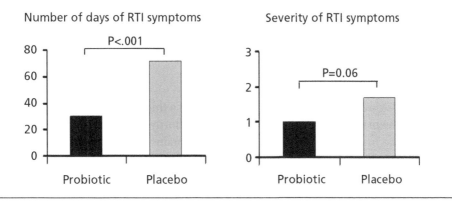

L. rhamnosus GG (LGG, $N = 61$) or placebo ($N = 58$) daily for a three-month training period and then participated in a marathon race with a two-week follow-up of illness symptoms (Kekkonen *et al.* 2007). There were no differences in the number of respiratory infections or gastrointestinal (GI) symptom episodes. Nevertheless, in their conclusions, the authors mentioned that the duration of GI symptom episodes in the LGG group tended to be shorter than in the placebo group during the training period (2.9 compared with 4.3 days) and was significantly shorter during the two weeks after the marathon (1.0 compared with 2.3 days). Caution is needed when interpreting these data, as the percentage of runners who actually suffered GI symptom episodes during the two weeks after the marathon was, as one might expect, low (4% in each group). As such, the sample the authors base their rather speculative conclusion on was small (only two to three runners in each group). In a study on the effect of a *L. casei* probiotic supplement on respiratory tract infection and immune and hormonal changes in soldiers participating in three weeks of commando training followed by a five-day combat course, no difference in infection incidence between groups receiving daily probiotic or placebo was reported (Tiollier *et al.* 2007). Among the immune parameters investigated, the major finding was a significant decrease in salivary SIgA concentration after the combat course in the placebo group, with no change over time in the probiotic group. Another randomised, placebo-controlled trial in 64 university athletes reported a lower incidence of URTI episodes during a four-month winter training period in athletes receiving daily probiotic (*L. casei Shirota*) compared with placebo and this study also reported better maintenance of salivary SIgA in the probiotic group (Gleeson *et al.* 2011b). A meta-analysis using data from both athlete and non-athlete studies involving 3,451 participants concluded that there is a probable benefit in reducing URTI incidence (Hao *et al.* 2011). Further large-scale studies are needed to confirm that taking probiotics can reduce the number of training days lost to infection and to determine the most effective probiotics, as their effects are strain-specific.

From the research reviewed here, one cannot reach a solid conclusion of probiotic benefit for sportspeople but there is now sufficient understanding of the mechanism of action of certain probiotic strains and enough evidence from trials with athletes and sportspeople to signify that this is a promising area of research. Given that some probiotics appear to provide some benefit (Table 9.1), with no evidence of harm and are low cost, there is currently no reason why athletes should not take probiotics, especially if they are travelling abroad or are illness-prone.

Bovine colostrum

Bovine colostrum is the first collection of a thick creamy-yellow liquid, produced by the mammary gland of a lactating cow shortly after birth of her calf, usually within the first 36 hours. Bovine colostrum contains antibodies, growth factors, enzymes, gangliosides (acid glycosphingolipids), vitamins and minerals and is commercially available in both liquid and powder forms. Numerous health claims have been made for bovine colostrum, ranging from performance enhancement to preventing infections, but well-controlled studies in athletes are rare. The gangliosides in bovine colostrum may modify the gut microbial flora and act as decoy targets for bacterial adhesion, as well as having some direct immunostimulatory properties (Rueda 2007). A few studies suggest that several weeks of bovine colostrum supplementation can elevate levels of antibodies in the circulation and saliva. In a study of 35 middle-aged distance runners who consumed a supplement of either bovine colostrum or placebo for 12 weeks, median levels of salivary SIgA increased by 79% in the bovine colostrum group after the 12-week intervention, with no change in the placebo group (Crooks *et al.* 2006). While this result was statistically significant, its physiological interpretation must be viewed with caution, owing to the small numbers in this study and the large variability in salivary SIgA levels. A more recent study reported that four weeks of daily bovine colostrum supplementation prevented exercise-induced falls in salivary lysozyme and speeded the recovery of neutrophil function after two hours of strenuous cycling in healthy men compared with placebo (Davison and Diment 2010). Further studies are needed to confirm and extend these observations of effects on immune responses to exercise and to establish whether bovine colostrum can reduce the incidence of URTIs in athletes (Table 9.1).

CONCLUSIONS AND RECOMMENDATIONS

There are many nutritional supplements on the market that are claimed to 'boost' immunity (see Table 9.1). Unfortunately, the claims for these supplements are often based on selective evidence of efficacy in animals, *in vitro* experiments, children, the elderly or clinical patients in severe catabolic states and direct evidence for their efficacy for preventing the more modest, exercise-induced decrease in immune function or for improving immune function in otherwise healthy athletes is lacking. Some scientists even question the value of using immunonutrition support for athletes because blunting the immune, inflammatory and free radical perturbations that occur during exercise might interfere with the important signalling mechanisms that promote training adaptations (Ristow *et al.* 2009). Nevertheless, exercise training increases the body's requirement for most nutrients and, in most cases, these increased needs are met by increased food consumption. However, some athletes adopt an unbalanced dietary regimen and the poor nutritional status of some athletes very likely predisposes them to immunodepression. Although countering the effects of all of the factors that contribute to exercise-induced immunodepression is impossible, minimising many of the effects is possible and should be a goal for the athlete and support staff. Athletes can help themselves by eating a well-balanced diet that includes adequate carbohydrate, protein and micronutrients. Other factors that may help the athlete maintain immune function and avoid infection include appropriate scheduling of heavy training, competition and rest (Chapter 8), reducing other life stressors and obtaining adequate sleep (Chapter 2) and practising good hygiene and avoiding sick people (Chapter 10).

KEY POINTS

- Decreased nutrient availability during prolonged high-intensity exercise and poor dietary practices during training may be involved in the aetiology of exercise-induced immune depression.
- Whether the immune depression associated with nutrient deficiencies translates into the increased incidence of URTI symptoms observed in athletes remains unclear.
- To maintain immune function, athletes are advised to eat a well-balanced diet with sufficient energy intake to maintain energy balance. This should also ensure an adequate intake of micronutrients.
- Athletes are advised to consume sufficient fluids during exercise and recovery to limit the potential detrimental effects of dehydration on immune function.
- Carbohydrate ingestion during exercise (30–60 g/hour) or shortly after exercise can attenuate some of the immune impairment.
- A high carbohydrate diet will not only optimise athletic performance but may also decrease the immunosuppressive effect of stress hormones.
- Athletes on energy-restricted diets should consider a low-dose multivitamin supplement. Care is needed though because megadoses of some vitamins and minerals can reduce immune responses.
- Current evidence supporting the use of dietary supplements (coined 'immunos-timulants') to prevent or treat common infections in athletes is limited.

FURTHER READING

Albers, R., Antoine, J. M., Bourdet-Sicard, R., Calder, P. C., Gleeson, M., Lesourd, B., Samartin, S., Sanderson, I. R., Van Loo, J., Vas Dias, F. W. and Watzl, B. (2005) Markers to measure immunomodulation in human nutrition intervention studies. *British Journal of Nutrition* 94: 452-481. [This review provides a critical account of the measures used in nutritional immunology studies.]

Walsh, N. P., Gleeson, M., Pyne, D. B., Nieman, D. C., Dhabhar, F. S., Shephard, R. J., Oliver, S. J., Bermon, S. and Kajeniene, A. (2011) Position statement. Part two: Maintaining immune health. *Exercise Immunology Review* 17: 64–103. [Information found on pages 69–73 relates specifically to nutritional countermeasures to exercise-induced immune perturbations.]

10 Practical guidelines on minimising infection risk in athletes

Stéphane Bermon, Michael Gleeson
and Neil P. Walsh

LEARNING OBJECTIVES

After studying this chapter, you should be able to:

- describe the value of monitoring the immune system status of athletes;
- describe some practical guidelines for minimising the risk of developing immunodepression in athletes;
- describe some practical guidelines for minimising exposure to pathogens and reducing the risk of infection in athletes;
- describe some practical guidelines on vaccination and medicines for the travelling athlete;
- describe some practical guidelines about training when suffering from infection and recovery from infection.

INTRODUCTION

Athletes dread the thought of catching a cold or the flu. Infections can interfere with training, impair performance and even prevent an athlete from competing. As you will have realised from the preceding chapters, the functioning of the immune system is affected by stress. There are many different forms of stress: strenuous exercise is one; psychological challenges, under-nutrition and environmental extremes are others. A combination of some of these may be experienced by elite athletes and an accumulation of stress may lead to chronic immunodepression and hence increased susceptibility to opportunistic infections. Although impairment of immune function sometimes leads to the reactivation of a latent virus, the development of a new infection generally requires exposure to a pathogen and there are many situations in which the athlete's exposure to pathogens is increased. Hence, athletes, coaches and their medical support personnel seek guidelines on the ways to reduce the risk of illness, which, when it occurs, is likely to compromise training and competitive performance. This chapter begins by describing the potential value of immune monitoring in athletes and then provides an explanation of the current guidelines that can be given to athletes to minimise the risk of picking up unwanted infections. Although some general guidelines can be given on practical strategies to reduce exposure to pathogens and minimise the degree of stress-induced immunodepression, much current advice is based on speculation. Future experimental studies are required to evaluate and confirm the effectiveness of these strategies in reducing the incidence and severity of illness in athletes.

MONITORING IMMUNE SYSTEM STATUS IN ATHLETES

Blood analysis can serve a useful purpose for athletes as it can sometimes give answers as to why performance has declined for no other obvious reason. It can also serve as a health check and give an indication of an individual's likely susceptibility to infection. A blood test can be used to assess the status of many organ systems, including the heart, liver, kidneys and endocrine glands. However, perhaps the most common tests are those designed to assess the numbers of red and white blood cells and the body's iron status. Some normal values for blood parameters in adult men and women are shown in Table 10.1 and this section explains what these values mean and what the consequences of values outside the normal range can mean. Since red blood cell count and haemoglobin concentration are not directly linked to immune function, these parameters will not be described here.

Table 10.1 Blood test results showing normal ranges for adult men and women

BLOOD MEASURE	MALES	FEMALES
Red blood cell count ($\times 10^{12}$/L)	4.5–6.5	3.8–5.8
Haemoglobin concentration (g/dL)	13.4–17.0	11.5–16.5
Serum ferritin concentration (μg/L)	40–180	12–190
Serum B12 concentration (μg/L)	160–1,100	160–1,100
Serum folate concentration (μg/L)	1.5–20.0	1.5–20.0
Haematocrit percentage (%)	40–50	37–47
White blood cell count ($\times 10^9$/L)	4.0–11.0	4.0–11.0
Neutrophil count ($\times 10^9$/L)	2.0–7.5	2.0–7.5
Lymphocyte count ($\times 10^9$/L)	1.0–3.5	1.0–3.5
Monocyte count ($\times 10^9$/L)	0.2–0.8	0.2–0.8
Eosinophil count ($\times 10^9$/L)	0–0.4	0–0.4
Creatine kinase activity (U/L)[1]	15–110	15–90

[1] U = unit of enzyme activity

Metals

Transition metals such as iron, zinc, manganese and copper have numerous biological roles as both structural and catalytic co-factors for proteins. Therefore these metals are essential for life and it is suggested that approximately 30% of all proteins interact with a metal co-factor. In keeping with the strict requirement for metals in a variety of cellular processes, transition metals are essential for proper immune function (Kehl-Fie *et al.* 2010).

Iron

Iron is an important component of the oxygen-carrying pigment haemoglobin. As an iron deficiency can lead to anaemia (below-normal blood haemoglobin concentration), it is important to maintain normal iron stores. A serum ferritin value below the normal range (Table 10.1) indicates iron deficiency, which is likely to result in the development of anaemia. Ferritin is a serum protein that is used in the tissues of the body to store iron and its concentration (which can be measured by enzyme-linked immunosorbent assay, ELISA) gives a good indicator of the size of the body's iron stores.

Moreover, iron deficiency depresses certain aspects of cell-mediated immunity as well as cytokine secretion/production whereas humoral immunity is unaffected (Munoz *et al.* 2007). On the other hand, iron can be toxic to cells, when present at high concentrations, because of its ability to promote the formation of damaging oxidative radicals. In such situations, several organs tissues (e.g. heart, liver, brain, gonads, skin) can be affected by the iron excess leading to either haemosiderosis or haemochromatosis, which are potentially lethal diseases. Therefore, iron, which is sold over the counter at most chemists, should only be taken on medical advice. It is possible to measure the serum free-iron concentration.

Iron is a key immune regulator of the host-pathogen interaction and its associated morbidity. Indeed, iron is essential for the growth and virulence of most microbial pathogens and one of the host's defence strategies is to reduce iron availability and to deprive micro-organisms of this vital element. The increased expression of hepcidin that accompanies inflammation is also generally viewed as part of the strategy of pathogen iron deprivation, since it leads to a decrease in serum iron levels. In addition, the host produces molecules that directly compete with the infecting micro-organism for iron. One of these molecules is lactoferrin, an iron-binding glycoprotein that is abundantly expressed in mucosal secretions of the respiratory, gastrointestinal and mammary epithelia. Therefore, one can say that there is a real struggle for iron at the host–pathogen interface (Nairz *et al.* 2010).

Magnesium and other minerals important for immune function

The serum concentrations of other minerals important for immune function and exercise performance, such as magnesium and zinc and cooper, can also be determined. Although deeply involved in muscle physiology, magnesium also plays a key role in the immune response. It is a co-factor for immunoglobulin synthesis, C3-convertase, immune-cell adherence, antibody-dependent cytolysis, immuno-globulin (Ig)-M lymphocyte binding, macrophage response to lymphokines and T helper–B cell adherence (Tam *et al.* 2003). Magnesium concentrations can be measured in serum and in erythrocytes. Zinc is critically important for proper immune function, as even a mild zinc insufficiency results in widespread defects in both innate and adaptive immunity (Wintergest *et al.* 2007). There is increasing evidence suggesting that the host actively sequesters zinc during infection to hinder microbial growth. The concentration of zinc in erythrocytes is thought to provide a better measure of body zinc status than the serum zinc concentration, as the latter is more readily influenced by recent food intake. Manganese is essential to normal immune function but, fortunately, manganese deficiency is rare.

Copper is also essential to a normal immune function, including proliferative response and normal phagocytic function of neutrophils and macrophages. Copper status can be assessed by measuring blood copper and its transport protein, cerulo-plasmin, but the first is decreased by concomitant zinc intake and the latter is influenced by inflammation, pregnancy and oral contraceptives.

Serum B12 and folic acid

Vitamin B12 and folic acid are two water-soluble B vitamins that are required for the production of DNA. Hence, they are important for cells (immune cells) that are dividing at rapid rates. This is true of the stem cells of the bone marrow, which are the precursors of both red and white blood cells. A deficiency of B12 and/or folic acid can result in the development of megaloblastic anaemia (lowered blood haemoglobin concentration with increased mean red cell volume).

Vitamin D status

In recent years, it has been recognised that vitamin D is important in maintaining immunity (Kamen and Tangpricha 2010) and several studies indicate that vitamin D status can be suboptimal in both the general population and athletes (Larson-Meyer and Willis 2010), particularly in conditions where exposure to sunlight is limited. Ensuring that the individual has adequate vitamin D status may therefore be helpful and this can be assessed using blood tests to measure the plasma concentration of 25-hydroxy vitamin D.

White blood cells

White blood cells (leukocytes) are the cellular part of the immune system and are very important in surveying the body for infection. They find, trap, neutralise and kill invading pathogens. There are many different types of white blood cells which have specific functions in protecting you against developing infections as described in Chapter 2. Endurance training causes the body to release hormones such as cortisol that can reduce the number and function of white blood cells in the blood. Cortisol is released when the body is stressed; it is known as a 'stress hormone' and the body perceives exercise as a stressor just as it does, for example, in situations such as examinations, moving house, redundancy, bereavement (Khansari *et al.* 1990).

Cortisol levels can become high; for example, if training has been particularly hard, the athlete has been doing very long exercise sessions or many competitions, not eating enough carbohydrate at meals or during training or having inadequate sleep. In contrast, the plasma concentration of testosterone tends to fall during periods of stress. Hence, the plasma ratio of cortisol to testosterone is promoted by some sports scientists as a useful indicator of stress in athletes.

If the total white blood cell count is high, it may be that the athlete has not recovered properly from a training session or that an infection of some kind is present. It is never advisable to train hard with a cold or infection of any kind; essentially, the body's immune system is fighting to keep you healthy, so it does not make sense to stress it more (see section entitled 'Should athletes train during periods of infection?') The best advice is to take a few days off from training until the symptoms of illness have gone. In the long term, fewer days training will be missed by stopping training altogether during illness than keeping training and risking the development of further complications such as post-viral fatigue and overtraining syndrome. These complications may stop an athlete training completely for very long periods of time or ultimately force him or her to retire from their sport.

Neutrophils

Neutrophils are the most abundant white blood cell in the blood circulation, they make up approximately 60% of the total white blood cell count. They act as a first line of defence against invading pathogens (micro-organisms capable of causing illnesses) by destroying them and by stopping them from multiplying in the body. During exercise, more neutrophils enter the bloodstream from the bone marrow and help to clear up damaged muscle fibres. Hence, an individual undergoing endurance training may use up bone marrow reserves of neutrophils faster than a non-training individual and thus low neutrophil levels (quite common in endurance athletes) may affect how the body deals with an invading pathogen. This could leave an individual more susceptible to catching colds and infections. An elevated neutrophil count is usually indicative of an acute bacterial infection.

Lymphocytes

Lymphocytes make up approximately 20–25% of the white blood cell count. They have many functions in the immune system. Lymphocytes are important for producing antibodies (killing agents) against invading pathogens. These cells exhibit a 'memory' capability so that, if the body is invaded again by the same pathogen (e.g. chicken pox, measles), the immune system can react immediately to fight the illness so that symptoms do not normally develop a second time.

More sophisticated (and expensive) tests can distinguish the different types of lymphocytes present which include B cells, T cells and natural killer (NK) cells. There is some value in measuring these subsets, as this may identify individuals who have low numbers of NK cells and therefore tend to be more susceptible to viral infections. Indeed, several studies indicate that susceptibility to infections and cancer is greater

Figure 10.1 Numbers of circulating natural killer (NK) cells among a first team squad of professional football players (English Premier League); blood samples were obtained at rest at the start of preseason training and at the end of the season; horizontal bars represent the mean values

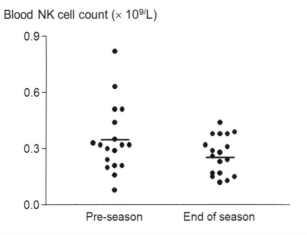

in individuals who possess low NK-cell activity compared with individuals with moderate-high NK-cell activity (Levy *et al.* 1991; Imai *et al.* 2000; Ogata *et al.* 2001). Figure 10.1 illustrates the range in NK-cell counts (CD3-CD56+ cells) among a squad of elite professional soccer players; clearly, among these 25 individuals, there are some that can be identified as having rather low NK-cell counts. Ideally, both NK-cells counts and cytolytic activity should be measured but the latter still remains a non routine laboratory analysis.

Another marker of immune system status that can be obtained from lymphocyte subset analysis is the T-helper/suppressor (CD3+CD4+/CD3+CD8+) ratio. A low value is associated with impaired immunity and increased risk of infection. Quantifying markers of activation such as the expression of CD38, CD69, HLA-DR on T cells can identify individuals who are currently infected. During viral infections, the numbers of cells expressing CD38, HLA-DR and CD45RO are usually increased, as are the numbers of NK cells.

Monocytes

Monocytes make up approximately four to five per cent of the white blood cell count. They have an important role in controlling immune responses and in killing pathogens, including bacteria and viruses. An elevated monocyte count tends to be indicative of a chronic infection.

Eosinophils

Eosinophils are white blood cells involved in reactions to allergies. A higher than normal number of these cells in the circulation generally indicates the presence of an allergic condition (this may include asthma or hay fever). This is especially likely to show up in the summer months when the pollen count is high.

Creatine kinase

Creatine kinase is an enzyme used as an indicator of muscle damage. Damage to skeletal muscle (e.g. by unaccustomed downhill running, weight training, endurance cycling) results in the release of increased levels of creatine kinase into the blood. The normal reference range for the sedentary population (Table 10.1) is frequently exceeded in athletes because regular exercise training involves a certain degree of muscle damage and rebuilding. However, if levels are extremely high (e.g. more than 500 U/L) this can be taken as an indication that training should be reduced before a competition to ensure that the muscles have properly recovered from the last training session. On a week-to-week basis, it is important to incorporate adequate rest days. The minimum recommendation is one day per week where you do only very light training or no exercise at all. It is worth remembering that it is during recovery periods that the body adapts to the training sessions, muscle fibres regenerate and glycogen stores are replenished and, ultimately, with an appropriate period of tapering, the desired 'training effect' of improved performance is gained.

How much do these blood tests cost?

Red cell counts, haemoglobin, haematocrit and a differential white blood cell count can be performed on a single 5-mL blood sample and should cost about €6–12. Measures of serum ferritin, B12, folic acid, free iron, magnesium, zinc and creatine kinase will cost about €12 each. Thus, for the list of parameters shown in Table 10.1, the cost should be about €60. Measuring lymphocyte subsets is more expensive and requires access to a flow cytometer. A lymphocyte subset analysis that gives percentages of NK cells, B cells, T cells and the CD4/CD8 ratio should cost about €35. Measurement of immune cell functions (e.g. neutrophil oxidative burst, mitogen-stimulated lymphocyte proliferation, NK-cell cytolytic activity) is time consuming and expensive (around €60 per test). Furthermore, most immune cell functions have to be measured within a few hours of blood collection. Hence, these measures are usually restricted to research studies and are not really practical for routine monitoring of athletes in training.

Salivary immunoglobulins

The monitoring of changes in the salivary concentrations of immunoglobulins (IgA and IgM) during training has been conducted with some success in elite athletes. Studies on elite Australian swimmers have shown that low levels of saliva secretory IgA (SIgA) are associated with increased incidence of upper respiratory tract infections (URTI; Gleeson 2000b). These studies have also shown that SIgA levels may fall acutely after a training session and that over the course of a seven-month training season, SIgA in saliva samples obtained at rest falls progressively. Hence, this indicator of mucosal immunity can be a useful practical measure that can be used to identify individuals who may be at higher risk of URTI and to monitor the effects of individual and repeated training sessions on mucosal immunity (Neville *et al.* 2008). Salivary IgA values can vary quite markedly between individuals (as illustrated in Figure 10.2) but, as you can see in Figure 6.5, when SIgA is expressed as a percentage of the athlete's known healthy baseline value, the salivary SIgA concentration falls significantly before an URTI episode and hence its regular (e.g. weekly) measurement can aid in the prediction of infection risk among different individuals. Salivary SIgA concentration can be measured by ELISA and some microwell plate kits are commercially available. These cost about €350 for a 96-well kit sufficient for the analysis of 40 samples (and a range of standards) in duplicate. Further developments in technology may soon allow the measurement of salivary SIgA (and possibly cortisol and testosterone as well) using rapid response analysers and possibly even hand-held analysers, which would greatly assist this type of monitoring in field situations (e.g. at the training ground).

Figure 10.2 Salivary IgA concentration measured in samples taken at rest in professional footballers (two first team squads in English premier league), elite swimmers (GB national squad; males: closed circles, females: open circles) and national standard cyclists

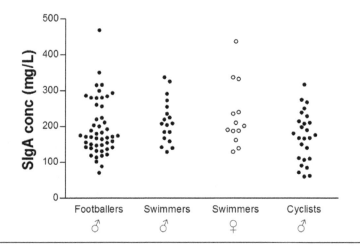

Other salivary antimicrobial proteins

To date, the majority of exercise studies have assessed salivary SIgA as a marker for monitoring immune status in athletes (Gleeson *et al.* 2000b; Neville *et al.* 2008) but, more recently, the importance of other antimicrobial proteins in saliva, including α-amylase, lactoferrin and lysozyme has gained greater recognition (Bishop and Gleeson

2009). These antimicrobial proteins could soon be used for athlete monitoring purposes.

Cytokines

Cytokines modulate post-exercise changes in immune function, possibly increasing the risk of infection or the appearance of inflammatory symptoms mimicking URTI. A study demonstrated decreased anti-inflammatory plasma cytokines (IL-8, IL-10, IL-1ra) at rest and after exercise and increased proinflammatory cytokines (IL-6) in illness-prone distance runners when compared with runners who did not suffer frequent episodes of URTI symptoms (Cox *et al.* 2007). A cytokine gene polymorphism study by the same group (Cox *et al.* 2010a) identified an underlying genetic predisposition to high expression of the proinflammatory IL-6 in athletes prone to frequent URTI symptoms. These studies suggest that not only infections but dysregulated inflammation can cause the symptoms of 'sore throat' (Bermon 2007). The value of measuring circulating or possibly even salivary cytokines for monitoring immune status in athletes has yet to be determined.

TRAINING AND RECOVERY GUIDELINES TO MINIMISE THE RISK OF INFECTION

Infections can interfere with training, impair performance and even prevent an athlete from competing (Reid *et al.* 2004). Unfortunately, athletes engaged in heavy training programmes (e.g. exercising for more than two hours per day at greater than 70% of maximum heart rate), particularly those involved in endurance sports, appear to be more susceptible than normal to infection (see Chapter 1). The most common form of infection in athletes are those that affect the upper respiratory tract. As described in detail in previous chapters the functioning of the immune system is affected by stress and there is some convincing evidence that the increased susceptibility to URTI in athletes actually arises from a depression of immune function. Furthermore, other stressors, including extreme environmental conditions (see Chapter 7), improper nutrition (see Chapter 9), psychological stress and lack of sleep (see Chapter 2) can compound the negative influence of heavy exertion on immunocompetence. An accumulation of stress may lead to chronic immunodepression and hence increased susceptibility to opportunistic infections in athletes (Figure 10.3).

Although impairment of immune function sometimes leads to the reactivation of a latent virus, the development of a new infection generally requires exposure to a pathogen and there are many training and competitive situations in which the athlete's exposure to pathogens is increased (Figure 10.3). During exercise, exposure to airborne pathogens will be increased, owing to the higher rate and depth of breathing. A study in adolescent male soccer players showed that, following a one-hour indoor training session, the colony count of *Staphylococcus aureus* (a bacteria associated with URTI) was significantly increased in the nasal passages (Figure 10.4;

Figure 10.3 Factors contributing to infection incidence in athletes

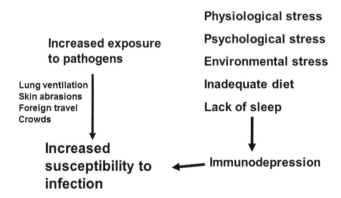

Figure 10.4 Colony count of *Staphylococcus aureus* on the surface of the nasal passages, inner ear and skin and before and after a 1-hour indoor soccer training session in male Malaysian adolescents * *P* < 0.05 compared with before exercise (data from William *et al.* 2004)

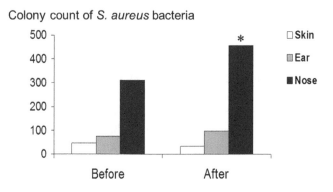

William *et al.* 2004). An increase in gut permeability may also allow increased entry of gut bacterial endotoxins into the circulation, particularly during prolonged exercise in the heat (Bosenberg *et al.* 1988). Some of the lifestyle strategies and training strategies that can be adopted by athletes to minimise the risk of developing immunodepression are listed in Box 10.1 and Table 10.2. Dr David Pyne also discusses strategies for modifying training to limit the risk of immunodepression in the *Exercise Immunology Review* Position Statement (see Recommended reading Walsh *et al.* 2011a).

Box 10.1 Lifestyle strategies for athletes to minimise the risk of immunodepression

- Keep life stress to a minimum.
- Get regular and adequate sleep (at least seven hours per night).
- More rest may be needed after travel across time zones to allow circadian rhythms to adjust.
- Avoid crash dieting and rapid weight loss.
- Ensure adequate total dietary energy, carbohydrate and protein intake.
- A good well-balanced diet should provide all the necessary vitamins and minerals but, if fresh fruit and vegetables are not readily available, multivitamin supplements should be considered.
- Consume carbohydrate drinks (approximately 6% weight by volume) before, during and after prolonged workouts appears to reduce some of the adverse effect of exercise on immune function (around 30–60 grams of carbohydrate per hour during exercise).
- Wear proper outdoor clothing and avoid getting cold and wet after exercise.

Table 10.2 Training strategies to limit immunodepression

TRAINING DESCRIPTOR	COMMENT
Frequency	Increase the frequency of shorter training sessions rather than enduring fewer but longer sessions.
Volume	Reduce the overall weekly training volume and/or volume of individual training sessions.
Intensity	Avoid prolonged intensive training sessions or activities. Employ shorter sharper (spike) sessions mixed with lower-intensity work.
Load (volume x intensity)	Systematically manipulate either the training volume and/or intensity to manage the degree of training load.
Load increments	Reduce the size of increments in frequency, volume, intensity and load of training e.g. increases of 5–10% per week rather than 15–30%.
Load sequencing – weekly microcycle	Undertake two or three easy to moderate training sessions after each high-intensity session rather than the traditional pattern of simply alternating hard with easy sessions.
Load sequencing – multi-week macrocyle	Plan an easier recovery or adaptation week every second or third week rather than using longer 3–6 week cycles with increasing loads.
Recovery – session/week	Implement recovery activities immediately after the most intensive or exhaustive training sessions.
Recovery – season	Permit athletes at heightened risk of illness a longer period of passive and active recovery (several weeks) after completion of a season or major competition.

Source: reproduced with permission from Walsh *et al.* (2011b)

▊ FACTORS DIRECTLY ASSOCIATED WITH EXERCISE TRAINING

As explained in Chapters 4 and 5, the functional capacities of leukocytes may be decreased by acute bouts of prolonged strenuous exercise: the mechanism(s) for which probably involve, amongst other factors, stress hormones (see Chapter 2). Thus, an acute bout of physical activity is accompanied by a temporary depression of several immune cell functions that may provide a temporary period of increased suscepti- bility to infection: the so-called 'open window' hypothesis.

For exercise lasting less than one hour, exercise intensity is the most critical factor in determining the degree of exercise-induced immunosuppression (Nieman *et al.* 1993b, 1994). When subjects cycled for a fixed duration of 45 minutes, immune system perturbations were greater at an intensity of 80% $\dot{V}O_2$ max compared with 50% $\dot{V}O_2$ max (Nieman *et al.* 1993b, 1994). However, others have shown that exercising for three hours at 55% $\dot{V}O_2$ max produced greater changes in leukocyte trafficking, plasma cortisol concentration and neutrophil function than exercising to fatigue in less than an hour at 80% $\dot{V}O_2$ max (Robson *et al.* 1999b). Furthermore, 24 hours after exercise, neutrophil function had recovered to pre-exercise levels after the shorter, higher-intensity bout but neutrophil function was still significantly depressed at this time after the longer bout. Hence, very prolonged exercise sessions, as well as high intensity bouts of shorter duration, appear to threaten the proper immune function of athletes.

Exercise training also modifies immune function, with most changes on balance suggesting an overall decrease in immune system function, particularly when training loads are high, as discussed in Chapter 8. Furthermore, even in well-trained individuals, sudden increases in the training load are accompanied by signs of more severe immunodepression. Given that many reports have linked heavy training with impaired immune function, any training programme should be appropriate to the individual athlete's physical condition and the athlete's responses to the training stress including performance, mood, fatigue, muscle soreness, perception of effort should be monitored closely. Training strategies to minimise the risk of immunodepression need to consider the management of training volume and intensity, training variety to overcome monotony and strain, a periodised and graded approach to increasing training loads, how the training is spread over the course of the day and provision of adequate rest and recovery periods. This implies the use of some means to measure the training load in terms of intensity, as well as duration or distance covered. The availability of heart-rate monitors or power-meters (cycling) makes this possible, so it should be a relatively simple task for the athlete or coach to record and upload to a personal computer a daily log of the time spent by the athlete in specified heart rate zones. A summary of the various methods that can be used to monitor the training load is given in Table 10.3.

Many factors can increase the stress hormone response to exercise and some of these are listed below and have been discussed in detail elsewhere in this textbook:

- fasting (Chapter 9)

- low glycogen stores (Chapter 9)
- dehydration (Chapter 9)
- hypoglycaemia (Chapter 9)
- heat (Chapter 7)
- cold (Chapter 7)
- altitude (hypoxia) (Chapter 7)
- psychological stress (Chapter 2)
- sleep deprivation (Chapter 2)
- jet-lag and travel across time zones (Chapter 2).

Since these factors may therefore increase the degree and duration of exercise-induced immunodepression, it is important that the impact of these factors is kept to a minimum. Training has to be hard if athletes are going to compete successfully but the training should be managed to avoid the risk of immunodepression (see 'load increments' and 'load sequencing' in Table 10.2). On days where the training load is high, training should be split into two or more sessions. Prolonged immunodepression is more likely to develop if all the exercise on a hard training day is done in a single session. When an increase in the weekly training load is planned, it is probably advisable to limit the increase to no more than 5–10% above the previous week's load.

Monitoring the athlete for signs of impending overtraining

Given that overtraining is commonly associated with recurrent infections, it is important that this condition is prevented from developing. Ways of monitoring athletes for signs of impending overtraining have received increasing attention and several markers were discussed in Chapter 8. Heart-rate monitoring could be used to help detect the early stages of overtraining and the most commonly observed features are increased resting heart rate and/or decreased maximal heart rate and/or altered heart rate variability (Baumert *et al.* 2006). Sleep disturbance is a common symptom in overtrained athletes (Budgett 1990) and chronic lack of sleep is itself associated with impaired immunity (see Chapter 2 and Walsh *et al.* 2011a). Athletes should be encouraged to get adequate sleep and seven hours sleep per night is probably the minimum required by most. Some studies have reported lower blood lactate responses during submaximal exercise tests in overtrained athletes. The reduced blood lactate response to exercise in the overtrained state contrasts with the elevated blood lactate response to exercise following exercise-induced muscle damage described by Gleeson *et al.* (1995c, 1998) and may offer a means of distinguishing between overtraining and overreaching.

The immune system is extremely sensitive to stress – both physiological and psychological – and thus, potentially, immune variables could be used as a sensor of stress in relation to exercise training (see Chapter 8 for further details). Regular monitoring of immune variables (e.g. salivary SIgA) could provide a diagnostic window for evaluating the impact of acute and chronic exercise on health (Pedersen

Table 10.3 Practical tools to monitor training adaptation and progression into the underperformance syndrome

TOOL	DESCRIPTION	EVIDENCE FOR EFFICACY/ LIMITATIONS	RATING[1]
Diaries, questionnaires, sleep and resting HR: Diaries, POMS, DALDA, TQR and RESTQ-Sport. Sleep and HR_{rest}	A variety of self-report questionnaires for monitoring mood, exertion, life demands and recovery. Simple monitors (e.g. Actigraph) can assess sleep quantity and quality.	Limited information on predicting progression to UPS. Issues with compliance, particularly for lengthy questionnaires. Remains unclear whether the quantity and quality of sleep identifies progression into UPS. Probably most effective when used in conjunction with other tools listed.	●●●○○
Training load: Distance, time, speed, power etc. HR zones, TRIMP,[2] session RPE	Some simple, yet descriptive, tools now easily monitored with GPS/power meters etc. HR, TRIMP and session RPE provide more specific information about training stress.	Training load assessment can be subjective (e.g. session RPE). Nevertheless, session RPE may be useful when HR monitors are unavailable. TRIMP provides information beyond HR alone but has limited utility for exercise above the anaerobic (lactate) threshold. Probably most effective when used in conjunction with other tools listed.	●●●○○
Exercise and performance testing: Sub-maximal and maximal exercise testing	Assess blood lactate and other neuroendocrine responses (e.g. plasma ACTH, cortisol) to an exercise test.	Maximal lactate response is reduced in UPS. Utility of lactate and neuroendocrine responses to exercise tests to track progression into (and recovery from) UPS is mixed. Probably most effective when used in conjunction with other tools listed.	●●○○○
Exercise performance tests:	Exercise performance tests are essential to diagnose UPS.	Useful to identify recovery from intensified training. Less useful to confirm recovery from UPS as fitness will likely decrease during UPS. Exercise performance tests should be sport specific. Probably most effective when used in conjunction with other tools listed.	●●●●○

Notes:
[1] Rating is based upon supporting evidence and utility of the tool for implementation on a continuum where: ○○○○○ indicates no supporting evidence/utility and ●●●●● indicates very strong supporting evidence/utility.
[2] TRIMP (training impulse) is calculated using training duration, maximal heart rate (HR), resting HR and average HR during the training session
ACTH = adrenocorticotrophic hormone; DALDA = daily analysis of life demands for athletes; POMS = profile of mood state; RPE = rating of perceived exertion; TQR = total quality recovery; UPS = unexplained underperformance syndrome

and Bruunsgaard 1995; Gleeson 2000b; Neville *et al.* 2008) and identifying athletes who are most at risk of developing infections. The main drawback here is that measures of immune function are expensive and usually limited to just one aspect of what is a multi-faceted system containing much redundancy. Hormones have also been suggested as potential markers of overtraining but no consistent and reproducible hormonal changes have been reported in overtrained athletes. A summary of the potential value of various biochemical, haematological and immuno-logical markers as indicators of training stress, overreaching and impending overtraining is shown in Table 10.4.

Nutritional factors (see Chapter 9)

Athletes can help themselves by eating a well-balanced diet that includes adequate intake of energy, carbohydrate, protein and micronutrients. Consumption of carbohydrate drinks during training is recommended, as this practice appears to attenuate some of the immunosuppressive effects of prolonged exercise, provided that exercise is not continued to the point of fatigue. Results for most nutritional supplements tested as countermeasures to exercise-induced inflammation, oxidative stress and immune dysfunction following heavy exertion have been disappointing. Athletes may benefit from an increased intake of antioxidants but the dangers of excessive over-supplementation of micronutrients should be highlighted. Many micronutrients given in quantities beyond a certain threshold can reduce immune responses, impair the absorption of other micronutrients or have toxic effects. Moreover, the real benefit of immuno-nutritional support for athletes has been challenged because it is suspected to interfere with important signalling mechanisms for training adaptations (Ristow *et al.* 2009), by partially blocking immune changes, oxidative stress and inflammation. Hence, in general, supplementation of individual micronutrients or consumption of large doses of simple antioxidant mixtures is not recommended. The most effective nutritional strategies to maintain robust immune function during intensive training are to avoid deficiencies of essential micronu-trients, to ingest carbohydrate during exercise and ingest Lactobacillus probiotics on a daily basis. When cold symptoms begin, there is some evidence that taking zinc lozenges at this time (greater than 75 mg zinc/day; high ionic zinc content) can reduce the number of days that illness symptoms last. Ensuring that the individual has adequate vitamin D status may also be helpful and this can be assessed using blood tests to measure the plasma concentration of 25-hydroxy vitamin D.

Psychological factors (see Chapter 2)

Although acute psychological stressors can evoke a temporary increase in some aspects of immune function, various forms of chronic psychological stress very clearly have the opposite effect. Traumatic life events such as bereavement, divorce and prolonged care of an aged or disabled relative are perceived as stressful and generally result in depressed immune function and increased incidence of infection. Elite athletes have

Table 10.4 Biochemical, haematological and immunological tools to monitor training adaptation, progression into the unexplained underperformance syndrome and immune health in athletes

TOOL	DESCRIPTION	EVIDENCE FOR EFFICACY/ LIMITATIONS	RATING[1]
Biochemical:			
Free testosterone: cortisol ratio	May provide an indicator of anabolic/catabolic balance; can be assessed in both blood and saliva.	May indicate response to training but cannot identify UPS. A low free testosterone: cortisol ratio (>30% below normal) indicates over-reaching. Unclear how these changes relate to performance. Costly and time consuming.	●●○○○
Plasma glutamine	Non-essential amino acid; important fuel for immune cells; ratio to glutamate may indicate training stress.	Plasma glutamine decreases in response to intensified training, over-reaching and UPS. Ratio to glutamate has been shown to indicate training intolerance. Requires blood sample. Costly and time consuming.	●●●○○
Blood CK and CRP	Indicators of muscle damage and inflammation.	Not suitable to indicate training adaptation, overreaching or UPS. Some utility to exclude other explanations for underperformance. Requires blood sample. Costly and time consuming.	●○○○○
Serum iron, ferritin and transferrin	Indicators of inflammation and chronic recovery; iron deficiency can lead to anaemia.	May be reduced in chronically exercising individuals, particularly during high intensity training. Decrease may negatively affect performance. Requires blood sample. Costly and time consuming.	●●○○○
Haematological:			
Red blood cell count, haemoglobin and haematocrit	Standard clinical laboratory tests.	Normal clinical ranges established. These tests cannot detect over-reaching or UPS. Useful for determining overall health status. Can be performed on finger prick rather than venous blood sample.	●●○○○
Immunological:			
Blood leukocyte counts	Standard clinical laboratory test provides total leukocytes and differential counts (neutrophils, lymphocytes, monocytes etc.).	Normal clinical ranges established. Some evidence of lowered leukocyte counts during intensified training, over-reaching and UPS. May indicate response to training but cannot identify UPS. Altered differential counts may indicate infection. Costly and time consuming.	●●○○○
Blood lymphocyte subset counts	Flow cytometric analysis of lymphocyte subsets (e.g. T-helper/suppressor CD4+/ CD8+ ratio).	A low T-helper/suppressor lymphocyte ratio is associated with impaired immunity and increased risk of infection. Some T-lymphocyte markers (CD38, CD69, HLA-DR) can identify individuals who are currently infected. Cannot identify UPS. Extremely costly and time consuming limits utility.	●●○○○

Table 10.4 continued			
TOOL	DESCRIPTION	EVIDENCE FOR EFFICACY/ LIMITATIONS	RATING[1]
Functional immune assays	Well-equipped laboratories can make measurements of immune function (e.g. neutrophil phagocytic activity, natural killer cell activity etc).	Typically requires a fresh blood sample. Extremely costly and time consuming limits utility.	●○○○○
Blood cytokines	Well-equipped laboratories use ELISA to assess cytokines in plasma and possibly saliva.	Preliminary evidence that illness prone athletes have higher plasma inflammatory (e.g. IL-6) and lower anti-inflammatory (e.g. IL-1ra) cytokines. *In vitro* vaccine-stimulated cytokine response also used. Extremely costly and time consuming limits utility.	●●○○○
Saliva AMPs	Assessment of saliva IgA and other AMPs important for host defence using ELISA.	Good evidence that decreases in salivary IgA track infection during training and competition. Less is known about salivary AMPs and infection in athletes. Not suitable as markers of over-reaching or UPS. Highly variable both within and between participants. Variability likely owing to poor standardisation of saliva collection, handling and reporting. Costly and time consuming.	●●●○○
In vivo immune tests	Blood antibody response to influenza vaccination. Skin DTH tests including recall antigens (e.g. Mantoux) and novel antigens (e.g. DPCP).	Represents a co-ordinated, integrated immune response. Clinically relevant and responsive to stress. Cannot identify UPS. Limited data in athletes. Blood antibody measurements are costly and time consuming which limits utility. DPCP skin test is cheap, quick and skinfold response (skin thickening) is easy to measure. Temporary erythema (reddening) at skin site and slight itchiness may discourage some participants.	●●●○○

Notes:
[1] Rating is based upon supporting evidence and utility of the tool for implementation on a continuum where: ○○○○○ indicates no supporting evidence/utility and ●●●●● indicates very strong supporting evidence/utility
AMP = antimicrobial protein; CK = creatine kinase; CRP = C-reactive protein; DPCP = diphenylcyclopropenone; DTH = delayed type hypersensitivity; ELISA = enzyme-linked immunosorbent assay; IgA = immunoglobulin A; IL = interleukin; UPS = underperformance syndrome

to train hard to compete successfully, so some degree of physical training stress is unavoidable. In addition, there is the added psychological stress of competition, team and commercial pressures, international travel, selection pressures, funding pressures and other major life events. The aim of the coach, working with a sport psychologist, should be to anticipate these additional stressors and, through appropriate evaluation and planning, eliminate or minimise as far as possible their impact upon the athlete.

During training, psychological profiling may be undertaken to some effect using self-scored profiles of mood states (POMS); some scientists believe that the best gauge of excessive training stress is how the athlete feels. The abbreviated POMS scale (Morgan *et al.* 1987) or the Daily Analysis of Life Demands in Athletes (Figure 10.5; Rushall 1990) are examples of simple questionnaires that can be used on a daily basis to assess the impact of training on the athlete's psyche. Gauging sensations of muscle soreness and fatigue during and after each training session has also been recommended (Noakes, 1992) and may be an effective way of monitoring the recovery from deliberate overreaching and identifying early development of overtraining syndrome.

Figure 10.5 Daily analyses of life demands in athletes (DALDA) questionnaire (from Rushall 1990)

Part A Sources of stress

	A	B	C	
1				Diet
2				Home life
3				School/College/Work
4				Friends
5				Sport training
6				Climate
7				Sleep
8				Recreation
9				Health

A = Worse than normal; **B** = Same as normal; **C** = Better than normal

Total **A** response _____

Total **B** response _____

Total **C** response _____

Part B Symtoms of stress

	A	B	C	
1				Muscle pains
2				Techniques
3				Tiredness
4				Need for a rest
5				Supplementary work
6				Boredom
7				Recovery time
8				Irritability
9				Weight
10				Throat
11				Internal
12				Unexplained aches
13				Technique strength
14				Enough sleep
15				Between sessions recovery
16				General weakness
17				Interest
18				Arguments
19				Skin rashes
20				Congestion
21				Training effort
22				Temper
23				Swellings
24				Likability
25				Running nose

A = Worse than normal; **B** = Same as normal; **C** = Better than normal

Total **A** response _____

Total **B** response _____

Total **C** response _____

Travel, jetlag and sleep disruption

With frequent international competitions now being the norm in many sports, competitors are faced with regular air travel, with the associated problems of sleeplessness and jetlag. Travelling for many hours in a confined space, with several hundred other individuals (a certain proportion of which are bound to have infections) and rebreathing the same dry air in hypobaric conditions is highly conducive to the spread of infection. Precautions including the wearing of a filter mask, maintaining hydration, avoiding alcohol and trying to get some sleep are recommended. As far as sleep disruption is concerned, studies involving athletes are lacking; although, one study has shown that sleep quality (percentage of time spent in bed asleep) but not sleep quantity was poorer in athletes than age and sex matched non-athletic controls (Leeder *et al.* 2012). The authors show the benefit of using simple wristwatch actigraphy to monitor the quantity and quality of sleep in athletes that Walsh and colleagues highlighted recently (Walsh *et al.* 2011a). Another interesting rhinovirus nasal inoculation study reported a three-fold higher common cold incidence in humans sleeping less than seven hours per night when compared with those sleeping more than eight hours per night. In this study, sleep quality was also inversely correlated with the infection rate (Cohen *et al.* 2009).

Environmental factors (see Chapter 7)

Athletes are often required to compete in extremes of heat or cold. For many endurance athletes, periods of training at altitude may be required. Exercising in these environmental extremes is associated with an increased stress hormone response and perception of effort. For cold, the limited evidence does not support the contention that athletes training and competing in cold conditions experience a greater reduction in immune function than those exercising under thermoneutral conditions. As far as altitude is concerned, some evidence supports the belief that high-altitude exposure increases URTI and decreases cell-mediated immunity. There has been substantial interest in the effects of heat exposure on immune function for many years. It is well known that the growth and replication rates of certain bacteria, viruses and fungi are impaired by high temperatures. Of course, our own body reacts to infections by increasing body core temperature after production of the endogenous pyrogens, including IL-6, which enhance the individual's resistance to infection. Body temperature also increases a few degrees during strenuous exercise and might lead to exertional heat illness (core temperature above 40°C). With the exception of this condition, laboratory studies showed that exercising in the heat does not impair immune function when compared to thermoneutral conditions (Walsh *et al.* 2011a).

HYGIENE PRACTICE AND MEDICAL SUPPORT

Other behavioural lifestyle changes, such as good hygiene practice, may limit transmission of contagious illnesses by reducing exposure to common sources of infection, including airborne pathogens and physical contact with infected individuals. Some simple strategies that athletes can use to minimise the potential for transmission of infectious agents are listed in Box 10.2. The most important of these are good hand hygiene and avoiding close contact with people who are infected. Hand washing (with the correct technique to ensure all parts of hands are cleaned effectively) with soap and water (Figure 10.6) is effective against most pathogens but does not provide continuous protection. Hand gels containing over 60% alcohol disinfect effectively but the protection they provide does not last long (only a few minutes), so they need to be applied frequently and this can cause skin drying and irritation. Other sanitisation methods include the use of non-alcohol based antimicrobial hand foams (e.g. Byotrol™ products, which contain a mixture of cationic biocides and hydrophobic polymers) that are claimed to disinfect hands for up to six hours. However, individuals need to be aware that these products are removed by hand washing and excessive sweating and so really need to be reapplied every few hours.

Figure 10.6 Hand disinfection technique: ensure that all parts of hands are effectively washed

HAND DISINFECTION TECHNIQUE

Whichever method is used, ensure *all* of the hand is covered

Pay attention to finger tips and back of hands!

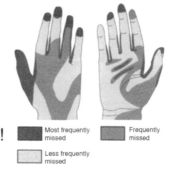

Most frequently missed

Frequently missed

Less frequently missed

Other simple, commonsense practical strategies to limit pathogen exposure include avoiding touching hands to the eyes, nose and mouth, as microbes often gain entry at these sites if hands are contaminated, and limiting contact with surfaces such as door handles that may have been contaminated by others (Figure 10.7). Personal items, such as drinks bottles and towels (Figure 10.8) should not be shared with others, to reduce the risk of cross-contamination.

> **Box 10.2** Practical guidelines for prevention of transmission of infections among athletes (from Walsh *et al.* 2011b)
>
> - Check that your athletes are up-to-date on all vaccines needed at home and for foreign countries, should they travel abroad for training and competition.
> - Minimise contact with infected/sick people, young children, animals and potentially contaminated objects.
> - Avoid self-inoculation by not touching the eyes, nose and mouth. Microbes often gain entry at these sites if hands are contaminated.
> - Keep at distance (over one metre) from people who are coughing, sneezing or have a 'runny nose' and, when appropriate, wear or ask them to wear a disposable mask.
> - Wash hands regularly, before meals and after direct contact with potentially contagious people (e.g. after shaking hands), animals, blood, secretions, public places and bathrooms.
> - Carry hand sanitising gel or foam (e.g. Byotrol™) with you where lavatories are not available or not clean enough.
> - Do not share drinking bottles, cups, towels, etc.
> - While competing or training abroad, choose cold drinks from sealed bottles, avoid crude vegetables and meat. Wash and peel fruits before eating.
> - Quickly isolate a team member with infection symptoms and move out his/her roommate.
> - Protect airways from being directly exposed to very cold and dry air during strenuous exercise, by using a face mask.
> - Wear flip-flop or thongs when going to the showers, swimming pool and locker rooms to avoid dermatological diseases.
> - Maintain good oral hygiene; brush teeth regularly and consider using an antiseptic mouthwash morning and evening.
> - Remember that good personal hygiene and thoughtfulness are the best defences against infection.

Although impairment of immune function sometimes leads to reactivation of a latent Epstein-Barr virus (EBV; Eichner 1987, Gleeson 2000b), which is widely prevalent in the young population, the development of clinical infection generally involves exposure to an external pathogen. The most frequent pathogens are viruses such as rhinovirus, influenza A and B, parainfluenza, adenovirus, EBV (primo-infection or reactivation) and coronavirus (Walsh *et al.* 2011b).

Medical support, including regular check-ups, appropriate immunisation and prophylaxis may be particularly important for athletes who are at high risk of succumbing to recurrent infection. Athletes should ensure that their schedule of immunisation is updated regularly (Table 10.5 and see www.cdc.gov/vaccines [USA]; http://immunisation.dh.gov.uk/category/the-green-book and www.nhs.uk/Planners/vaccinations/Pages/Adultshub.aspx [UK]), paying particular attention to the viruses which are prevalent at venues of international competition. Influenza vaccines are available each year and these are probably most effective if given in the autumn for

Figure 10.7 Avoiding infection: avoid touching hands to the eyes, nose and mouth. Microbes often gain entry at these sites if hands are contaminated. Limit contact with surfaces that may have been contaminated by others (e.g. door handles)

AVOIDING INFECTION

Avoid touching these (your own!) as much as possible

- Eyes

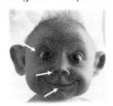

- Nose

- Mouth

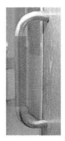

Door handles
- Avoid contact with the most frequently touched area
- Avoid using whole hand

Figure 10.8 Avoiding infection: avoid sharing personal items

AVOIDING INFECTION

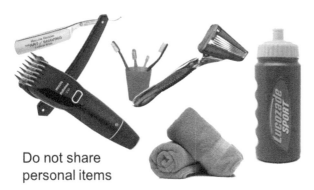

Do not share personal items

athletes who will be competing in the winter months when the prevalence of flu is generally highest.

Table 10.5 Recommended immunisations for adults	
VACCINE	SCHEDULE
Hepatitis B	3 doses (0, 1–2 and 4–6 months)
Influenza	1 dose annually before influenza season
Diptheria, tetanus, pertussis	1 dose and booster every 10 years
Human papilloma virus	3 doses
Measles, mumps, rubella	1 or 2 doses
Varicella (chickenpox)	2 doses (0, 4–8 weeks)
Hepatitis A	2 doses (0, 1–2 and 4–6 months)
Meningococcal	1 dose

Source: US Centers for Disease Control and Prevention, 2012; updates can be found at www.cdc.gov/vaccines

MEDICATION FOR COUGHS, COLDS AND FLU

Colds and influenza (flu) are caused by viruses that are transmitted from person to person. Colds and flu are three to four times more common in the winter months. The symptoms of a cold are sneezing, runny nose and headache and will usually last for a few days. A sore throat may also develop which can make eating, swallowing and even talking difficult. The runny nose is caused by the increased mucous secretion of inflamed nasal passages and the headache results, at least in part, from blockage of the sinuses, leading to sinus pressure and pain above and below the eyes. The mucous membranes of the nose and upper respiratory tract can become irritated by cold, flu or allergies. This causes them to become inflamed and produce excess mucous.

With more severe colds, a fever may develop that is accompanied by shivering, tiredness and aches and pains. Flu usually lasts longer than a cold and the symptoms, although similar in nature, are often more severe. Flu is often associated with feelings of weakness and fatigue and these sensations probably arise, owing to the actions of cytokines on the brain.

A vast variety of medicines are available to treat colds and flu when they do occur. The most common cause is a viral infection and so antibiotics will generally be ineffective. Most cold remedies do not require a prescription and contain one or more pain-killers with anti-inflammatory actions (e.g. aspirin, paracetamol, ibuprofen), decongestants (e.g. phenylephrine, oxymetazoline, menthol) and stimulants (e.g. caffeine). It is important to keep in mind that some over-the-counter cold and flu remedies (those that contain ephedrine, pseudoephedrine, methylephedrine, thuaminoheptane) are included in the current World Anti Doping Agency (WADA) list of banned substances (WADA 2013). Athletes and support staff are recommended to check the medication status before using it. The WADA prohibited list changes frequently and can be found online (www.wada-ama.org) and a particularly useful website allows searches by brand name (www.globaldro.com). Sore throats can be eased by sucking lozenges that contain compounds with local anaesthetic and antiseptic actions (e.g. hexylresorcinol and benzalkonium). For the treatment of extremely painful throats, sprays containing the local anaesthetic lidocaine are available.

Coughing is a reflex reaction to irritation at the back of the throat or to congestion in the lungs and helps clear congestion. A dry or tickly cough is when you have an itchy or tickly feeling at the back of your throat and no phlegm or mucous is produced when coughing. This type of cough can lead to a dry and sore throat and can be treated by a dry cough syrup, liquid or pastilles containing dextromethorphan. Inhaling steam can help to break up phlegm or mucous in the lungs for a chesty cough.

Once the athletes have obtained advice from their doctor concerning the remedies that they can take without contravening the doping laws, it is advisable for athletes to carry a supply of these with them when travelling away from home. The presence of ulcers on the tonsils or a chesty cough producing a yellow/green mucous may indicate the presence of a bacterial infection (note that both viral and bacterial infections can be present simultaneously). A five- to seven-day course of antibiotics (e.g. penicillin, erythromycin, tetracycline, ciprofloxacin) is likely to be the most effective treatment for this and in some countries (including the UK) can only be obtained with a prescription issued by a qualified doctor. Quinolones (an antibiotic family including ciprofloxacin) should be used with caution in high-level athletes, since they can induce severe and lasting Achilles tendinopathies (Melhus 2005).

Antibiotics are ineffective against viral illness. One double-blind, placebo-controlled cross-over trial study examined the effectiveness of prophylactic administration of the antiviral agent valaciclovir for control of EBV reactivation and upper respiratory symptoms in elite distance runners (Cox *et al.* 2004). Although valaciclovir treatment resulted in an 82% reduction in the detectable EBV load in saliva for EBV seropositive runners compared with the placebo treatment, salivary SIgA concentration and the incidence of upper respiratory symptoms were unchanged over the course of the study.

Dietary supplements that are claimed to 'boost' immune function seem to be a popular choice with athletes (see Chapter 9). Unfortunately, the evidence supporting the use of dietary supplements to prevent or treat the common cold is weak. A Cochrane meta-analysis has shown that therapy with megadoses of vitamin C that was initiated after the onset of cold symptoms had no effect on cold duration. The authors concluded that the failure of vitamin C supplementation to reduce the duration of colds in the normal population indicates that megadose vitamin C treatment for the common cold is not generally justified (Douglas *et al.* 2007). There is some evidence, albeit patchy, that suggests taking zinc supplements can reduce the incidence of URTI (Veverka *et al.* 2009). In the studies that have reported a beneficial effect of zinc lozenges in treating the common cold (i.e. reduction of symptom duration, severity or both) zinc lozenges (with high ionic zinc content and ingesting greater than 75 mg zinc/day) had to be taken within 24 hours of the onset of symptoms to be of any benefit (Hemila 2011). Some herbal medicines (e.g.

Pelargonium sidoides, Kaloba®) seem to be reasonably effective in reducing severity and/or duration of symptoms of sinusitis, bronchitis and the common cold but are probably not any more effective than the usual over-the-counter cold remedies that can be purchased from the local pharmacy. The daily ingestion of probiotics may also confer some benefit to immune function and reduce the risk of both respiratory and gastrointestinal infections (Gleeson *et al.* 2012c; Hao *et al.* 2011). Further discussion of these and other dietary immunostimulants can be found in Chapter 9.

SHOULD ATHLETES TRAIN DURING PERIODS OF INFECTION?

When an athlete is suffering from an infection some deterioration in performance is to be expected (Reid *et al.* 2004). It is important for the team doctor to determine whether there is a systemic viral infection present. A simple URTI requires no more than some reduction in training load, with the use of a symptomatic treatment ensuring that the prescribed medication does not breach the anti-doping rules. If the individual has developed a systemic viral illness (e.g. with symptoms below the neck, including swollen glands, aching joints and muscles, vomiting, diarrhoea, fatigue, chesty cough), exercise should be stopped for several days (Budgett 1990). Heavy training can increase the severity and duration of such disease. Iron supplements should not be taken during periods of infection. Although rare, enteroviral infections of muscle and myocarditis have been known to result, with incapacitating and life-threatening consequences. A summary of the advice that can be given to athletes and coaches regarding training when infection is present is provided in Box 10.3. Advice for exercise training upon return from infection is provided in Box 10.4.

Box 10.3 Guidelines for exercise during episodes of upper respiratory tract or gastrointestinal infections in athletes (from Walsh *et al.* 2011b)

First day of illness:

- No strenuous exercise or competitions when experiencing URTI symptoms such as sore throat, coughing, runny or congested nose. No exercise when experiencing symptoms like muscle/joint pain and headache, fever and generalised feeling of malaise, diarrhoea or vomiting. Drink plenty of fluids, keep from getting wet and cold, and minimise life stress.
- Consider use of topical therapy with nasal drainage, decongestants and analgesics if feverish. Report illness to a team physician or health care personnel and keep away from other athletes if you are part of a team training or travelling together.

Second day of illness:

- If body temperature above 37.5–38 degrees Celsius or increased coughing, diarrhoea or vomiting: no training. If no fever or malaise and no worsening of 'above the neck' symptoms: light exercise (pulse less than 120 beats per minute) for 30–45 minutes, indoors during winter and by yourself.

Third day of illness:

- If fever and upper respiratory tract or gastrointestinal symptoms are still present, consult your physician. In gastrointestinal cases, antibiotics should be taken if unformed stools occur more than four times a day or for fever, blood, pus or mucus in stools. If no fever or malaise and no worsening of initial symptoms: moderate exercise (pulse less than 150 beats per minute) for 45–60 minutes, preferably indoors and by yourself.

Fourth day of illness:

- If no symptom relief, do not try to exercise but make an office visit to your doctor. Stool cultures or examination for ova and parasites should generally be reserved for cases that last beyond 10–14 days. If first day of improved condition, follow the guidelines in Box 10.4.

Box 10.4 Guidelines for return to exercise after infections (from Walsh et al. 2011b)

- Wait one day without fever and with improvement of upper respiratory tract or gastrointestinal symptoms before returning to exercise.
- Stop physical exercise and consult your physician if a new episode with fever or worsening of initial symptoms or persistent coughing and exercise-induced breathing problems occur.
- Use the same number of days to step up to normal training as spent off regular training because of illness.
- Observe closely your tolerance to increased exercise intensity and take an extra day off if recovery is incomplete.
- Use proper outdoor clothing and specific cold air protection for airways when exercising in temperatures below 10°C the first week after URTI.

KEY POINTS

- Monitoring of selected immune variables may help to identify individual athletes who may be at higher risk for URTI. Blood monitoring can also be useful to pick up deficiencies of some micronutrients (e.g. iron, zinc, magnesium, vitamin B12, folic acid) that could impair both immune function and exercise performance.
- The immune system is extremely sensitive to stress – both physiological and psychological – and athletes fail to perform to the best of their ability if they become infected or stale. Excessive training with insufficient recovery can lead to recurrent infections and a debilitating syndrome in which performance and wellbeing can be affected for months.
- Training strategies to minimise the risk of immunodepression need to consider the management of training volume and intensity, training variety to overcome monotony and strain, a periodised and graded approach to increasing training loads and provision of adequate rest and recovery periods.

- Nutritional considerations should emphasise the need for adequate intakes of energy, fluid, carbohydrate, protein and micronutrients. Ensuring the recovery of glycogen stores on a day-to-day basis and consuming carbohydrate during exercise appear to be ways of minimising some of the immunodepression associated with an acute bout of exercise.
- To limit the effects of psychological stress athletes should be taught self-management and coping skills and benefit may be gained from monitoring athletes' responses to the psychological and psychosocial stresses of high-level training and competition.
- Limiting initial exposure when training or competing in adverse environmental conditions (heat, humidity, cold, altitude, sleep disruption), and acclimatising where appropriate will reduce the effects of environmental stress.
- Other behavioural, lifestyle changes such as good hygiene practice, may limit transmission of contagious illnesses by reducing exposure to common sources of infection. Medical support including regular check ups, appropriate immunisation and prophylaxis may be particularly important for athletes who are at high risk of succumbing to recurrent infection.

FURTHER READING

Ronsen, O. (2005) Prevention and management of respiratory tract infections in athletes. *New Studies in Athletics* 20: 49–56.

Walsh, N. P., Gleeson, M., Pyne, D. B., Nieman, D. C., Dhabhar, F. S., Shephard, R. J., Oliver, S. J., Bermon, S. and Kajeniene, A. (2011) Position statement. Part two: Maintaining immune health. *Exercise Immunology Review* 17: 64–103.

11 Allergy in sport

Paula Robson-Ansley

LEARNING OBJECTIVES

After studying this chapter, you should be able to:

- describe the allergic response to inhalant allergens such as grass, dust house mites;
- explain the classification of allergens;
- discuss the potential impact of exercise on T-helper cell polarisation and the allergic response;
- describe the clinical tests which are used to identify sensitisation to allergens;
- understand effective management recommendations for the treatment of allergy in athletes;
- understand the rare condition of exercise-induced anaphylaxis.

INTRODUCTION

This chapter discusses immunoglobulin (Ig)E-mediated allergy in the context of sport and exercise. IgE-mediated allergy is the most common type of allergic disease, although allergy may involve other immunological mechanisms as seen in contact allergies (affecting the skin) and allergic alveolitis (affecting the lungs). It is important to define common terms used within the allergy literature to avoid confusion as often terms are used interchangeably. If an individual is classified as 'atopic' then they have an exaggerated IgE response to allergens. Atopy is associated with a predisposition to develop allergic disease. Whereas, if a person is 'allergic' to an allergen then they will have a heightened IgE level and also display clinical symptoms when in the presence of the allergen (e.g. itchy eyes, running nose). Allergy is the clinical expression of atopic disease such as asthma, rhinitis, eczema, food allergy. Between 30% and 40% of individuals in developed countries are atopic whereas only a proportion will have allergic diseases such as rhinitis (10–20%) and asthma (5–10%) (Sunyer *et al.* 2004). This chapter focuses on inhalant, airborne allergens to which athletes are most exposed in their training environment; the scope of this chapter does not extend to discussing food, drug or insect allergies.

UPPER RESPIRATORY TRACT SYMPTOMS IN ATHLETES

It is a commonly held belief that the frequency of upper respiratory tract (infection-type) symptoms (URTS) is increased following single bouts of ultra-endurance exercise and excessive exercise training. To date, the evidence to support this supposition is inconclusive. Temporary modulations in innate and adaptive immune system function may contribute to the increase in susceptibility to infection reported during times of high volume-training and competition (Nieman 1994b) and numerous research studies have demonstrated that excessive exercise can transiently suppress markers of immune function (Robson *et al.* 1999b; Nieman *et al.* 1989b). However, studies demonstrating a direct relationship between the temporal suppression of immune function following excessive exercise and incidence of upper respiratory tract infection have not been forthcoming. Whether the URTS commonly reported in athletes are a consequence of infection and/or inflammatory conditions is an area of current debate. South African scientists (Schwellnus *et al.* 1997) demonstrated that use of an anti-inflammatory nasal spray significantly reduced self-reported episodes of URTS in runners following a 56-km marathon, indicating that some symptoms are related to localised inflammation in the airways.

The diagnosis of infection as the cause of URTS by physicians has come under scrutiny. Research suggests that athletes with recurrent URTS require further clinical investigation to rule out non-infection, inflammatory based causes. One study analysed nasopharyngeal and throat swabs from athletes reporting URTS (Cox *et al.* 2008). Swabs were analysed for bacterial, viral, chlamydial and mycoplasmal respiratory pathogens. A total of 37 episodes from 28 athletes over a five-month period were reported but pathogens were identified in only 30% of cases with bacterial infections, accounting for about five per cent of episodes. Herpes group viruses and Epstein-Barr virus reactivation have been associated with URTS reported by elite athletes (Reid *et al.* 2004); however, anti-herpes virus treatment was not effective in reducing the frequency of URTS episodes in these athletes, again indicating other non-infective causes for URTS in athletes.

These and other data have led to the development of the 'non-infectious' hypothesis for upper respiratory tract illness, where self-reported episodes of 'infection' may be more related to other factors including allergy-related symptoms, local inflammation in the airways and bronchospasm from cold dry air inhalation. Data suggest that a 'rule of thirds' could be applied to the cause of URTS in athletes, where one-third is attributable to non-infectious conditions (allergy, exercise-induced bronchospasm), one-third to infection and one-third to inflammatory based disorders (Figure 11.1). The current consensus is that the cause of URTS in athletic populations is uncertain and symptoms should only be referred to as infection-based if a pathogen is identified (Walsh *et al.* 2011a). Inflammation from non-infective causes is common in athletes and some conditions are treatable and can be well managed if diagnosed correctly.

As this chapter is concerned with allergy in sport, it is worth considering that some of the commonly reported symptoms (e.g. itchy and running nose, sneezing and

Figure 11.1 'Rule of thirds' for aetiology of upper respiratory tract symptoms in athletes based on the position statement from the International Society of Exercise and Immunity, 2011 (Walsh *et al.* 2011); EIB = Exercise-induced bronchospasm

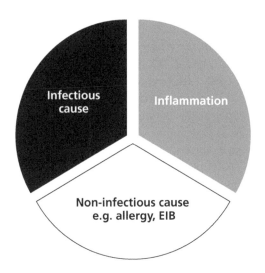

ocular irritation) are more likely to be allergic (Dijkstra and Robson-Ansley 2011). Allergies are highly treatable and can be well managed, so identification of allergens provoking allergic responses in individuals is desirable, especially for high-performance athletes competing over spring and summer months when pollen counts are at their peak (Helenius and Haahtela 2000).

THE ALLERGIC RESPONSE

Allergies are the result of an immune system dysfunction; they are a normal immuno-logical process mounted against an inappropriate stimulus. In simple terms, the immune system believes that it is being invaded by a parasite rather than a harmless allergen present in the environment. Hence, the development of the allergic response is similar to the development of an anti-parasitic immune response.

The majority of pathogens with which the immune system usually has to deal with are microscopic, single-unit organisms, such as viruses and bacteria, but a parasite is substantially larger and often visible to the eye. To eradicate a large parasite, the immune system will need to use alternative methods, as a cell-mediated approach alone is not going to be effective in winning this battle. One option is to make the environment hostile to the parasite and then annihilate it. The primary response is led by mast cells, which contain a large variety of preformed mediators including histamine, enzymes (tryptase and chymase) and heparin proteoglycans that cause vasodilation, oedema and itching, which is recognised as the early phase of the allergic response.

Allergy symptoms, such as a running nose and watery eyes, associated with airborne allergens result in an increase in the watery, mucous barrier on mucosal surfaces which reduces the ability of a parasite to take a hold on the host; localised itching from neural stimulation by histamine aids removal of the parasite from the skin by initiation of scratching of the skin; in addition, oedema and swelling of the tissues raises the temperature of the affected area and facilitates leukocyte entry to the site. The mast cell-driven response is followed by the development of allergic inflammation primarily caused by the recruitment of eosinophils into the local environment. This is achieved by the production and release of proinflammatory cytokines by mast cells and T-helper 2 cells which stimulate synthesis of eosinophils by the bone marrow and their migration into the tissues.

On reaching the target tissues, eosinophils degranulate, release protein mediators (i.e. major basic protein, eosinophil cationic protein and eosinophil derived neurotoxin) on to the surface of the parasite. These mediators, whilst extremely effective at annihilating parasites, are highly toxic for human tissues and can cause extensive tissue damage. For example, eosinophilic-derived proteins irritate the nerve terminals inducing nerve hyperreactivity, destroy collagen fibres in the basal membrane and induce the death of epithelial cells. The integrity of the epithelium is then disrupted leading to exposure of basal membranes to allergens and irritants resulting in chronic allergic inflammation.

The reason for the apparent immune system confusion resulting in an allergic, yet anti-parasitic response to an innocuous common protein requires explanation. To gain entry into the host, parasites secrete digestive enzymes onto the skin and mucosal tissues to digest the bonds between mucosal and skin cells resulting in tissue breakdown and entry into the host domain. In response to the parasitic digestive enzymes, the host's immune system mounts an anti-parasitic response; however, the proteins that trigger an allergic response (allergens) are also enzymes. Unfortunately, the antigen-presenting cells (dendritic cells) are unable to differentiate between parasite-derived and non parasite-derived enzymes and initiate an immune response to the supposed aggressor which is recognised as allergic symptoms to the allergen.

Most allergens are proteins or glycoproteins, although the glycan moiety of the glycoprotein does not stimulate IgE production. Sources of allergen are diverse and include pollens, house dust mites, fungal spores, animal hairs, drugs and foods (Table 11.1). As most allergens are proteins, some allergens are destroyed during exposure to heat and digestive enzymes. For example, pollens do not cause gut-derived allergic reactions, as they are denatured by digestive enzymes if orally ingested and so are restricted to causing an allergic response in the oral cavity/respiratory tract. The biochemical and physiochemical properties of the allergen influence the site of allergic reaction. Indeed, allergens that are resistant to heat and digestive enzymes may facilitate systemic allergic responses (e.g. those involved in nut allergies). It is not fully understood why some atopic individuals are sensitive to some allergens, whereas these allergens have no effect on other atopic individuals. It is thought that genetic make-up is important, as are extrinsic factors (e.g. viruses, tobacco smoke, and

ALLERGEN	EXAMPLES OF ALLERGEN	PREVALENCE
Inhalant:		
Pollens (tree, weeds, grass)	Birch, oak, timothy grass, mugwort, plantain	Seasonal: pollen calendars can be used to determine months of high pollen load
Moulds/fungi	Aspergillus	Variable/perennial
Animal dander	Cat, dog, horse, hamster	Perennial
Bird feathers	Duck, chicken, pigeon	Perennial
House dust mite	Dermatophagoides pteronyssinus (found in UK)/farina (non-UK)	Perennial: high load in warm houses during winter months when ventilation is low
Insects	Cockroach, fly, midge	Seasonal
Oral:		
Food	Peanuts, seafood, soya, eggs, chocolate	Non-seasonal
Drugs	Penicillins, antibiotics	Non-seasonal
Injected:		
Insects	Bee, wasp	Summer
Drugs	Blood products, vaccines, antibiotics	Non-seasonal

Table 11.1 Common sources of allergen

Source: adapted from Holgate *et al.* (2006)

pollutants), which may also contribute to allergen recognition by the immune system by altering normal homeostatic defence mechanisms.

Genes associated with IgE regulation, inflammation and production of allergen-specific IgE have been studied in some detail. Studies have shown that genes coding for proteins associated with major histocompatibility class (MHC) I and II genes which will influence presentation of antigen and allergen peptides to T helper cells are involved in development of allergic disease.

The most common allergens are those in the environment and most individuals are exposed to a mix of allergens rather than single allergens at any one time (unless in a specific workplace). Allergen exposure may occur in domestic and occupational settings and are often referred to as indoor or outdoor allergens to reflect the origin of their source. Typical outdoor allergens that may affect the outdoor training atopic athlete include pollens and fungi, whereas indoor training athletes may encounter animal dander or house dust mite faeces. Indeed, all athletes at some point in their day will encounter both indoor and outdoor allergens, although, depending on where they train, they may be exposed to greater levels of allergen.

To summarise, an allergic response has a very similar pattern to a parasite-killing response, a mast-cell dominated early-phase response followed by the later infiltration of eosinophils, driving the development of allergic inflammation. The latter is caused primarily by the eosinophilic-derived proteins, which are highly toxic for human tissues causing severe damage, if this response is present in the respiratory system, owing to inhalation of allergens such as pollens, dust house mites, animal dander, and this can result in the development of chronic allergic conditions such as asthma and rhinitis.

Cytokines and the allergic response

The allergic immune response involves production of IgE antibodies by B cells that is elicited by signalling between T cells and B cells with accompanying signals from cytokines. T helper cells are the main T-cell population involved in the development of the allergic response, consisting of a balance between the activation and response of T helper 1 (Th1), T helper 2 (Th2), T regulatory (Treg) and possibly T helper 17 (Th17 cells).

As discussed in previous chapters, in a Th1-dominant immune response, the production of the cytokine, interferon gamma (IFN-γ) results in the activation of macrophages and enhanced microbial killing. B cells are then stimulated to produce complement binding and opsonising antibodies increasing chemotaxis and recruitment of phagocytic cells to remove foreign organisms. In a Th2-dominant immune response, the production of the cytokines IL-4 and IL-13 induces the production of IgE antibodies by B cells. On primary exposure to an allergen, IgE binds to mast cells via specific receptors including the high-affinity FcεRI and, on a subsequent exposure to a triggering antigen, the IgE is cross-linked with the allergen resulting in mast cell degranulation and release of mediators such as histamine, enzymes (tryptase and chymase) and heparin proteoglycans (Figure 11.2). The production of IL-5 causes activation and proliferation of eosinophils leading to an inflammatory response. Th1 and Th2 responses are mutually antagonistic but can also be regulated by Treg cells. There are different types of Treg cells, which secrete different combinations of cytokines, the two main ones being IL-10 and TGF-β.

T cells recognise an antigen as a complex of a peptide fragment presented to them bound to a self-MHC molecule (MHC class II) whereas B cells can recognise intact antigen. B cells are able to produce different classes of antibodies dependent upon the cytokines in the environment in which they initially encounter antigen. To switch the type of antibody produced by the B cell to the production of IgE antibodies, both IL-4 and IL-13 are required in the local milieu.

Hygiene hypothesis

Data indicate that there has been an increase of allergic symptoms such as allergic asthma and rhinitis in the general population, which can result in long-term health problems (Bousquet *et al.* 2008; O'Connell, 2004). One reason for this has been attributed to keeping young children in extremely clean conditions, resulting in a lack of early childhood exposure to pathogens and thus a lack of priming for the development of a healthy immune system; this is known as the hygiene hypothesis (Strachan 2000). During pregnancy, the fetus and mother's immune system response is polarised in a Th2 direction and exposure to pathogens develops a Th1-polarised

Figure 11.2 Mechanisms of immunoglobulin (Ig)E-mediated atopic disease (source: *Journal of the American Pharmacological Association* 2008)

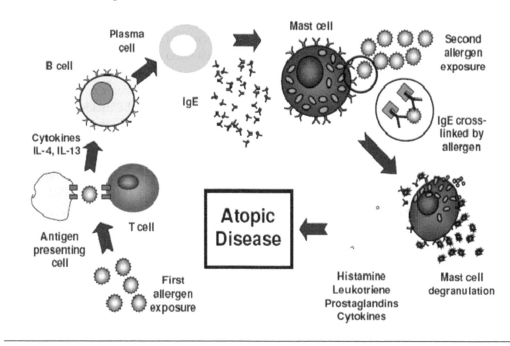

response early in life, reducing the risk of developing Th2-associated diseases such as allergy. Studies indicate that exposure to rural environments is associated with a lower incidence of allergy and asthma; indeed, farm children have a lower incidence of allergic disease than the general population (Alm *et al.* 1999). Furthermore, exposure to dogs during early childhood has also been shown protective against the development of allergic disease and it is thought this is due to exposure to a high endotoxin load that induces a Th1- polarised immune response (Simpson and Custovic 2005).

IFN-γ is a key cytokine in driving a Th1-polarised immune response, it prevents viral replication and has a proinflammatory effects. This cytokine produced predominantly by T cells and NK cells and, importantly, inhibits Th2 cells and blocks the effect of IL-4 on the production of IgE by B cells. IFN-γ is produced in response to viral infection and forms the basis of the theory that reduced exposure to infection (lower IFN-γ levels) leads to increased allergic sensitisation as proposed in the hygiene hypothesis.

However, the immune response will not be entirely polarised in the direction of a Th1 or Th2 response and relative amounts of cytokines present in any environment will determine the overall response to a foreign agent. It is important to recognise that rarely is a response purely of one type or another and that regulatory factors play a large part in determining the balance and overall outcome.

Atopy and allergy in athletes

A study by a team of researchers from Northumbria University endeavoured to address the relationship between self-reported URTI and atopy/allergy in runners of the 2010 London Marathon (Robson-Ansley *et al.* 2012). This involved the screening of a cohort of runners who competed in the marathon distance for atopy and allergic disease using the Allergy Questionnaire for Athletes (AQUA) and specific serum IgE concentrations in response to a panel of common inhalant allergens (including tree, grass, and weed pollen, cat, house dust mite) as well as the incidence of upper-respiratory tract infection-like symptoms in the runners for two weeks following the marathon. The results showed that atopy was present in a high proportion of the marathon runners (almost one in two) which was in agreement with current prevalence data from elite long distance runners (49%) (Helenius *et al.* 1998) and is higher than that reported for randomly selected adults in the UK (34–44%) (Sunyer *et al.* 2004). Furthermore, 40% of the runners were classified as being allergic to one or more of the selected inhalant allergens. Interestingly in this study, a strong association between a positive AQUA and the incidence of post-race URTS in runners was found and similarly atopy was significantly predictive of URTS, which indicates that a high proportion of these symptoms may be related to allergy rather than to infection.

There is considerable evidence indicating an increased incidence of exercise-induced bronchospasm and atopy in highly trained athletes compared with non-athletic controls (Helenius *et al.* 1998). In a study on elite Finnish ice hockey players, 58% of the athletes, compared with 36% of the control subjects, were atopic (Lumme *et al.* 2003). In another study, 50% of potential Australian Olympic and Paralympic athletes who were screened prior to the 2000 Olympics had symptoms of allergic rhinoconjunctivitis and 56% had a positive skin-prick test to at least one inhalant allergen (Katelaris *et al.* 2000).

Exercise-induced Th1/Th2 polarisation and allergy in athletes

Immunological data suggest that chronic exercising training can lead to a polari-sation of T-helper lymphocytes toward the Th2 phenotype (Steensberg *et al.* 2001b; Lakier 2003), which may predispose athletes to greater frequency of reported URTS, such as allergic rhinitis and asthma. A Th2-polarised response involves an increase in production of Th2 archetypical cytokines such as IL-4, IL-5 and IL-13, resulting in an upregulation of IgE antibody formation via B lymphocytes. In turn, this results in an increase in IgE production as well as recruitment of mast cells and eosinophils which, as previously described, play a key role in the induction of allergic sympto-mology. Data indicating alterations in archetypical Th2 cytokines in response to exercise is sparse, as much research has focused on the Th1 proinflammatory cytokine response to exercise.

Studies indicate, however, that IL-6 can drive Th2 differentiation of naïve T-helper lymphocytes (Dienz and Rincón 2009) and deletion of the IL-6 gene promotes Th1 differentiation (Munegowda *et al.* 2012). Strenuous, prolonged exercise has consistently been shown to increase circulating concentrations of IL-6, which is produced in greater amounts than any other cytokine (Ullum *et al.* 1994a; Nieman *et al.* 1998b). Indeed, it may be proposed that, in chronic exercise training, the repeated exercise-induced elevations in IL-6 play a role in the reported increased incidence of atopy and allergic disease in athletes by driving Th2 differentiation (Figure 11.3).

Figure 11.3 Exercise-induced interlukin (IL)-6 shifts the T helper lymphocyte (Th)1/Th2 balance towards Th2 by inhibiting Th1 differentiation and promoting Th2 (adapted from Diehl and Rincón 2002)

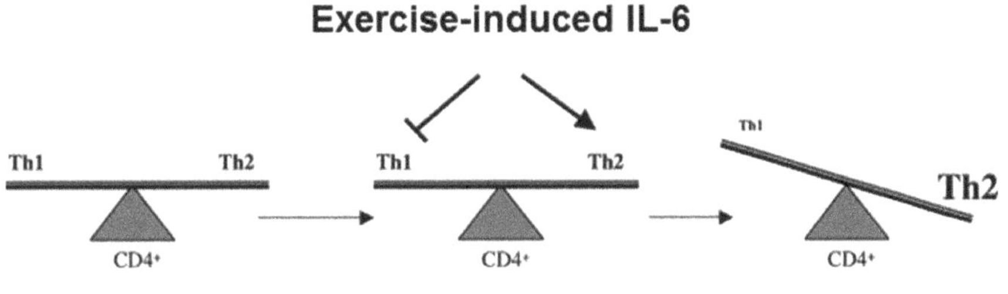

IL-6 promotes the differentiation of Th2 cells and simultaneously inhibits Th1 polarisation through two independent molecular mechanisms (Diehl and Rincón 2002). Firstly, IL-6 activates nuclear factor of activated T cells, which leads to the production of IL-4 by naïve CD4+ cells. Following the initial stimulus by IL-6, the IL-4 secreted from CD4+ T cells acts in an autocrine fashion by upregulating additional IL-4 production from CD4+ cells. The increased IL-4 in the local milieu inhibits IFN-γ production, thereby inhibiting Th1 polarisation but promoting Th2 differentiation. Secondly, IL-6 inhibits Th1 differentiation by inducing the expression of suppressor of cytokine signalling (SOCS)-1, which interferes with IFN-γ, thus, inhibiting the signalling for the differentiation of naïve CD4+ cells into Th1 cells.

Research indicates that endurance exercise, in particular, is associated with elevations in both IL-6 and its soluble receptor (which acts to amplify the IL-6 signalling) (Robson-Ansley *et al.* 2009; Walshe *et al.* 2010), which may result in the increased incidence of atopy and IgE-mediated disease in endurance trained athletes compared with the general population. As yet, the role of exercise-induced IL-6 in the development allergy/atopy in athletes remains untested but this could provide a fruitful avenue of potential investigation.

IMPACT OF ALLERGY ON HEALTH, WELLBEING AND ATHLETIC PERFORMANCE

The physical effects of untreated allergy will influence athletes' health and wellbeing as well as potentially having a detrimental effect on athletic performance. Endurance athletes are at particular risk as they have extensive exposure to many outdoor inhalant allergens during the pollen season. The shifting of breathing from nose to combined mouth and nasal breathing results in a greater deposition of airborne allergens to the lower airways (McFadden *et al.*, 1985). It has been previously proposed that athletes who are repeatedly and excessively exposed to outdoor inhalant allergens may develop symptoms of allergic asthma and rhinitis (Bermon 2007), which are often misdiagnosed as infections (Cox *et al.* 2008). The physical effects of untreated allergy can affect a variety of tissues and organs in the body, resulting in chronic allergic inflammation, those areas most affected by airborne/inhalant allergens include the lungs, nose and eyes.

The lungs

In the lungs, untreated allergy can trigger and exacerbate underlying asthma. As the rate and depth of breathing increases during exercise, the athlete's exposure to various airborne elements is magnified, which intensifies the contact between the respiratory system and the environment. It is worth bearing in mind that not all athletes with exercise-induced bronchospasm (EIB) are atopic and not all atopic athletes have EIB.

Several mechanisms, which may act in together or alone, are involved in the development of EIB in elite athletes and these are comprehensively reviewed elsewhere (Anderson and Kippelen 2005):

- Airway drying: high lung ventilation rates induce a loss of water via evaporation, resulting in drying of the airways. The epithelial cells within the respiratory tract become hyperosmolar, which provides an osmotic stimulus for the movement of water from any cell in the locality, resulting in cell shrinkage and the release of proinflammatory mediators. The proinflammatory mediators, including histamine, neuropeptides, cysteinyl leukotrienes and prostaglandins produce contraction of bronchial smooth muscle and a degree of airway obstruction.
- Airway cooling: in cold weather, high volumes of cold air will enter the lungs which will be rapidly rewarmed. The process of rapid rewarming may induce vascular hyperaemia of the bronchial microvascular, airway oedema and a degree of airway narrowing/obstruction. Indeed, epithelial injury and airway remodelling does occur in some athletes, in particular endurance athletes, which results in a sensitised airway smooth muscle and the development of airway hyper-responsivity.
- Allergy: endurance athletes, more specifically track and field athletes, are exposed to vast number of pollen allergens throughout the spring and summer. High lung ventilation rates, often exceeding 100 L/minute, result in a shift of breathing from

the nose to combined mouth and nasal breathing. In atopic athletes, there will be a high deposition of airborne allergens (together with unconditioned air and other inhaled particles) in the lower airways inducing an allergic response, airway hyper-responsivity and subsequent narrowing of airways. In addition to pollen allergy, the indoor training environment can also be highly allergenic for some individuals. Indeed, Helenius *et al.* (2005) reported high levels of dog, cat and house dust mite allergens within indoor arenas in Finland.

EIB is relatively common in high-performance athletes, which is understandable considering the exercise-related aetiological factors. Poor air quality, cold temperatures and exposure to aeroallergens can exacerbate EIB, which can severely impact on athletic performance. Unfortunately, EIB is often misdiagnosed and poorly treated (Ansley *et al.* 2012; Hull *et al.* 2009), which can result in the development of asthma with longer-term health implications. More recently, owing to the provision of continuing education programmes for sport team support staff and the development of mobile EIB screening equipment, recognition and correct treatment for the condition is on the increase.

The nose

In the nose, allergy will result in allergic rhinitis. Allergic rhinitis is characterised by nasal congestion, sneezing, itching of nose, postnasal drip and chronic allergic rhinitis can lead to sleep disturbance, cough and fatigue. Allergic rhinitis can be confused with nasal infections, highlighting the importance of allergy screening to permit appropriate treatment of symptoms. It can disrupt sleep because of night-time congestion and dry mouth. Research indicates that long-term sleep disturbance affects physical and cognitive performance as well as resulting in the suppression of immune function, potentially increasing susceptibility to infectious episodes. There is a convincing link between sleep disturbance and allergic rhinitis, supported by a study investigating the impact of rhinitis symptoms on sleep in a large cohort of individuals (Young *et al.* 1997). Participants with frequent rhinitis symptoms (more than five nights per month) were significantly more likely to experience chronic excessive daytime sleepiness and/or non-restorative sleep.

Other research has determined that allergic rhinitis can be detrimental to reaction time, attention and vigilance, which are key elements of sporting performance. Severe rhinitis can lead to cytokine release and exogenous administration of IL-6 (a key inflammatory cytokine) to athletes has been shown to significantly impair ten-kilometre time trial performance and increase sensation of fatigue during exercise (Robson-Ansley *et al.* 2004). Of clinical significance, poorly treated or undiagnosed rhinitis can lead to the development of EIB and asthma (Bousquet *et al.* 2001). Indeed, allergic inflammation in one area of the respiratory tract (the nasal passages) can result in inflammation further down the airways (EIB/asthma) and this is known as the 'united airways' hypothesis. The correct management of rhinitis in asthmatics significantly reduces the incidence of hospital admission with asthma. It is of utmost importance that allergic rhinitis is not considered to be a trivial symptom but is treated appropriately to prevent the subsequent development of EIB or exacerbation of underlying asthma. Allergic rhinitis in sport is comprehensively reviewed by Dijkstra and Robson-Ansley (2011).

The eyes

In the eye, untreated allergy will result in allergic conjunctivitis. This is a common disorder affecting 21% of the adult population in the UK. It can develop in the conjunctiva, the mucous membrane lining the eye. In mild cases, the conjunctiva becomes inflamed in response to an allergen, producing itchy, watery and sticky eyes and visual disturbance. The condition is mild and is generally caused by excessive tear and mucous production (Katelaris *et al.* 2003). The onset and time course is determined by the duration of exposure to the allergen (e.g. grass pollen) season. Allergic conjunctivitis could impair athletic performance, in particular for those whose sports require excellent vision (such as rifle shooting or archery).

TESTING FOR SENSITISATION TO AEROALLERGENS

Obtaining objective evidence of sensitisation to common aeroallergens is key in the confirmation of allergic disease in association with positive allergy history. There are two main proposed 'gold-standard' methods: skin-prick testing and serum allergen-specific IgE (see Technique box 11.1 for details).

Tests to avoid for allergy screening

There are many alternative methods proposed by alternative therapists as diagnostic for allergies but these tests must be viewed with caution and are not recommended. These tests are of unproven value, often expensive and can be misleading on allergy diagnosis. They include hair analysis, the 'Vega' electrical test where an allergen (often food) is placed in a chamber contained within an electrical circuit completed by the person, auricular cardiac reflex testing (based essentially on changes in heart rate), applied kinesiology (where the proposed allergen is placed in one hand and muscle appears weaker if the individual has an allergy to the allergen). Blood tests for IgG are also advertised for diagnosis of allergy but high IgG indicates that an individual has been exposed to a protein recently and is not indicative of IgE-mediated disease.

Team screening for inhalant allergic disease in sport

The diagnosis of IgE-mediated disease is dependent upon both the allergy history taken from an individual and the results of skin-prick or radioallergosorbent (RAST) tests (see Technique box 11.1). The allergy history should be taken by a trained professional, asking pertinent questions on frequency and severity of symptoms and

Technique box 11.1

Testing for sensitisation to aeroallergens

Obtaining objective evidence of sensitisation to common aeroallergens is key in the confirmation of allergic disease in association with positive allergy history. There are two main proposed 'gold-standard' methods: skin-prick testing and serum allergen-specific IgE.

Skin-prick testing

Skin-prick is a painless and bloodless procedure to determine sensitivity to a common allergen. The test involves placing a drop of an allergy extract solution (e.g. a solution containing an extract of tree pollen, dust house mite or grass pollen), which is pressed into the skin using a lancet. After a 15-minute period, the size of wheal (reaction) is measured and compared against a negative control (containing the allergy diluent only). A positive test is determined when the wheal is 2 mm or greater in diameter than the negative control. A wheal 6 mm or greater in diameter tends to be of greater clinical relevance but this is not always the case, hence the size of the wheal does not indicate the degree of sensitivity, just that the individual is sensitised to the specific allergen.

Serum allergen-specific IgE determination

This involves the collection of a whole blood sample into a vacutainer tube, from which the serum/plasma is separated. The serum/plasma is then tested against a panel of common aeroallergens using radioimmunoassay, enzyme-linked immunosorbent assay or chemiluminescence methods. The most widely known test for allergen-specific IgE testing is the radioallergosorbent (RAST) test; this technology can measure up to 650 different types of specific IgE. Rapid-result, specific IgE tests are also available that use finger-prick blood sampling but these tests are limited to ten predetermined allergens per panel and can be costly if screening in large numbers.

In general, for inhalant allergies, skin prick tests tend to be more sensitive than RAST tests, which have a sensitivity (true positive) between 60–80%, whereas RAST tests have a greater specificity (true negative) than skin-prick tests, often as high as 90% (Calabria et al. 2009). Skin-prick tests are inexpensive but require a trained professional to conduct the testing; they provide immediate results and have good educational value to the individual. The RAST test is completely safe and is able to identify a wider range of possible allergens, although testing can become expensive. In some instances, total IgE levels have been used to identify atopy but this is not informative for identifying specific allergens.

The measurement of total IgE concentration requires sensitive tests for its determination, as the total serum IgE concentration is approximately 10,000 times less than that of IgG. Total IgE will determine whether the levels lie within normal reference ranges but the predictive value of the test is limited, as approximately 50% of individuals with allergies will have total IgE concentrations within the normal range. Some sport-related allergy studies have measured total IgE concentration but this is not a particularly useful method of determining allergen sensitivity and specific IgE or skin-prick tests are preferable. Despite this, IgE measurement is relatively inexpensive and it can be performed in a standard laboratory. Elevated IgE concentrations should warrant further specific IgE tests to determine the specific allergen, so that an appropriate management plan may be developed.

potential allergic triggers. However, clinically testing all athletes in a team for the presence of allergic disease using gold-standard clinical methods is neither practical nor cost effective and a more practical method of initiating an allergy screening programme for large groups of athletes may be done using an athlete-specific questionnaire such as the AQUA (Bonini *et al.* 2009).

The AQUA has been validated as a reliable tool for assessing the prevalence of allergy in a group of athletes. The AQUA was derived from the European Community Respiratory Health Survey Questionnaire and adapted to the target population using open interviews with athletes, team physicians and coaches. It was administered for validation to professional football players, alongside allergy diagnosis using skin-prick testing/specific IgE determination and comprehensive allergy history. A total AQUA score of five or more had the best predictive value for allergy (0.94) with a specificity of 97% and a sensitivity of 58%. The AQUA has been used in several studies to assess allergic symptoms in athletes and also provides a useful tool for highlighting athletes with allergic symptoms who require further specialist clinical support and advice on managing their allergies.

Sports medicine practitioners have used the questionnaire approach to screening on the Great Britain Track and Field Team at the 2006 Gothenburg European Championships to identify self-reported prevalence of allergy and asthma symptoms (Dijkstra and Robson-Ansley 2011). The questionnaire was completed by 63 team members, of whom 38 (60%) athletes gave a positive response to the question 'Have you ever suffered from hay fever?', with only five (8%) of these positive responders reported having had specific clinical allergy tests to confirm the diagnosis (Dijkstra, unpublished data). The data indicated that, despite experiencing symptoms of inhalant allergy, the majority of UK track and field athletes did not pursue further clinical confirmation, which might have put them at risk of poor management of their condition which could not only affect performance but also their health and wellbeing. This initial questionnaire-based screening lead to the implementation of an active allergy screening and management programme. UK Athletics has produced a set of practical guidelines for both athletes and support staff to advise on allergy management for athletes (see Box 11.1).

In summary, the AQUA questionnaire may be used to highlight athletes at risk of allergy who require further clinical investigation. This should be followed up with clinical allergy diagnosis, which is dependent on clinical allergy history and objective tests of IgE sensitivity (skin-prick test or specific IgE measurements). Once a positive diagnosis of allergy is made, a treatment and management plan can be developed to reduce or eliminate the impact of the allergy on athlete performance and wellbeing.

PRACTICAL GUIDELINES FOR DIAGNOSIS AND MANAGEMENT OF ALLERGY IN SPORT

When an allergen is identified through objective screening procedures, the athlete is advised to reduce exposure to the allergen, which can often reduce symptoms

> **Box 11.1** Advice on allergy management for athletes
>
> Source: UK Athletics medical considerations for travel and competition, UKA Guidelines (Dijkstra and Robson-Ansley 2011).
>
> - Know your own allergy risk.
>   a. What time of year are you affected?
>   b. What causes your allergies? (blood/skin-prick tests may be necessary to determine this).
>   c. What are your normal symptoms?
> - Know your training and competition environment.
> - Minimise exposure to pollens (training venue, time of day training) and rinse your nose with salt water washes after training.
> - Preventive use of corticosteroid nasal spray and/or non-sedating antihistamine is very important and are permitted by the World Anti-Doping Agency (WADA). A corticosteroid nasal spray is the most effective treatment. We do not advise the use of non-sedating anti-histamines around competition, as these may be detrimental to performance in both sprinters and endurance athletes.
> - Asthmatics should take their inhalant medication regularly and according to instructions in potentially polluted environments. You may need additional medication or changed doses in high pollen or polluted environments.
> - If you have allergies, your doctor should assess you before leaving for the holding camp or soon after arriving, to ensure that you have an optimal management strategy.

(Custovic *et al.* 1998). For example, in an individual with cat allergy, removal of the offending animal from the household will reduce symptoms. A reduction in dust house mites, a common allergen, can be achieved by removal of curtains and carpeting, washing bed linen at a temperature higher than 60°C and killing mites using pesticides such as acaricides. For pollen allergy sufferers, the shutting of car and bedroom windows during high pollen days and washing of hair and clothing after being outside can help to reduce allergen load. However, if an athlete is required to exercise outside during high pollen days, allergen avoidance is not going to prove a viable option and other management plans need to be set in place.

Pharmacological treatment

Unfortunately, the use of any pharmacological treatments for allergy and asthma by recreational endurance athletes with allergic disease is extremely low (23%), with athletes reporting that they do not wish to take preventative medication for fear of affecting performance (Robson-Ansley *et al.* 2012). Furthermore, fewer than 50% of the runners who took part in the previously described London Marathon study who had diagnosed asthma reported using their prescribed medication. The risk of untreated allergy and asthma on long-term health is considerable and is associated with a higher risk of hospitalisation (Crystal-Peters *et al.* 2002). Hence, educational plans should be developed to inform recreational level athletes of the risk of untreated/poorly managed allergic conditions on long-term health and to ensure optimum management of their condition by clinical practices.

Reassuringly, a greater proportion of elite athletes although still modest, take allergy medications (50% of Finnish elite athletes) and this may be due to the clinical provision for athletes at that level of participation (Alaranta *et al.* 2005). In general, elite athletes are reluctant to take any medication and this may be attributed to an impact on performance but also to the overt awareness of World Anti-Doping Agency (WADA) regulations and concern about infringing drug regulations. Intranasal corticosteroids are highly recommended as the management drug of choice, in conjunction with second-generation antihistamines (severity dependent) and, where practicable, allergen avoidance (Alaranta *et al.* 2005). Immunotherapy should also be considered as a potential therapy for pollen-allergic individuals. Increased awareness and education of both the athlete and clinical support team is needed, as the majority of pharmacological allergy and asthma treatments are permitted for competing athletes by WADA through use of therapeutic use exemption procedures (Dijkstra and Robson-Ansley 2011).

Pollen calendars

Knowledge of environmental conditions (climate, season, type of pollen) to which an athlete may be exposed during training and competition is key to managing allergy and minimising any negative impact on sporting performance.

Pollen calendars are widely available on the Internet and through the National Pollen Bureau in the UK (Figure 11.4). These should be used to determine risk periods for an allergy-prone athlete to ensure that appropriate allergy management plans are in place to manage their condition. With athletes travelling internationally to competition or training camps, it is possible to obtain common seasonal aeroallergens for their specific country of competition (e.g. common Mediterranean grasses, olive pollen) in advance of travel and advise susceptible athletes or screen entire teams as a precautionary action.

If an athlete is competing overseas, it is also important to remember seasonal differences will be apparent, especially if travelling to a different hemisphere. For example, pollen counts could be high in the country of destination compared with those that the athlete has left (e.g. travelling from the UK in December to Australia). Many countries measure and provide reports on pollen counts; hence, athletes should be able to obtain pollen counts for their destination. Furthermore, the non-UK strain of house dust mite (*Dermatophagoides farinae*) may cause symptoms in athletes who do not react to the house dust mite whilst residing in the UK (*D. pteronyssinus*) so attention to bedding and sleeping environment is of importance.

Figure 11.4 UK Pollen Calendar (National Pollen and Aerobiology Research Unit, University of Worcester). The exact timing and severity of pollen seasons will differ from year to year depending on the weather and also regionally depending on geographical location

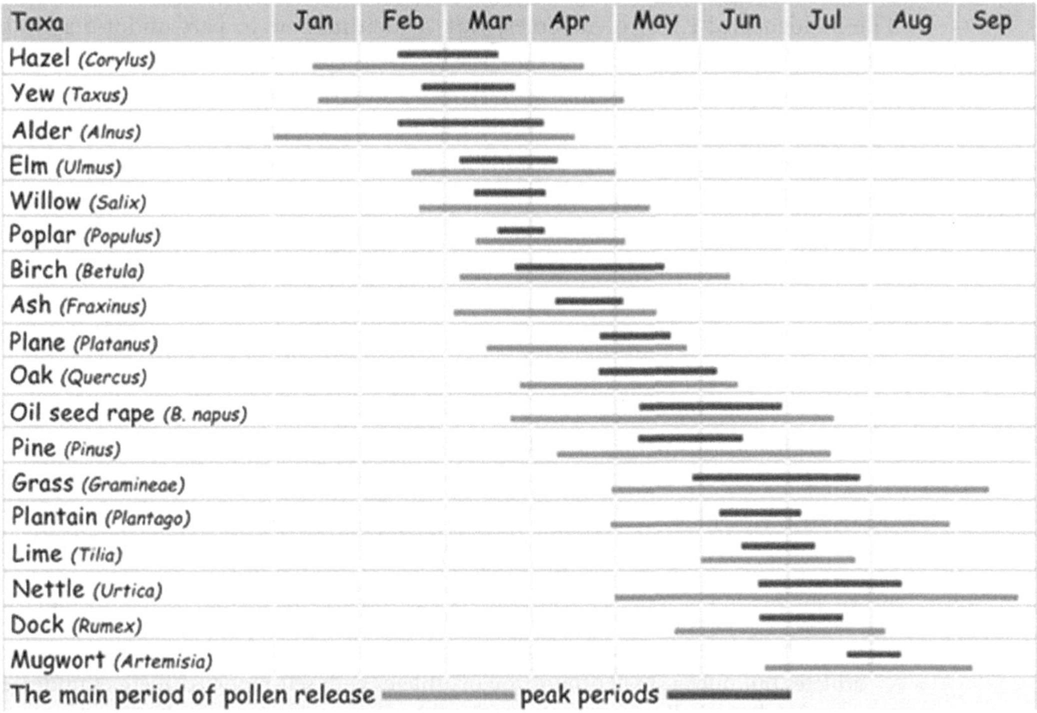

Taxa	Jan	Feb	Mar	Apr	May	Jun	Jul	Aug	Sep
Hazel (Corylus)									
Yew (Taxus)									
Alder (Alnus)									
Elm (Ulmus)									
Willow (Salix)									
Poplar (Populus)									
Birch (Betula)									
Ash (Fraxinus)									
Plane (Platanus)									
Oak (Quercus)									
Oil seed rape (B. napus)									
Pine (Pinus)									
Grass (Gramineae)									
Plantain (Plantago)									
Lime (Tilia)									
Nettle (Urtica)									
Dock (Rumex)									
Mugwort (Artemisia)									

The main period of pollen release ━━━━━━ peak periods ━━━━━━

EXERCISE-INDUCED ANAPHYLAXIS

Another exercise-related allergic condition that affects some exercising individuals is exercise-induced anaphylaxis (EIAn) (Robson-Ansley and Toit 2010). EIAn is a rare syndrome previously described in high-performance athletes and in individuals undertaking only very occasional exercise. It often occurs only in association with the ingestion of a food allergen around the time of exercise, when it is referred to as food-dependent exercise-induced anaphylaxis (FDEIA). The onset of EIAn is generally reported following submaximal exercise of a relatively short duration. There are no consistent exercise-associated factors, such as extreme ambient temperature or humidity although some pharmacological agents (aspirin, anti-inflammatories) and alcohol ingestion has been associated with increased incidence. Several hypotheses have been proposed to explain the pathophysiology of FDEIA and these include alterations in plasma osmolality and pH, tissue enzyme activity and gastrointestinal permeability. Evaluation of these hypotheses in the context of exercise physiology renders the majority of these inappropriate. More recently, it has been suggested that, at the onset of exercise the redistribution of blood from the gut, which has specific resident mast cells, transports recently ingested allergens to areas of phenotypically different mast cells where a transient loss of tolerance or an intensification of low-grade allergy manifests as anaphylaxis (Robson-Ansley and Toit 2010). The incidence of EIAn is extremely rare, which may be in part under-diagnosis because of its rarity but also individuals who have experienced EIAn symptoms may well have stopped any physical activity to avoid reoccurrence. However, there are reports of athletes with a sudden onset of EIAn and any athletes with suspected exercise-induced anaphylaxis should be managed according to standard clinical anaphylaxis guidelines and later referred to a specialist allergy centre for further assessment.

KEY POINTS

- URTS are commonly reported in athletes particularly following periods of intense training and following prolonged bouts of exercise.
- Current research has led to the development of the 'non-infectious' hypothesis for upper respiratory tract symptoms in athletes, suggesting that many of the symptoms reported post-exercise include itchy and running nose, sneezing and ocular symptoms are more likely allergic in origin than infectious.
- Atopy in highly trained athletes is higher than compared with non-athletic controls with recreational marathon runners reporting a similar prevalence as elite athletes but only a small proportion of athletes with self-reported allergies undergo specific clinical allergy tests to confirm the diagnosis or optimally manage their allergies.
- Atopy and allergic disease is higher in athletes than the general population and, if unmanaged, can impact upon athletic performance as well as future wellbeing.

FURTHER READING

Alaranta, A., Alaranta, H., Heliovaara, M., Alha, P., Palmu, P. and Helenius, I. (2005) Allergic rhinitis and pharmacological management in elite athletes. *Medicine and Science in Sports and Exercise* 37: 707–11.

Bermon, S. (2007) Airway inflammation and upper respiratory tract infection in athletes: is there a link? *Exercise Immunology Review* 13: 6–14.

Cox, A.J., Gleeson, M., Pyne, D.B., Callister, R., Hopkins, W.G. and Fricker, P.A. (2008) Clinical and laboratory evaluation of upper respiratory symptoms in elite athletes. *Clinical Journal of Sport Medicine* 18: 438–45.

Dijkstra, H.P. and Robson-Ansley, P. (2011) The prevalence and current opinion of treatment of allergic rhinitis in elite athletes. *Current Opinion in Allergy and Clinical Immunology* 11: 103–8.

Helenius, I., Lumme, A. and Haahtela, T. (2005) Asthma, airway inflammation and treatment in elite athletes. *Sports Medicine* 35: 565–74.

Robson-Ansley, P. and Toit, G.D. (2010) Pathophysiology, diagnosis and management of exercise-induced anaphylaxis. *Current Opinion in Allergy and Clinical Immunology* 10: 312–17.

Robson-Ansley, P., Howatson, G., Tallent, J., Mitcheson, K., Walshe, I., Toms, C., Du Toit, G., Smith, M. and Ansley, L. (2011) Prevalence of allergy and upper respiratory tract symptoms in runners of London marathon. *Medicine and Science in Sports and Exercise* 44: 999–1004.

12 Exercise and the prevention of chronic diseases: the role of cytokines and the anti-inflammatory effects of exercise

Michael Gleeson

LEARNING OBJECTIVES

After studying this chapter, you should be able to:

- describe the effects of exercise on plasma cytokines;
- discuss the evidence that interleukin(IL)-6 is secreted from contracting muscle;
- describe the metabolic and immunoregulatory roles of IL-6;
- describe the effects of exercise on cytokine production by leukocytes;
- understand the link between chronic disease risk and chronic inflammation;
- describe the effects of a sedentary lifestyle and obesity on inflammation in adipose tissue;
- describe the long-term health benefits of performing regular exercise;
- discuss the anti-inflammatory actions of IL-6 and IL-10;
- appreciate other mechanisms by which exercise can exert anti-inflammatory effects.

INTRODUCTION

The different types of cytokines and some of their main roles were described in Chapter 2 but a short recap is provided here. The word 'cytokine' derives from the Greek, *cyto* meaning cell and *kine* meaning movement. Cytokines are peptides or proteins typically defined as 'molecules that are produced and released by cells of the immune system and mediate the generation of immune responses'. This definition of cytokines does not tell the whole story, however. It is more accurate to state that 'cytokines are secreted molecules that may exert specific effects both on the cell from which they are secreted (autocrine affects) and on other cells (paracrine affects)'. The important distinction between these definitions is that, while cytokines were initially identified as molecules released by cells of the immune system, their origins and influence spread far beyond that of the immune system alone. Indeed, exercise has proved to be a fascinating example of how cells of non-immune origin are able produce and release specific cytokines. The first part of this chapter therefore discusses the mechanisms by which exercise stimulates the production of cytokines and examines the functional roles played by exercise-induced cytokines. Despite recent research demonstrating that cytokines are secreted from and act upon non-immune cells, cytokines are primarily viewed as immunoregulatory molecules. Indeed, the production of cytokines by specific immune cells is critical to many aspects of the host response to infection. The second part of this chapter focuses on how exercise influences the production of cytokines from immune cells. Finally, we examine how cytokine responses to exercise, together with other mechanisms, contribute to the anti-inflammatory effects of exercise, and why this may have important health implications, particularly in the prevention of chronic metabolic and cardiovascular diseases.

EXERCISE-INDUCED ACTIVATION OF CYTOKINE SECRETION

One of the earliest reports on the effects of exercise on cytokines observed an elevation in the circulating levels of several cytokines following the completion of a marathon (Northoff and Berg 1991). Some years later, several reports on the effects of exercise on cytokines began to appear in the scientific literature – the impetus behind this increase was probably the development of sensitive, specific, commercially available, assays for the detection of a large number of cytokines. One the earliest and most consistent findings has been that of an elevation in the circulating level of IL-6 following prolonged strenuous exercise. In an important study, Nehlsen-Cannarella *et al.* (1997) demonstrated that the plasma IL-6 concentration was dramatically increased following 2.5 h of high-intensity running. Furthermore, it was shown that when subjects consumed a carbohydrate (CHO) beverage during exercise, the increase in the circulating IL-6 concentration was decreased compared with subjects who consumed a placebo. While these studies provide no mechanistic insight into the source of the exercise-induced increase in the circulating IL-6 concentration, or its biological purpose, this study acted as a stimulus for subsequent investigations into the effects of exercise on cytokines. Indeed, many subsequent studies have demonstrated an increase in the circulating concentration of several cytokines following prolonged strenuous exercise. Increases in the circulating concentrations of both proinflammatory cytokines (e.g. IL-1β, tumour necrosis factor alpha (TNF-α) and anti-inflammatory cytokines (e.g. IL-6 and IL-10; Ostrowski *et al.* 1998a, 1999) cytokine inhibitors (e.g. IL-1 receptor antagonist and soluble TNF receptors) (Ostrowski *et al.*, 1998a), chemokines (e.g. IL-8, macrophage inflammatory protein and monocyte chemotactic protein-1; Ostrowski *et al.* 2001; Suzuki *et al.* 2002, 2003), and colony-stimulating factors (Suzuki *et al.* 2003) have been reported following endurance exercise. However, the finding of an increase in the circulating IL-6 concentration following prolonged exercise is the most marked and consistent exercise-induced response of any cytokine so far examined (Figure 12.1).

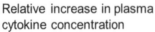

Figure 12.1 The cytokine response to prolonged strenuous exercise; IL = interleukin, TNF-α = tumour necrosis factor alpha (adapted from Febbraio and Pedersen 2002)

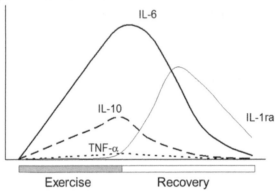

The IL-6 response to exercise

The main sources of IL-6 *in vivo* are activated monocytes/macrophages, fibroblasts and endothelial cells (Akira *et al.* 1993); however, numerous other cellular sources of IL-6 have been identified, including T cells, B cells, neutrophils, eosinophils, osteoblasts, keratinocytes and myocytes (Akira *et al.* 1993). An early study indicated that monocytes were unlikely to be the source of the exercise-induced increase in the plasma IL-6 concentration (Ullum *et al.* 1994a) as one hour of strenuous exercise caused no changes in the amount of IL-6 mRNA detected in peripheral blood mononuclear cells despite an elevation in the plasma IL-6 level. This finding was later confirmed by Starkie *et al.* (2000), who demonstrated that monocyte intracellular IL-6 protein expression was unchanged following a bout of prolonged strenuous exercise; importantly, Starkie *et al.* (2001a) also demonstrated that exercise had no significant effects on TNF-α or IL-1β production from monocytes. Several possible sites of origin were suggested for the exercise-induced increase in the circulating level of IL-6, with contracting skeletal muscle receiving the most attention. Specifically, the intriguing finding that mRNA for IL-6 was elevated in the previously contracting skeletal muscle following prolonged exercise led to the hypothesis that strenuous exercise – marathon running in this case – caused the destruction of contracting myofibres, triggering an inflammatory response and the subsequent release of IL-6 into the systemic circulation (Ostrowski *et al.* 1998b).

Although initial studies supported the hypothesis that an increase in the plasma level of IL-6 was related to exercise-induced muscle damage (Bruunsgaard *et al.* 1997a), it soon became apparent that muscle damage itself was only a minor contributor to the exercise-induced rise in the circulating level of IL-6. Firstly, although many of the initial studies examining the effects of exercise on cytokines used running as an exercise model, several studies have also examined the cytokine response to prolonged bicycle exercise. While prolonged cycling induces only a minimal degree of muscle damage (if any) and consequently does not trigger an inflammatory response, cycling exercise does result in a considerable elevation (typically three- to ten-fold higher than resting values) in the circulating IL-6 concentration. Specifically, in a recent study, Starkie *et al.* (2001b) demonstrated that 60 minutes of either running or cycling, at mode-specific lactate threshold, resulted in a similar elevation in the plasma IL-6 concentration. However, perhaps the strongest evidence that muscle damage is not a prerequisite for an increase in the systemic IL-6 concentration in response to exercise came from Croisier *et al.* (1999). In this study, subjects performed two bouts of eccentric muscle contractions separated by a period of three weeks. After the initial exercise bout, the expected elevation in serum myoglobin (a marker of muscle damage) and delayed onset muscle soreness was observed, in addition to a rise in the circulating IL-6 concentration. Importantly, it is well known that following a period of recovery from an initial bout of muscle damaging exercise a second exercise bout identical to the first causes a much lower level of muscle damage. Therefore, and as expected, the second exercise bout resulted in minimal increases in serum myoglobin and muscle soreness, yet the increase in the circulating IL-6 concentration was very similar to that observed in response to the initial bout of exercise. These studies provide compelling evidence that the increase in the circulating IL-6 concentration following exercise is not primarily related to muscle damage.

However, it is important to note that, in response to prolonged running, the plasma IL-6 kinetics appear to be bimodal. During both prolonged cycling and running, the plasma IL-6 concentration rises gradually and generally peaks at the cessation of exercise. However, after a rapid decline in the circulating IL-6 concentration post-exercise, prolonged running causes a sustained elevation in the IL-6 concentration that is observed for several days. While the increase in the plasma IL-6 concentration that occurs during exercise is not related to muscle damage, the low, sustained elevation in the plasma IL-6 concentration that is observed after prolonged running may be related to muscle damage. The inflammatory response triggered by muscle-damaging exercise is well characterised and results in the sequential infiltration of neutrophils and macrophages into the damaged tissue at between 6–48 hours post-exercise. Activated macrophages release IL-6 as part of the inflammatory response and, although speculative, it would seem a likely scenario that the sustained elevation in the circulating IL-6 concentration in response to prolonged running is attributable to the presence of activated macrophages in the damaged skeletal muscle.

Although later studies confirmed earlier findings of an increased IL-6 mRNA in skeletal muscle following prolonged exercise (Ostrowski *et al.* 1998b; Starkie *et al.* 2001b), these studies do not demonstrate that the skeletal muscle is the source of the exercise-induced increase in the systemic IL-6 concentration. In this regard, a study by Adam Steensberg, a student of Professor Bente Pedersen from the Copenhagen

Muscle Research Centre, is very important. In this study, catheters were placed into the femoral artery of one leg and the femoral vein of both legs and subjects performed five hours of single-legged knee extensor exercise, a purely concentric exercise model (Steensberg *et al.* 2000). The results of this study were intriguing and demonstrated that the contracting leg releases IL-6 and that this release almost exclusively accounts for the elevated systemic IL-6 concentration. Importantly, despite the same supply of various hormones, metabolites and other potential mediators of IL-6 production from the femoral arteries to the resting and exercising legs, no release of IL-6 was detected from the resting leg. This demonstrates that IL-6 release from the muscle is absolutely dependent upon muscle contraction and that secreted factors (e.g. adrenaline) do not play an important role in the exercise-induced increase in the systemic IL-6 concentration. Importantly, this study did not conclusively demonstrate that skeletal muscle was the source of the exercise-induced increase in the systemic IL-6 concentration. The arteriovenous difference technique is only able to measure the net uptake or release of a given molecule (in this case IL-6) over a specific region of tissue (in this case the upper leg). Therefore, although this study does provide strong evidence that IL-6 is released from the exercising limb, it is possible that other cellular sources within the upper leg, such as resident tissue macrophages, fibroblasts in connective tissue, the endothelium of the muscle capillary bed, adipose tissue or bone may have contributed to increased release of IL-6 from the upper leg during exercise.

One of the most interesting findings of this study was the kinetics that the IL-6 concentration/release displayed during the exercise period. In Figure 12.2A, we can see that, during the first three hours of exercise, the systemic IL-6 concentration is only modestly elevated but during the last two hours of exercise the IL-6 concentration rapidly increases. Similarly, although the release of IL-6 from the resting leg is unaffected by exercise, IL-6 release from the exercising leg is greatly increased during the final two hours of exercise (Figure 12.2B). It therefore appears that the release of IL-6 from the contracting muscles and subsequent accumulation in the systemic circulation is closely related to the duration of the exercise bout. It is well known that, during prolonged exercise, the level of muscle glycogen in the contracting skeletal muscles decreases and it was therefore hypothesised that, during prolonged exercise, IL-6 is released from skeletal muscles in response to an energy crisis, specifically a reduction in muscle glycogen stores, within the contracting myofibres. As muscle glycogen levels decrease, the contracting muscles' reliance on blood glucose as a substrate for energy increases. Thus, IL-6 released from the contracting muscles may signal the liver to increase its glucose output and prevent a drastic, exercise-induced, fall in the blood glucose concentration (Steensberg *et al.* 2000) as illustrated in Figure 12.3. This hypothesis is supported by the observation that carbohydrate ingestion during exercise, which provides an exogenous source of glucose and helps to maintain the blood glucose concentration, attenuates the systemic IL-6 concentration (Nehlsen-Cannarella *et al.* 1997; Starkie *et al.* 2001b). Later studies confirmed that the IL-6 response to exercise was mostly dependent on exercise duration and to a somewhat lesser extent on exercise intensity (Fischer 2006).

Figure 12.2 (A) Systemic interleukin (IL)-6 concentration during 5 hours of single-legged knee extensor exercise. (B) Release of IL-6 from resting and exercising legs during 5 hours of single-legged knee extensor exercise (from Steensberg *et al.* 2000)

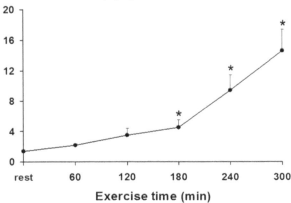

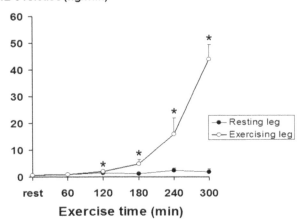

With prolonged exercise (over 2.5 hours), IL-6 levels can increase over 100-fold, although more modest increases are reported with shorter duration exercise (Fischer 2006). Increases have also been noted using intermittent exercise protocols when the exercise duration was relatively short (Meckel *et al.* 2009). With exercise, the increase in IL-6 is transient, normally returning to resting levels within one hour after exercise. The plasma IL-6 concentration increases exponentially with exercise duration and a major stimulus of its synthesis and release appears to be a fall in muscle glycogen content (Keller *et al.* 2005; Pedersen and Fischer 2007). Increases in intracellular calcium and increased formation of reactive oxygen species are also capable of activating transcription factors known to regulate IL-6 synthesis (Fischer 2006).

Figure 12.3 An energy crisis in the contracting muscle – most likely glycogen depletion – stimulates the production of interleukin (IL)-6 by the working muscles. IL-6 is then released from the muscle, resulting in an elevation in the systemic IL-6 concentration. IL-6 also stimulates adrenocorticotrophic hormone (ACTH) and cortisol secretion and may also be involved in the development of central fatigue; CRP = C-reactive protein, T_b = body temperature

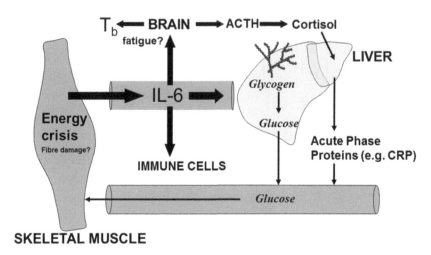

To test the hypothesis that muscle glycogen concentration is indeed a critical factor mediating the release of IL-6 from contracting muscles, Steensberg *et al.* (2001a) performed a study in which pre-exercise muscle glycogen levels were manipulated. To do this, the day before the experimental trial, subjects performed one hour of one-legged cycling exercise to reduce the level of muscle glycogen in one leg only. On the day of the experimental trial, catheters were placed into the femoral artery of one leg and the femoral vein of both legs and subjects performed five hours of two-legged knee extensor exercise. Just before the exercise began, the muscle glycogen concentration of the depleted leg (the leg that was exercised on the day before the experimental trial) was around 50% lower than that of the control (non-exercised) leg and during the first three hours of exercise, the release of IL-6 was significantly greater in the glycogen-depleted leg compared with the control leg. Towards the end of the five-hour exercise period, the release of IL-6 was not different between the control and depleted leg; however, by this time, the muscle glycogen levels were not significantly different. These data provide strong evidence that muscle glycogen is an important regulator of IL-6 production in skeletal muscle during exercise and support the hypothesis that IL-6 is released from contracting muscle in response to an 'energy crisis'.

As discussed above, the detection of an increased amount of IL-6 mRNA in post-exercise compared with pre-exercise muscle biopsies and an increased release of IL-6 protein from a contracting leg as determined via the arteriovenous difference technique, does not provide definitive information on the actual cellular source of the exercise-induced increase in the systemic IL-6 concentration. Similarly, muscle biopsies contain many other cell types in addition to myocytes (e.g. endothelial cells and macrophages) and therefore the increase in IL-6 mRNA detectable in post-exercise muscle biopsies could be caused by an increased production of IL-6 in numerous cell types. To conclusively determine the cellular source of the exercise-induced increase in IL-6, Hiscock *et al.* (2004) obtained muscle biopsies at rest and following 120 minutes of cycling exercise. Biopsies were sectioned and IL-6 protein and mRNA expression within myofibres was determined by immunohistochemistry (staining with fluorescence-labelled monoclonal antibody to IL-6) and *in situ* hybridisation, respectively. The expression of IL-6 protein in myocytes at rest was not detectable but it was present following two hours of low-intensity exercise and was mostly located at the periphery of individual myofibres. Furthermore, an increase in the level of IL-6 mRNA was also observed in post-exercise muscle biopsy samples compared with pre-exercise. These data provide compelling evidence that the source of exercise-induced increase in the systemic IL-6 concentration is indeed the contracting skeletal myocytes. Many of the studies described above were carried out at Copenhagen University by Dr Bente Klarlund Pedersen and colleagues and she was the first to suggest (Pedersen *et al.* 2003) that muscle derived cytokines should be termed 'myokines' (see Box 12.1).

Box 12.1 Dr Bente Klarlund Pedersen PhD FACSM

Bente Klarlund Pedersen is Professor of Integrative Medicine and a specialist in infectious diseases and internal medicine. She is the Director of the Danish National Research Foundation's Centre of Inflammation and Metabolism (www.inflammation-metabolism.dk). She has served as President for The International Society of Exercise and Immunology and President for the Danish Society of Infectious Medicine, Chairman for the research council at Rigshospitalet, coordinator of the Muscle Research Cluster at the Medical Faculty, University of Copenhagen, and as president for the National Council for Public Health in Denmark. Her research has established the importance of muscle-derived cytokines (myokines) such as interleukin-6 in metabolism, obesity and chronic disease (Febbraio and Pedersen 2002; Pedersen 2009; Pedersen and Febbraio 2008; Steensberg *et al.* 2000, 2001a, 2003) and she is one of the most prolific researchers in the field of exercise immunology.

Possible biological roles of IL-6

Despite an increase in our understanding of the mechanisms regulating the release of IL-6 and the sources of the exercise-induced IL-6, the biological role of the exercise-induced increase in the systemic IL-6 concentration has, until very recently, been unknown. In an elegant study, Febbraio *et al.* (2004) tested the hypothesis that IL-6 released from the contracting muscles during exercise signals to the liver to stimulate hepatic glucose production. In this study, subjects performed three experimental trials consisting of two hours of cycling exercise. In one trial, subjects exercised at 70% $\dot{V}O_2$ peak, in a second trial subjects exercised at 40% $\dot{V}O_2$ peak and, in a third trial, subjects exercised at 40% $\dot{V}O_2$ peak and received a constant infusion of recombinant human (rh) IL-6 at a rate intended to match the elevated systemic IL-6 concentration seen during the high-intensity exercise trial. To calculate the endogenous glucose production (hepatic glucose production), subjects were infused with a glucose stable isotope tracer during all trials. Importantly, endogenous glucose production was significantly greater in the 40% $\dot{V}O_2$ peak + rhIL-6 trial compared with the 40% $\dot{V}O_2$ peak trial and was very similar to the endogenous glucose production observed during the 70% $\dot{V}O_2$ peak trial. The main regulator of hepatic glucose production *in vivo* is the glucagon to insulin ratio but, additionally, cortisol and catecholamines also modulate hepatic glucose production. Crucially, in the study by Febbraio *et al.* (2004), no differences were observed between the 40% $\dot{V}O_2$ peak + rhIL-6 trial and the 40% $\dot{V}O_2$ peak trial for insulin, glucagon, cortisol, growth hormone, adrenaline or noradrenaline. Therefore, this study provides compelling support for the hypothesis that IL-6 released during exercise stimulates glucose production from the liver.

Exercise-induced elevations of plasma IL-6 may also influence fat metabolism. When rhIL-6 was infused into resting humans, increasing the plasma IL-6 concentration to levels observed during prolonged exercise, the rates of lipolysis and fat oxidation were increased (van Hall *et al.* 2003). It has also been shown that IL-6-deficient mice develop mature-onset obesity and that when these mice were treated with IL-6 for 18 days, their body weight decreased (Wallenius *et al.* 2002). These studies identify IL-6 as a possible regulator of fat metabolism and support the hypothesis that contracting muscles release IL-6 in a hormone-like manner to increase substrate mobilisation (Figure 12.4).

Strenuous exercise increases plasma concentrations of cortisol, glucagon, adrenaline and noradrenaline. Infusion of rhIL-6 into resting humans to mimic the exercise-induced plasma levels of IL-6 increases plasma cortisol in a similar manner (Steensberg *et al.* 2003). In contrast, the same rhIL-6 infusion does not change plasma adrenaline, noradrenaline or insulin levels in resting, healthy, young subjects. Therefore, muscle-derived IL-6 may be partly responsible for the cortisol response to exercise (Figure 12.3), whereas other hormonal changes cannot be ascribed to IL-6. Stimulation of cortisol secretion by IL-6 may be caused by an effect of IL-6 on the hypothalamus, stimulating the release of ACTH from the anterior pituitary gland or by a direct effect of IL-6 on cortisol release from the adrenal glands; evidence for both mechanisms exists.

In addition, it was demonstrated by Steensberg *et al.* (2003) that relatively small increases in plasma levels of IL-6 induce the two anti-inflammatory cytokines IL-1ra and IL-10 together with C-reactive protein. During exercise, the increase in IL-6 precedes the increase in the these two cytokines, arguing circumstantially for muscle-derived IL-6 to be the initiator of this response. IL-6 and IL-4 stimulate monocytes and macrophages to produce IL-1ra, which inhibits the effect of IL-1. Type-2

Figure 12.4 Some biological actions of muscle-derived interleukin (IL)-6; FFA = free fatty acids, TG = triacylglycerol (adapted from Pedersen *et al.* 2001)

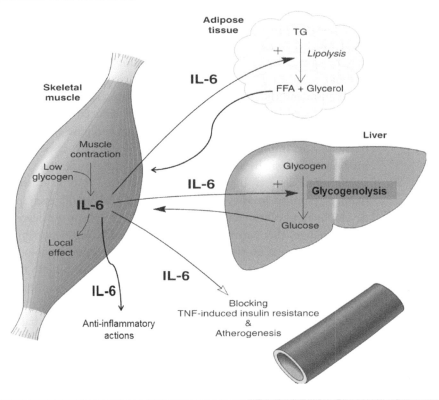

T lymphocytes, monocytes and B cells are the main producers of IL-10 and, together with IL-4, it can inhibit type-1 T-cell cytokine production. In accordance with this, strenuous exercise decreases the percentage of type-1 T cells in the circulation, whereas the percentage of type-2 T cells does not change. Both cortisol and adrenaline suppress the type-1 T cell cytokine production, whereas IL-6 directly stimulates type-2 T cell cytokine production. As discussed in Chapter 2, type-1 T cells drive the immune system towards protection against intracellular pathogens such as viruses; therefore, exercise, possibly working through muscle-derived IL-6, may decrease virus protection in the host and thus may account for athletes appearing to be more prone to acquire upper respiratory tract infection. However, it is very important to stress that the shift toward type-2 T-cell dominance might be beneficial, because it also suppresses the ability of the immune system to induce tissue damage. In addition, in autoimmune diseases such as type-1 diabetes mellitus, autoimmune thyroid disease and Crohn's disease, the balance is turned toward type-1 T-cell dominance. Therefore, by shifting the T-lymphocyte balance toward type-2 T cells, exercise may improve the symptoms of these disorders (Elenkov and Chrousos 2002).

Exercise induces highly stereotypical changes in leukocyte subpopulations. Thus, the number of neutrophils increases during and after exercise. Infusion of rhIL-6 results in similar changes and this effect is likely to be mediated by cortisol. Blood lymphocytes initially increase during exercise and decrease post-exercise. Although these initial changes can be ascribed to catecholamines, the prolonged lymphopenia may be caused by exercise-induced elevations of plasma IL-6. Altogether, these findings suggest that muscle-derived IL-6 may play a role in regulating both fuel metabolism and the immune system during exercise.

As discussed later in this chapter, exercise-induced elevation of circulating IL-6 levels may provide a mechanism to explain how exercise either reduces the suscepti-bility to, or improves, the symptoms of diseases associated with low-grade inflammation, such as type-2 diabetes, atherosclerosis and possibly some autoimmune diseases. In addition, muscle-derived IL-6 may also reduce the inflam-matory response in the exercised muscles and could even play a role in the development of central fatigue (Gleeson 2000a; Robson-Ansley *et al.* 2004) and the mood changes that accompany overtraining. The latter possibility, known as the 'cytokine theory of overtraining', is considered in more detail in Chapter 8.

Intriguingly, other tissues have been shown to contribute to the exercise-induced increase in the systemic IL-6 concentration in addition to the contracting skeletal muscle. For example, the brain has been shown to release IL-6 during exercise (Nybo *et al.* 2002) and IL-6 gene expression within adipose tissue has been shown to be increased in response to exercise (Keller *et al.* 2003). However, the stimulus for the increased production and release of IL-6 from these tissues is presently unclear, although glycogen depletion in the brain during exercise is one possibility (Matsui *et al.* 2012).

EXERCISE AND OTHER CYTOKINES

To determine whether other cytokines exhibit a similar exercise-induced pattern to that of IL-6, Chan *et al.* (2004) and Nieman *et al.* (2003a) examined the mRNA expression of a number of cytokines in response to prolonged exercise. At rest, the mRNA for a number of cytokines, including IL-1β, IL-6, IL-8, IL-15, TNF-α, IL-12p35 and IFN-γ, is detectable in skeletal muscle. In contrast, mRNA for several other cytokines including IL-1α, IL-2, IL-4, IL-5, IL-10 and IL-12p40 is not detectable. In both studies, following exercise an increase in mRNA expression was observed for IL-6 and IL-8; however, in the study by Nieman and colleagues, an increase in mRNA expression was also observed for IL-1β. An exercise-induced increase in mRNA expression was not observed for any other of the measured cytokines. It is probable that the inconsistency in the IL-1β mRNA response is explained by differences in the exercise protocols used in the two studies. Specifically, in the study by Nieman *et al.* (2003a), three hours of running was used as the exercise model, whereas in the study by Chan *et al.* (2004), one hour of cycling exercise was used. It is possible that the increase in IL-1β mRNA expression observed following three hours of running exercise represents the initiation of an inflammatory response induced by muscle damage. In contrast, one hour of cycling, which is unlikely to cause any significant muscle damage, has no effect on IL-1β mRNA expression. In support of this notion, although carbohydrate ingestion during exercise significantly reduced the exercise-induced increase in IL-6 and IL-8 mRNA, supporting a metabolic role for these cytokines, no effect of carbohydrate ingestion was seen on IL-1β mRNA expression. While considerable evidence exists supporting the idea that the increase in IL-6 expression following exercise is from a metabolic 'crisis' within the contracting muscle, the studies by Chan *et al.* (2004) and Nieman *et al.* (2003a) provide the first evidence that IL-8 may have a similar biological profile to that of IL-6. As stated above, carbohydrate ingestion during exercise was shown to blunt the exercise-induced increase in IL-8 mRNA. In addition, the study by Chan and colleagues showed that, when subjects started the one-hour bout of exercise in a muscle glycogen-depleted state, the exercise-induced increase in IL-8 mRNA was significantly greater compared with the control (normal muscle glycogen) trial. However, an important difference exists between the effects of exercise on IL-6 and IL-8 expression: while exercise causes an increase in the expression of both IL-6 and IL-8 mRNA within the contracting muscle, only IL-6 is released. The biological role of the exercise-induced increase of IL-8 within the contracting muscle awaits future research.

The plasma concentration of IL-1ra is markedly increased in response to prolonged exercise. Interestingly, although the increase in the plasma concentration of IL-1ra is of a similar magnitude to that of IL-6, the peak plasma IL-1ra concentration occurs slightly later than that of IL-6 (see Figure 12.1); in fact, in many studies it is seen to peak in the post-exercise recovery period. Given that IL-6 is a potent inducer of IL-1ra, it is likely that the release of IL-6 from the contracting muscle during prolonged exercise stimulates the release of IL-1ra from blood mononuclear cells. In support of this notion, IL-1ra mRNA is increased in blood mononuclear cells obtained following prolonged strenuous exercise whereas IL-6 mRNA is not (Ostrowski *et al.* 1998b). Given that IL-1ra is an anti-inflammatory cytokine, it is likely the increase in the exercise-induced increase in the IL-1ra concentration acts as a negative feedback mechanism, controlling the magnitude and duration of IL-6 and IL-1 mediated effects.

In this first part of the chapter, we have discussed how exercise directly effects the production of cytokines in various tissues. The magnitude and duration of the IL-6 response to exercise initially marked it out for further investigation. Subsequent studies have demonstrated that exercise directly stimulates the production of IL-6 from contracting skeletal muscle and that IL-6 released from skeletal muscle during exercise acts in a hormone-like fashion to stimulate glucose output from the liver and lipolysis in adipose tissue. However, exercise induces an increase in the systemic concentration and muscle levels of numerous additional cytokines. Intriguingly, the functions of many of these cytokines, with respect to exercise, are poorly understood and many additional studies are required to more fully understand the biological role of these exercise-induced cytokines.

> **Box 12.2** Differences between the cytokine responses to sepsis and exercise
>
> Increases in circulating cytokines occur as a response to both sepsis (caused by infection) and exercise, and occasionally authors comment on the similarities between the two. However, there a number of important differences in the pattern, time course and magnitude of the response.
>
> - Certainly, strenuous exercise is accompanied by an increase in circulating cytokines, having some similarities with the response to sepsis and trauma. An inflammatory response represents a fundamental series of humoral and cellular reaction cascades in response to infection, tissue injury and related insults. An excessive response is commonly seen under the pathological conditions of trauma, sepsis and burns. Most, if not all, of the distinguishing features of a classical inflammatory response are detectable in an exercising individual, namely mobilisation and activation of granulocytes, lymphocytes and monocytes; release of inflammatory factors and soluble mediators; involvement of active phase reactants; and activation of the complement and other reactive humoral cascade systems.
> - In sepsis, there is a sequential release of substantial amounts of TNF-α, IL-1β and IFN-γ from activated immune cells. Particularly large increases in these circulating cytokines are observed in bacterial diseases. As the infection is cleared and inflammation subsides, there is a later secretion of inflammation responsive cytokines (e.g. IL-6) and anti-inflammatory cytokines such as IL-1 receptor antagonist (IL-1ra), IL-10 and soluble TNF receptors (sTNF).
> - In exercise, there is a rather small and sometimes undetectable rise in proinflammatory cytokines like TNF-α, IL-1β and IFN-γ. Rather, there is an increase in circulating IL-6 (released not from immune cells but from contracting muscle fibres) which induces increased secretion of IL-1ra, IL-10 and sTNF (Pedersen *et al.* 2009).
> - While the manifestation of many exercise-induced immune and related changes has been reported and confirmed repeatedly, several of the underlying mechanisms triggering and modulating the elicited immune responses are undoubtedly different. Sepsis-associated cytokine responses are largely initiated by activation of Toll-like receptors on antigen-presenting cells, while exercise-induced IL-6 release is activated by rises in intramuscular calcium and falls in glycogen. One similarity between exercise and sepsis is that the presence of endotoxin in the circulation can occur in some forms of exercise, owing to increased gut permeability, but endotoxin levels are generally much lower than observed in sepsis.
> - Although there are qualitative similarities between the immune responses to exercise and sepsis, the magnitude of the changes induced by most forms of exercise remains much smaller than in a typical inflammatory response (Shephard 2001).

INFLUENCE OF EXERCISE ON CYTOKINE PRODUCTION FROM LEUKOCYTES

As discussed briefly above, when cytokine production is examined in unstimulated leukocytes (leukocytes that have not been exposed to an activating agent such as lipopolysaccharide [LPS] or phorbol 12-myristate 13-acetate [PMA]), no cytokine so far examined is influenced by exercise. In two studies by Starkie *et al.* (2000, 2001a), prolonged exercise, either cycling or running, had no effect on the production of IL-1β, TNF-α or IL-6 from unstimulated monocytes. Similarly, Lancaster *et al.* (2005a) reported that prolonged exercise has no effect on the production of IL-4, IL-6 or IFN-γ from unstimulated lymphocytes. Thus, unlike skeletal muscle, exercise does not directly stimulate the production of cytokines from leukocytes.

Cytokine production by cells of the immune system is critical in the development of immune responses against invading pathogens. To date, studies that have examined the effects of acute or chronic exercise on cytokine production have primarily focused on monocytes and T lymphocytes, probably because of the important role that cytokine production from these cells plays in the development of immune responses. Specifically, the production of IL-1β, TNF-α and IL-6 by is an important component of the inflammatory response initiated by invading pathogenic microorganisms and tissue damage. You may recall from Chapter 2 that T lymphocytes are able to secrete numerous cytokines, including IFN-γ, IL-2, IL-4, IL-5 and IL-12. Specifically, T lymphocytes known as type-1 CD4+ lymphocytes (Th1 lymphocytes) secrete IFN-γ and IL-2, while type-2 CD4+ lymphocytes (Th2 lymphocytes) secrete IL-4, IL-5 and IL-12. The cytokines secreted by type-1 and type-2 T lymphocytes play critical roles in promoting both cell-mediated immunity (the activation of macrophages and CD8+ T cytotoxic lymphocytes, promotion of antibody class switching to IgG2a) and humoral immunity (B-cell activation and differentiation, promotion of antibody class switching to IgE and IgG1 and the activation of eosinophils), respectively.

While the effect of exercise on unstimulated monocyte cytokine production has received much attention – as initially it was believed that monocytes were likely to be the source of the exercise-induced increase in systemic cytokine concentrations – the effect of exercise on stimulated monocyte cytokine production has also been examined in several studies. For example, Starkie *et al.* (2001a) have shown that a competitive marathon suppresses the amount of IL-6, TNF-α and IL-1α produced by LPS-stimulated monocytes. Interestingly, it has been demonstrated that incubation of whole blood samples with adrenaline inhibits monocyte cytokine production, while the infusion of cortisol at either physiological or pharmacological concentrations similarly inhibits monocyte cytokine production. Exercise is a potent activator of the central nervous system, acting through motor centre stimulation of endocrine centres within the brain and blood-borne metabolic and peripheral neural feedback mechanisms. Thus, exercise causes a marked increase in the circulating concentration of several immunomodulatory hormones.

To examine the influence of exercise-induced increases in immunomodulatory hormones on monocyte cytokine production Lancaster *et al.* (2005b) carried out a study in which ten subjects performed bicycle exercise for 90 minutes in a 35ºC heat chamber supplemented with either a 6.4% (6.4 grams per 100 mL) carbohydrate beverage or a placebo. Importantly, supplementation with a carbohydrate solution during exercise results in a significant attenuation of the exercise-induced increase in the systemic concentration of numerous immunomodulatory hormones, including adrenaline and cortisol. The production of TNF-α and IL-6 by monocytes stimulated with either LPS or zymosan was determined in the pre- and post-exercise blood samples. Zymosan is a polysaccharide component of the cell wall of yeast and is recognised by specific receptors on the monocyte cell surface; of note, the receptors that recognise LPS are distinct from those that recognise zymosan. The results confirmed that exercise results in a decrease in the production of IL-6 and TNF-α by LPS-stimulated monocytes. Furthermore, the ingestion of carbohydrate during exercise, which resulted in an attenuation of the circulating concentration of several immunomodulatory hormones compared with placebo ingestion, attenuated the exercise-induced decrease in LPS-stimulated IL-6 and TNF-α production from monocytes. While these results certainly provide evidence that exercise modulates monocyte cytokine production via increases in the circulating concentrations of immunomodulatory hormones, they do not identify the specific hormones involved. While several studies have shown that LPS-stimulated monocyte cytokine production is impaired following prolonged strenuous exercise, few studies have examined monocyte cytokine production in response to stimuli other than LPS. Intriguingly, Lancaster et al. (2005b) found that in contrast to the observed suppressive effects of exercise on LPS-stimulated monocyte cytokine production, zymosan-stimulated monocyte cytokine production was augmented following exercise. While the reason for these divergent results are not yet clear, what they do emphasise is that exercise does not simply cause a general suppression of stimulated monocyte cytokine production.

As discussed above, type-1 and type-2 cytokine-producing T lymphocytes play very important roles in the development of immune responses and it is therefore not surprising that several studies have examined the influence of exercise on stimulated cytokine production from T lymphocytes. Several studies (Steensberg et al. 2001b; Ibfelt et al. 2002) have shown that prolonged exercise causes a decrease in the circulating concentration of IFN-γ-producing type-1 T lymphocytes and that this decrease is sustained for several hours post-exercise. In contrast, prolonged exercise has little effect on the number of circulating IL-4-producing type-2 T lymphocytes. However, these studies did not determine the amount of cytokine produced in response to stimulation.

The type-1 cytokine IFN-γ is very important in antiviral defence and several studies have demonstrated that the concentration of IFN-γ in the supernatant of stimulated whole blood is decreased following prolonged exercise. To examine the potential mechanisms involved in the exercise-induced suppression of IFN-γ production by T lymphocytes, Starkie et al. (2001c) performed a study in which subjects were given α- and β-adrenoreceptor antagonists (thus allowing the investigators to examine the influence of adrenaline and noradrenaline on exercise-induced alterations in T lymphocyte IFN-γ production) before completing a bout of strenuous exercise. The results of this study demonstrated that while α- and β-adrenoreceptor blockade abrogated the exercise-induced decrease in the number of circulating IFN-γ-producing T lymphocytes, it had no effect on the amount of IFN-γ produced by stimulated T lymphocytes. These results suggest that adrenergic stimulation is unlikely to be the mechanism causing the decrease in stimulated IFN-γ production following exercise.

To further explore the potential mechanisms regulating the exercise-induced suppression of stimulated IFN-γ production from T lymphocytes and the exercise-induced decrease in the number of circulating IFN-γ-producing T lymphocytes, Lancaster *et al.* (2005a) conducted a study in which subjects performed 2.5 hours of bicycle exercise supplemented with either a 6.4% carbohydrate solution, 12.8% carbohydrate beverage or placebo. The results of the study confirmed previous findings, demonstrating that stimulated IFN-γ production is decreased following exercise. The results showed that IFN-γ production in response to stimulation with PMA + ionomycin was decreased in both CD4+ T helper and CD8+ T cytotoxic lymphocytes following exercise. Interestingly, there was a dose-dependent effect of carbohydrate ingestion on stimulated IFN-γ production from T lymphocytes, although both the 6.4% and 12.8% carbohydrate beverages (the prescribed drinking regimen employed resulted in subjects receiving 38.4 g or 76.8 g of carbohydrate per hour) attenuated the exercise-induced suppression of stimulated T-lymphocyte IFN-γ production observed during the placebo trial. Furthermore, there was a significant correlation between the post-exercise CD4+ and CD8+ T-lymphocyte IFN-γ production and the post-exercise cortisol concentration. While not demonstrating cause and effect, these results suggest that cortisol plays a role in the post-exercise suppression of T lymphocyte IFN-γ production.

The finding of suppressed cytokine production from specific cells of the immune system has led to the hypothesis that defects in cytokine production may account for the reported increased sensitivity to upper respiratory tract infections (URTI) following prolonged strenuous exercise or during periods of intense training (Smith 2003). While the evidence strongly suggests that both monocyte and type-1 T-lymphocyte cytokine production is suppressed following endurance events, it is important to realise that these changes have not been shown to be a causative factor in the increased susceptibility to URTI that has been reported to occur following prolonged strenuous exercise and during periods of intensified exercise training. However, some evidence suggests that the balance of the proinflammatory to anti-inflammatory cytokines produced in response to stimulation of leukocytes with antigen may be an important determinant of illness risk (Gleeson *et al.* 2012b). It appears that athletes with a relatively high incidence of URTI (i.e. illness-prone individuals) exhibit a significantly higher IL-10 response to antigen stimulation of whole blood culture than athletes who are generally less susceptible to URTI. Furthermore, the IL-10 response to antigen stimulation is influenced positively by training load (Gleeson *et al.*, 2012a; Wang *et al.* 2012).

LINKS BETWEEN SEDENTARY BEHAVIOUR, CHRONIC INFLAMMATION AND CHRONIC DISEASE

The prevalence of obesity continues to rise worldwide and is being accompanied by proportional increases in a host of other medical conditions associated with derangements of immunometabolism (Mathis and Shoelson 2011) such as type-2 diabetes, cardiovascular diseases, chronic obstructive pulmonary disease, colon cancer, breast cancer, dementia and depression. Inflammation appears to be aetiologically linked to the pathogenesis of all these conditions (Ouchi *et al.* 2011) and the development of a chronic low-grade inflammatory state (as indicated by elevated levels of circulating inflammation markers such as IL-6, TNF-α and C-reactive protein) has been established as a predictor of risk for several of them (Pradhan *et al.* 2001). Importantly, physical inactivity and sedentary behaviour increase the risk of all these conditions (Pedersen and Saltin 2006; Hardman and Stensel 2009; Warren *et al.* 2010). An inactive lifestyle leads to the accumulation of visceral fat and, consequently, the activation of a network of inflammatory pathways that results in inflammation in adipose tissue, increased release of adipokines (peptides and proteins including some cytokines that are secreted from white adipose tissue) and the development of a low-grade systemic inflammatory state (Ouchi *et al.* 2011). Chronic inflammation promotes the development of insulin resistance, atherosclerosis, neurodegeneration and tumour growth and, subsequently, the development of several diseases associated with physical inactivity (Figure 12.5). Exercise has anti-inflammatory effects and therefore, in the long-term, regular physical activity can protect against the development of these chronic diseases, as well as having other benefits for health, functional capacity and quality of life (Pedersen and Saltin 2006; Hardman and Stensel 2009), which are summarised in Table 12.1. Furthermore, exercise can be used as a treatment for (or to ameliorate the symptoms of) many of these conditions which is increasingly being promoted as the concept that 'exercise is medicine'.

Obviously, exercise increases energy expenditure and burns off some of the body fat that would otherwise accumulate when individuals eat more dietary energy than they need. In that simple sense, exercise reduces the risk of developing obesity and excessive adiposity. Regular exercise also imbues cardiovascular health benefits by improving the blood lipid profile through decreasing the concentration of plasma triglycerides and small low-density lipoprotein particles and by increasing the concentration of protective high-density lipoprotein cholesterol (Kraus *et al.* 2002). These beneficial alterations in plasma lipids are presumed to limit the development of atherosclerosis. However, the protective effect of a physically active lifestyle against chronic inflammation associated diseases may, to some extent, be ascribed to an anti-inflammatory effect of exercise (Kasapis and Thomson 2005). This may be mediated not only via a reduction in visceral fat mass (with a subsequent decreased production and release of adipokines) but also by induction of an anti-inflammatory environment with each bout of exercise (Petersen and Pedersen 2005). The remainder of this chapter explains the possible mechanisms by which exercise exerts its anti-inflammatory effect and briefly discuss the implications for the use of exercise as medicine in the prevention and treatment of chronic disease.

Figure 12.5 Physical inactivity and positive energy balance lead to an accumulation of visceral fat which becomes infiltrated by proinflammatory macrophages and T cells. The proinflammatory M1 macrophage phenotype predominates and inflamed adipose tissue releases adipokines and tumour necrosis factor alpha (TNF-α) that lead to a state of persistent low-grade systemic inflammation. This promotes the development of insulin resistance, tumour growth, neurodegeneration and atherosclerosis. The latter is exacerbated by the deleterious changes in the blood lipid profile associated with a lack of physical activity; CRP = C-reactive protein, FFA = free fatty acids, HDL = high-density lipoprotein, IL = interleukin, LDL = low-density lipoprotein, MØ = macrophage, TLR = toll-like receptor

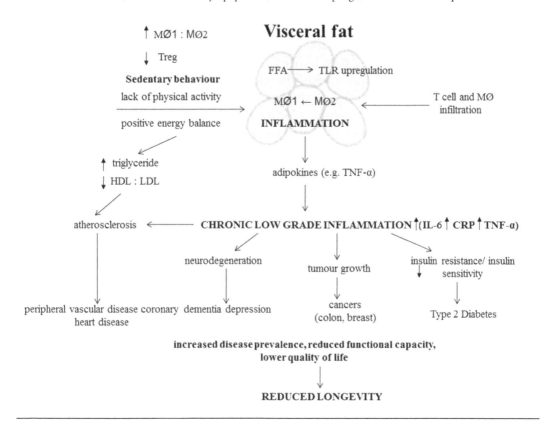

ANTI-INFLAMMATORY EFFECTS OF EXERCISE

The anti-inflammatory effects of exercise have mostly been ascribed to two possible mechanisms: (1) increased production and release of anti-inflammatory cytokines from contracting skeletal muscle (Mathur and Pedersen 2008); and (2) reduced expression of Toll-like receptors (TLRs) on monocytes and macrophages (Flynn and McFarlin 2006) with subsequent inhibition of downstream responses such as proinflammatory cytokine production, antigen presentation and co-stimulatory molecule expression (Gleeson et al. 2006). However, the anti-inflammatory effects of exercise arise not only from these two mechanisms but also other effects of exercise

Table 12.1 Summary of the interaction between physical activity and major diseases assessing evidence that exercise may: (A) lower disease risk and (B) have therapeutic value in treating disease	
DISEASE	EVIDENCE THAT PHYSICAL ACTIVITY MAY LOWER DISEASE RISK AND/OR HAVE THERAPEUTIC VALUE IN TREATING DISEASE
Coronary heart disease	A large body of epidemiological evidence demonstrates that high levels of PA and PF are associated with a lower risk of developing CHD. RCTs show that regular PA can favourably modify CHD risk factors including (but not limited to) dyslipidaemia, hypertension and obesity. RCTs also show that PA improves survival in CHD patients.
Stroke	Evidence that high levels of PA and PF reduce the risk of stroke is suggestive but not as compelling as that for CHD. RCTs show that PA can lower but not necessarily normalise blood pressure in hypertensive individuals.
Cancer	High levels of PA are associated with lower risk of colon and breast cancer. PA may lower cancer risk by systemic (reduced body fat and insulin levels, enhanced immune function) and site-specific (reduced sex steroid hormone levels for breast cancer, decreased bowel transit time for colon cancer) mechanisms. Some observational and RCT evidence supports a therapeutic role for PA in preserving mobility and function in cancer patients.
Type 2 diabetes mellitus	Observational epidemiological evidence consistently demonstrates an association between high levels of PA/PF and a reduced risk of developing type 2 diabetes. RCTs show that lifestyle intervention (diet and PA) can lower body mass, improve glucose tolerance and reduce the risk of developing T2D in high risk patients. In patients with type 2 diabetes, high levels of PA and PF are associated with a reduced risk of CHD and all-cause mortality.
Dementia	Observational epidemiological studies indicate that higher levels of PA are associated with a lower risk of cognitive decline and dementia in older adults. Some limited evidence is available from RCTs to suggest that PA induces modest improvements in cognition in people who are at increased risk of dementia and Alzheimer's disease.
Other	There is some evidence from observational and intervention studies to support a role for PA for enhancing physical function and improving quality of life in those suffering from chronic heart failure, chronic obstructive pulmonary disease, depression, intermittent claudication, osteoarthritis and osteoporosis.

CHD: coronary heart disease; PA: physical activity; PF: physical fitness; RCT: randomised controlled trial; T2D: type 2 diabetes

that have been established, such as the inhibition of monocyte/macrophage infiltration into adipose tissue (Kawanishi *et al.* 2010), phenotypic switching of macrophages within adipose tissue (Kawanishi *et al.* 2010), a reduction in the circulating numbers of proinflammatory monocytes (Timmerman *et al.* 2008) and an increase the circulating numbers of IL-10 secreting regulatory T cells (Yeh *et al.* 2006; Wang *et al.* 2012). The major focus of this part of the chapter is to explain these various mechanisms.

Reduction in visceral fat mass

The accumulation of body fat, particularly in the abdomen, liver and muscles, is associated with increased all-cause mortality (Pischon *et al.* 2008), the development of type 2 diabetes (Bays 2009), cardiovascular disease (Haffner 2007), dementia (Whitmer *et al.* 2008) and several cancers (Xue and Michels 2007). The production of proinflammatory adipokines is increased with adipose tissue expansion, whereas the amounts of anti-inflammatory cytokines produced are reduced. This leads to the development of a state of persistent system low-grade inflammation (Yudkin 2007). Regular exercise can reduce waist circumference and cause considerable reductions in abdominal/visceral fat, even in the absence of any loss of body weight, in both men and women regardless of age (Ross and Bradshaw 2009). Therefore, increased physical activity can bring about a reduction in systemic inflammation (Yudkin 2007) via a reduction in proinflammatory adipokine secretion as a direct result of lowering the amount of fat stored in abdominal depots.

Release of IL-6 from contracting muscle

As mentioned earlier in this chapter, during and after exercise of sufficient load, the active skeletal muscle will increase cellular and circulating levels of IL-6 (Pedersen 2009). When exercise is performed for about one hour, the increase in IL-6 is transient, normally returning to resting levels within one hour after exercise. IL-6 appears responsible for the subsequent rise in circulating levels of the anti-inflammatory cytokines IL-10 and IL-1ra and also stimulates the release of cortisol from the adrenal glands (Steensberg *et al.* 2003), as well as having previously mentioned metabolic effects. These actions and possible associated health effects are summarised in Figure 12.6. The causal role of IL-6 in stimulating IL-10, IL-1ra and cortisol secretion is substantiated by the observation that intravenous infusion of IL-6 totally mimics the acute anti-inflammatory effects of a bout of exercise both with regard to elevations of plasma IL-10, IL-1ra and cortisol (Steensberg *et al.* 2003) and with regard to suppression of endotoxin-stimulated increases in TNF-α levels (Starkie *et al.* 2003). The IL-6 half life is prolonged by combining with the soluble IL-6 receptor (sIL-6R) and it is this complex which is crucial in determining the biological activity of IL-6. The expression of IL-6R in tissues is limited to hepatocytes, leukocytes and adipocytes (Rose-John *et al.* 2006) with a relatively low expression in resting skeletal muscle (Keller *et al.* 2005). Exercise training increases the expression of IL-6R on the muscle membrane (Keller *et al.* 2005), removing some of the dependency on the circulating sIL-6 receptor.

IL-1ra is secreted mainly by monocytes and macrophages and inhibits the pro-inflammatory actions of IL-1β (Freeman and Buchman 2001). IL-10 is known to be produced primarily by regulatory T cells and monocytes but also by Th2 cells, macrophages, dendritic cells, B cells, CD8+ T cells, Th1 cells, and Th17 cells (Maynard and Weaver 2008). Irrespective of the cellular source, the principal role of IL-10 appears to be containment and suppression of inflammatory responses so as to

Figure 12.6 Biological role of muscle-derived interleukin (IL)-6 during exercise. Full lines represent acute effects of IL-6 infusion. Broken lines represent possible health effects of IL-6, and suggested effects of acute IL-6 infusion; CRP = C-reactive protein, TNF-α = tumour necrosis factor alpha (adapted from Steensberg 2003)

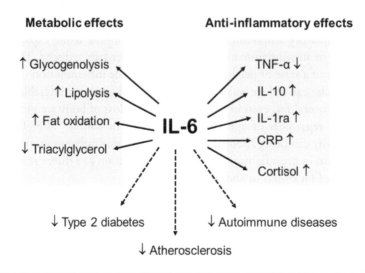

downregulate adaptive immune effector responses (Moore *et al.* 2001) and to minimise tissue damage in response to microbial challenges. Accordingly, IL-10 induces downregulation of major histocompatibility complex (MHC) antigens, the intercellular adhesion molecule-1, as well as the co-stimulatory molecules CD80 and CD86 on antigen presenting cells, and it has been shown to promote differentiation of dendritic cells expressing low levels of MHC class II, CD80 and CD86 (Maynard and Weaver 2008). In addition, IL-10 downregulates or completely inhibits the expression of several proinflammatory cytokines and other soluble mediators, thereby further compromising the capacity of effector T cells to sustain inflammatory responses.

Thus, IL-10 is a potent promoter of an anti-inflammatory state. Circulating levels of IL-10 are lower in obese subjects and acute treatment with IL-10 prevents lipid-induced insulin resistance (Hong *et al.* 2009). IL-10 increases insulin sensitivity and protects skeletal muscle from obesity-associated macrophage infiltration, increases in inflammatory cytokines and their deleterious effects on insulin signalling and glucose metabolism (Hong *et al.* 2009).

A limitation of the hypothesis that exercise-induced elevations of IL-6 are mostly responsible for the anti-inflammatory and long-term health benefits of regular exercise is that substantial increases in circulating IL-6 do not occur with short durations of low/moderate intensity exercise (Fischer 2006) despite the known health benefits (e.g. reduced risk of heart disease) associated with only very moderate increases in physical activity above that of a totally sedentary lifestyle (Miyashita *et al.* 2008).

Increased levels of circulating cortisol and adrenaline

Secretion of the adrenal hormones cortisol and adrenaline into the circulation is increased during exercise, owing to activation of the hypothalamic-pituitary-adrenal axis and the sympathetic nervous system (SNS), respectively. Impulses from the motor centres in the brain, as well as afferent impulses from working muscles, elicit an intensity-dependent increase in sympathoadrenal activity and in release of some pituitary hormones including adrenocorticotrophic hormone (ACTH; Galbo 1983). Increased SNS activity stimulates adrenaline and noradrenaline release from the adrenal medulla within seconds of the onset of exercise and ACTH stimulates cortisol secretion from the adrenal cortex within a matter of minutes. These hormonal responses usually precede the rises in circulating concentrations of cytokines. Thus, the magnitude of the elevations in plasma cortisol and adrenaline are related to the intensity and duration of exercise (Galbo 1983). Cortisol is known to have potent anti-inflammatory effects (Cupps and Fauci 1982) and catecholamines downregulate the LPS-induced production of TNF-α, IL-6 and IL-1β by immune cells (Bergmann *et al.* 1999). Cortisol secretion is also augmented by the aforementioned rise in circulating IL-6 (Steensberg *et al.* 2003). Thus, hormones, myokines and cytokines all contribute to the anti-inflammatory effect of exercise (Figure 12.7).

Inhibition of macrophage infiltration into adipose tissue

The expression of proinflammatory cytokines, chemokines and cell adhesion molecules in adipose tissue is increased in obese mice (Jiao *et al.* 2009). Macrophages and T cells, which infiltrate adipose tissue in obesity, are known to regulate the inflammatory state of adipose tissue (Kanda *et al.* 2006). Thus, the migration of peripheral blood mononuclear cells (PBMCs) towards sites of inflammation, including adipose tissue and damaged vascular endothelium, is central to the development of sustained tissue inflammation (Zeyda *et al.* 2011). It is thought that the size of the adipocytes triggers macrophage infiltration, rather than overall obesity, and that recruitment of the macrophages may be stimulated by the chemokines, monocyte chemotactic protein (MCP)-1 and macrophage inflammatory protein (MIP)-1α (Bruun *et al.* 2005).

Exercise might limit the movement of PBMCs into inflamed adipose tissue in a similar manner to its effect of reducing PBMC migration towards a virus-infected human bronchial epithelial cell line (Bishop *et al.* 2009). Migration of PBMCs from the circulation into the tissues is a tightly regulated process involving a gradient of release of chemokines from the inflamed tissue (including from immune cells residing within), the expression of complimentary chemokine receptors on PBMCs and the expression of adhesion molecules on both immune and endothelial cells. Acute bouts of exercise reduce T-cell migration towards the supernatants of human rhinovirus-infected human bronchial epithelial cells in a manner that is independent of any involvement of adhesion molecules or exercise-induced elevations of cortisol or catecholamines (Bishop *et al.* 2009). However, it is known that acute exercise stress

Figure 12.7 Potential mechanisms contributing to the anti-inflammatory effects of exercise. Activation of the hypothalamic-pituitary-adrenal axis (HPA) and sympathetic nervous system (SNS) lead to the release of cortisol and adrenaline from the adrenal cortex and medulla, respectively. These hormones inhibit the release of tumour necrosis factor alpha (TNF-α) by monocytes. Interleukin (IL)-6 produced by contracting skeletal muscle also downregulates the production of TNF-α by monocytes and may stimulate further cortisol release. Acute elevations in IL-6 stimulate release of IL-1 receptor antagonist (IL-1ra) from monocytes and macrophages, thus increasing the circulating concentrations of this anti-inflammatory cytokine. Exercise training mobilises TReg cells, a major source of the anti-inflammatory cytokine IL-10 and decreases the proportion of inflammatory (CD14lowCD16+) monocytes, compared with classical (CD14high) monocytes. Following exercise CD14high monocytes express less TLR4 and thereby induce a reduced inflammatory response, marked by lower levels of proinflammatory cytokines and reduced adipose tissue infiltration. Exercise also increases plasma concentrations of key inflammatory immune cell chemokines; repeated elevations of such chemokines may lead to a downregulation of their cellular receptors, resulting in reduced tissue infiltration. A reduction in adipose tissue mass and adipocyte size, along with reduced macrophage infiltration, and a switch from a M1 to M2 phenotype all may contribute to a reduction in pro-inflammatory cytokine release from adipose tissue, such as IL-6 and TNF-α, and an increase in anti-inflammatory cytokine release, such as adiponectin and IL-10; MØ = macrophage

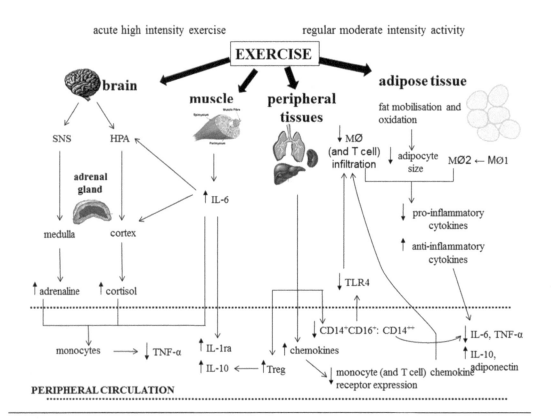

results in the release of chemokines into the circulation from multiple sources and sustained exposure of PBMCs to physiological concentrations of chemokines including MCP-1 results in chemokine receptor internalisation (Maffei *et al.* 2009).

This is thought to serve as a negative feedback mechanism to reduce migration and thereby terminate accumulation of PBMCs in inflamed tissue. It is therefore possible that an active lifestyle creates an environment of repeated short-lasting elevations in plasma chemokines that act over time to downregulate expression of their receptors on PBMCs and restrict migration of these cells towards adipose tissue. However, this potential mechanism needs to be explored further in humans.

Whether exercise acts to inhibit the release of chemokines from human adipose tissue and in this way reduce macrophage infiltration is not clear. Certainly, evidence from murine studies has shown that obese mice deficient in the macrophage chemokines MCP-1 and CXCL14 do not exhibit inflammatory responses such as macrophage infiltration, increased tissue expression of IL-6 and insulin resistance (Kanda *et al.* 2006). However, while exercise training reduces macrophage infiltration into adipose tissue in obese mice, it has little effect on adipose tissue MCP-1 and CXCL14 expression (Kawanishi *et al.* 2010), perhaps suggesting that these chemokines are not key to the exercise-induced restriction of macrophage infiltration of adipose tissue. Findings in humans do not report any independent effect of 12 weeks of exercise training on adipose tissue expression of MCP-1 (or MIP-1α, TNF-α and IL-6), despite falls in circulating concentrations of MCP-1 with exercise. Diet-induced weight loss, or weight loss in combination with exercise, were associated with non-significant falls in adipokine mRNA expression in adipose tissue and significant decreases in CD14 expression in adipose tissue were only found with diet alone).

In mice, training is reported to decrease the tissue expression of intercellular adhesion molecule-1 (ICAM-1) (Kawanishi *et al.* 2010), the expression of which is known to be increased in obesity in humans (Bosanská *et al.* 2010). Furthermore, antagonism of ICAM-1 in obese mice prevents macrophage infiltration into adipose tissue (Chow *et al.* 2005) and circulating ICAM-1 levels were reduced by six months of progressive aerobic exercise training in people with type 2 diabetes without changes in body mass and waist circumference (Zoppini *et al.* 2006). Further studies in humans are required to ascertain the role of exercise training on ICAM-1 in adipose tissue but ICAM-I might also play a role in the exercise-induced reduction of macrophage infiltration into adipose tissue.

Macrophage activation has been defined into two separate polarisation states, M1 and M2 (Martinez *et al.* 2008). The M1 macrophage produces TNF-α, IL-6 and nitric oxide while the M2 macrophage produces anti-inflammatory cytokines and arginase. Therefore, M1 macrophages induce a chronic inflammatory state and M2 macrophages subdue inflammation in adipose tissue. The inflammation state of adipose tissue also appears to be associated with a preferential recruitment of M1 macrophages and/or a phenotypic switch of macrophage polarisation in adipose tissue towards the M1 phenotype. Therefore, it is possible that the attenuated inflammatory state of adipose tissue associated with chronic exercise training occurs by both suppression of macrophage infiltration and acceleration of phenotypic switching from M1 to M2 macrophages. A study in mice fed a high-fat diet to induce obesity provided some evidence that exercise training induces the phenotypic switching from M1 to M2 macrophages in adipose tissue, as well as inhibiting M1 macrophage infiltration into adipose tissue (Kawanishi *et al.* 2010), although studies in humans are lacking.

DOWNREGULATION OF TLR EXPRESSION

TLRs are highly conserved transmembrane proteins that play an important role in the detection and recognition of microbial pathogens (described in more detail in Chapter 2) and they can also be activated by endogenous danger signals of tissue damage such as heat shock proteins (Kaisho and Akira 2006). The key product of TLR signalling in antigen-presenting cells is the production of proinflammatory cytokines and proteins and thus the TLR pathway plays an important role in mediating whole body inflammation (Takeda *et al.* 2003). Following a prolonged bout of strenuous exercise the expression of TLRs 1, 2 and 4 on monocytes is decreased for at least several hours (Lancaster *et al.* 2005b; Gleeson *et al.* 2006; Oliveira and Gleeson 2010; Figure 12.8). Prolonged exercise also results in a

Figure 12.8 Effect of 2.5 hours of cycling at 60% $\dot{V}O_2$ max in temperate (20°C) conditions on monocyte Toll-like receptor (TLR) expression (data from Oliveira and Gleeson 2010)

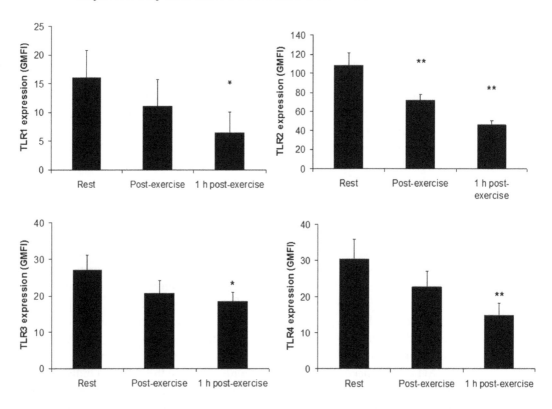

decreased induction of MHC class II, co-stimulatory molecules CD80 and CD86, and cytokines following stimulation with known TLR ligands (Lancaster *et al.* 2005b). Whether this reduction in cell surface expression of TLRs is due a downregulation of TLR gene expression, a shedding of TLRs from the cell surface or reinternalisation by the cell remains to be established.

Evidence is now emerging that TLRs may be involved in the link between a sedentary lifestyle, inflammation and disease. Exercise training studies and cross-sectional comparisons between physically active and inactive subjects have shown a reduced inflammatory response of blood monocytes to endotoxin stimulation *in vitro* and a lowered TLR4 expression at both the cell surface and mRNA level in physically active individuals (Flynn and McFarlin 2006; Gleeson *et al.* 2006; Figure 12.9), which is associated with decreased inflammatory cytokine production (Stewart *et al.* 2005) and has been shown to occur in both young and elderly adults (Figure 12.10). Over the long term, a decrease in TLR expression may represent a beneficial effect for health because it decreases the inflammatory capacity of leukocytes, thus altering whole body chronic inflammation and possibly reducing the risk of developing chronic disease. The precise physiological stimulus mediating an exercise-induced decrease in cell-surface TLR expression is not known; however, several possible signals have been implicated including anti-inflammatory cytokines, stress hormones and heat shock proteins (Gleeson *et al.* 2006).

Figure 12.9 Effect of exercise training and Toll-like receptor (TLR)4-mRNA and TLR4 expression. (A) A longitudinal study of 9 weeks of resistance training in elderly women (data from Flynn *et al.* 2003). (B) A cross-sectional study of trained and untrained elderly women; * = group difference (*P* < 0.05) (data from McFarlin *et al.* 2004)

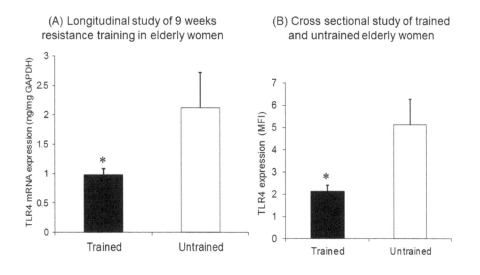

Figure 12.10 Effects of moderate exercise training and age on monocyte Toll-like receptor (TLR)4 expression. Data are for old and young subjects before and after a 12-week training intervention in the inactive groups or maintained activity level in the active groups; MFI = mean fluorescence intensity; * group difference ($P < 0.05$) (adapted from Stewart *et al.* 2005)

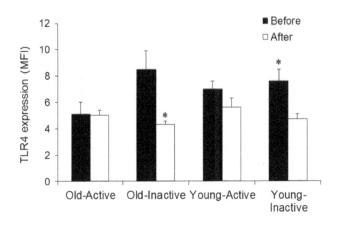

Reduced numbers of proinflammatory monocytes in blood

There are two main populations of monocytes, classical (CD14++) and inflammatory (CD14+CD16+), that differentially express cell-surface TLR4, with the inflammatory monocytes expressing 2.5 times more cell-surface TLR4 (Skinner *et al.* 2005). Despite constituting only ten per cent of the total monocyte population, inflammatory monocytes contribute significantly to the inflammatory potential of the monocyte pool as a whole (Belge *et al.* 2002). The circulating, inflammatory monocyte percentage is elevated in people with rheumatoid arthritis (Baeten *et al.* 2000), cardiovascular disease (Schlitt *et al.* 2004) and type 2 diabetes (Guiletti *et al.* 2007) and it has been suggested that inflammatory monocytes play a significant role in the pathogenesis of several diseases linked to inflammation. Transient increases in the inflammatory monocyte percentage after a single, acute bout of intense exercise have been observed (Simpson *et al.* 2009), followed by a rapid return to baseline during recovery, but regular exercise appears to reduce the proportion of inflammatory monocytes in the circulation in the resting state. For example, a cross-sectional comparison of healthy physically inactive elderly men and women with an age-matched physically active group indicated that sedentary people have a two-fold higher percentage of circulating, inflammatory monocytes (Timmerman *et al.* 2008). Furthermore, just 12 weeks of regular exercise training significantly reduced the percentage of inflammatory monocytes in the inactive group to the level of the active group (Figure 12.11) and endotoxin-stimulated TNF-α production was reduced significantly after the training intervention. Based on previous reports that glucocorticoid therapy selectively depletes CD14+CD16+ monocytes (Fingerle-Rowson *et al.* 1998), it is interesting to speculate that exercise-induced transient

Figure 12.11 Inflammatory monocyte subset (CD14+CD16+) percentage in physically active and sedentary subjects before and after 12 weeks of exercise training (for sedentary subjects) or continued physical activity (for active subjects); * = baseline group effect ($P < 0.05$). † = significant group × time effect ($P < 0.05$) (modified from Timmerman *et al.* 2008)

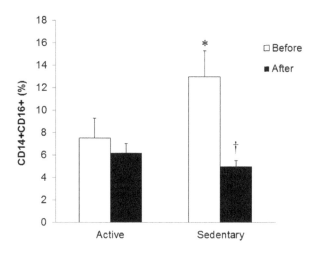

spikes in cortisol may have play a role in reducing CD14+CD16+ monocytes with exercise training.

Increased circulating numbers of regulatory T cells

CD4+CD25+ regulatory T cells specifically express the gene encoding forkhead/winged helix transcription factor (Foxp3) (Sakaguchi 2005) and suppress immune responses via cell contact-dependent mechanisms. Studies show that the depletion of these cells causes autoimmune disease and enhances the immune response to foreign antigens (Fernandez *et al.* 2008). Interestingly, one study showed that a 12-week programme of tai chi chuan exercise induced a significant increase in regulatory T cells (Yeh *et al.* 2006). Production of the regulatory T-cell mediators transforming growth factor alpha (TGF-α) and IL-10 in response to specific antigen stimulation (varicella zoster virus) was also significantly increased after this exercise programme. Furthermore, a study of people with type 2 diabetes showed that regular tai chi chuan exercise altered the Th1/Th2/Treg balance by increasing Foxp3 but not TGF-α expression (Yeh *et al.* 2009).

In a study that used a running mouse model, the responses of circulating regulatory T cells to moderate and high intensity exercise training were examined. Only the high-intensity training resulted in increases in regulatory T-cell numbers and activation and was also associated with reduced proinflammatory and increased anti-inflammatory cytokine expression (Wang *et al.* 2012). Intriguingly, the logical conclusion from these findings is that high-intensity exercise training might be more beneficial than moderate intensity in reducing risk of chronic cardiovascular and metabolic diseases via its anti-inflammatory effects. This notion is supported by another study which showed that the combination of high-intensity aerobic plus resistance exercise training, in addition to daily physical activity, is required to achieve a significant anti-inflammatory effect in people with type 2 diabetes (Balducci *et al.* 2010).

Other factors

During acute exercise there is also a marked increase in growth hormone, prolactin, heat shock proteins and other factors that have immunomodulatory effects (Pedersen and Hoffman-Goetz 2000). Taken together, it appears that each bout of exercise induces an anti-inflammatory environment. Various mechanisms can contribute to this (Figure 12.7) and it seems likely that their relative importance will vary dependent on the frequency, intensity and duration of the exercise performed. Intuitively, we might expect IL-6 to assume greater relative importance when the exercise is prolonged and glycogen-depleting, whereas catecholamine-mediated effects are likely to assume greater importance with shorter duration, high intensity exercise.

EXERCISE IS MEDICINE

In view of the anti-inflammatory effects of exercise described above and the role of inflammation in the pathogenesis of disease it is not surprising that exercise is now considered a prophylactic for preventing several major diseases as well as an effective therapy for many conditions/diseases (Table 12.1). Perhaps the strongest evidence for the role of exercise in disease prevention comes from randomised controlled trials evaluating the effectiveness of lifestyle intervention in preventing type 2 diabetes (for a review see Gill and Cooper 2008). These studies have demonstrated conclusively that lifestyle intervention (combined diet and exercise) is effective in preventing type 2 diabetes in groups of individuals who are at high risk of the disease by virtue of having impaired fasting glucose and/or impaired glucose tolerance, as well as being overweight or obese. A limitation of these studies is that they did not isolate the independent effects of exercise and diet in preventing type 2 diabetes but the effectiveness of exercise is supported by the finding in the Finnish Diabetes Prevention Study (Tuomilehto *et al.* 2001) that, among those in the intervention group who did not reach the goal of losing five per cent of their initial body mass but who achieved the goal of exercising for more than four hours per week, the odds ratio of diabetes was 0.2 (i.e. 80% lower) than in intervention participants who remained sedentary. Thus, although more needs to be learnt about the role of exercise in preventing type 2 diabetes, it is clear that exercise makes a valuable contribution to an overall lifestyle package for preventing this disease.

In addition, exercise appears to have major benefits for the treatment of type 2 diabetes. The findings of one non-randomised study (the Malmö Feasibility Study) showed that 54% of participants with early stage type 2 diabetes were in remission by the end of a five-year diet and exercise intervention (Eriksson and Lingärde 1991). Moreover, prospective observational studies indicate that high levels of physical activity and/or physical fitness are effective in reducing the risk of cardiovascular disease and/or all-cause mortality and there is evidence implicating inflammation in the pathogenesis of type 2 diabetes (Mathis and Shoelson 2011) and it is therefore likely that the therapeutic benefits of exercise for those with type 2 diabetes are due, at least in part, to the well established anti-inflammatory effects of regular exercise (Kasapis and Thompson 2005).

Aside from its role in preventing and treating type 2 diabetes, there is good evidence that exercise is effective in preventing several other major diseases particularly cardiovascular disease (Tanasescu *et al.* 2002), breast cancer (Eliassen *et al.* 2010) and colon cancer (Wolin *et al.* 2011) and there is some evidence to support a role of exercise in preventing dementia (Abbot *et al.* 2004). Moreover, while exercise should not be considered a panacea, there is evidence to support a role for exercise as a therapy for many diseases/conditions beyond those mentioned above, including chronic obstructive pulmonary disease, chronic kidney disease, asthma and osteoporosis (see Pedersen and Saltin 2006, for a comprehensive review).

THE ELITE ATHLETE PARADOX

As discussed in Chapter 1, although regular moderate intensity exercise is associated with a reduced incidence of URTI compared with a completely sedentary state, the long hours of hard training that elite athletes undertake appears to make them more susceptible to URTIs. This is also likely attributable to the anti-inflammatory effects of exercise inducing a degree of immunodepression. An increased risk of minor infections may be the (small) price to be paid for the long-term health benefits of regular exercise at high dosage.

A murine study indicated that intensive exercise training results in an increased anti-inflammatory cytokine (IL-10) response to antigen exposure (Wang *et al.* 2012) and a study on human endurance athletes revealed that those who were illness-prone during a four-month period of winter training had four-fold higher IL-10 production by antigen-stimulated whole blood culture compared with athletes who remained illness-free during the same period (Gleeson *et al.* 2012b). There is now extensive evidence from both murine and human studies that IL-10 production usually imposes some limits on the effectiveness of anti-pathogen immune responses, especially innate immunity and adaptive Th1 responses. These studies suggest that very high training loads induce a large enough anti-inflammatory state to increase the risk of picking up minor infections.

KEY POINTS

- Exercise results in an increase in the circulating and tissue levels of numerous cytokines.
- Exercise is capable of suppressing the production of specific cytokines from stimulated monocytes and T lymphocytes. Th1 cytokines are more affected than Th2 cytokines and exercise induces a decrease in the percentage of type-1 T cells with the possible consequence of a weakening of cell-mediated immune responses and increased susceptibility to viral infection.
- Release of IL-6 from contracting muscle appears to be the main source of the elevated plasma IL-6 concentration during exercise. The brain also releases IL-6 during exercise, whereas there is a net uptake of circulating IL-6 by the liver.
- Muscle damage is not primarily responsible for the elevated concentration of cytokines in the plasma during exercise. However, the production and/or release of some cytokines (notably IL-6) are increased when muscle glycogen content is depleted.
- IL-6 appears to act in a hormone-like manner and is involved in increasing substrate mobilisation (release of glucose from the liver and fatty acids from adipose tissue) during prolonged exercise. IL-6 also induces secretion of cortisol, IL-1ra, IL-10 and C-reactive protein and so has generally anti-inflammatory effects.
- Regular exercise reduces the risk of chronic metabolic and cardiorespiratory diseases, in part because exercise exerts anti-inflammatory effects.
- The anti-inflammatory effect of regular exercise may be mediated via both a reduction in visceral fat mass (with a subsequent decreased release of adipokines) and the induction of an anti-inflammatory environment with each bout of exercise.
- Various mechanisms may contribute to the anti-inflammatory effects of exercise including increased release of IL-6 from working skeletal muscle, increased release of cortisol and adrenaline from the adrenal glands, reduced expression of TLRs on monocytes/macrophages, inhibition of monocyte/macrophage infiltration into adipose tissue, phenotypic switching of macrophages within adipose tissue, a reduction in the circulating numbers of proinflammatory monocytes and an increase the circulating numbers of regulatory T cells.
- At present, we do not know what the relative importance of the different anti-inflammatory mechanisms that have thus far been identified are, although it seems likely that this will depend on the modes, frequencies, intensities and durations of exercise performed.
- The anti-inflammatory effects of exercise are also likely to be responsible for depressed immunity that makes the elite athlete more susceptible to common infections.
- High training loads may be needed to increase circulating numbers of regulatory T cells and maximise the anti-inflammatory effect but possibly at the cost of a small increase in infection risk.

FURTHER READING

Fischer, C. P. (2006) Interleukin-6 in acute exercise and training: what is the biological relevance? *Exercise Immunology Review* 12: 6–33.

Flynn, M. G. and McFarlin, B. K. (2006) Toll-like receptor 4: link to the anti-inflammatory effects of exercise? *Exercise and Sports Sciences Reviews* 34: 176–81.

Gleeson, M. (2007) Exercise and immune function. *Journal of Applied Physiology* 103: 693–9.

Gleeson, M., McFarlin, B. K. and Flynn, M. G. (2006) Exercise and toll-like receptors. *Exercise Immunology Review* 12: 34–53.

Kawanishi, N., Yano, H., Yokogawa, Y. and Suzuki, K. (2010) Exercise training inhibits inflammation in adipose tissue via both suppression of macrophage infiltration and acceleration of phenotypic switching from M1 to M2 macrophages in high-fat-diet-induced obese mice. *Exercise Immunology Review* 16: 105–18.

Pedersen, B. K. (2009) Edward F. Adolph distinguished lecture: muscle as an endocrine organ: IL-6 and other myokines. *Journal of Applied Physiology* 107: 1006–14.

Pedersen, B. K. and Saltin, B. (2006) Evidence for prescribing exercise as therapy in chronic disease. *Scandinavian Journal of Medicine and Science in Sports* 16 (Suppl 1): 5–65.

Timmerman, K. L., Flynn, M. G., Coen, P. M., Markofski, M. M. and Pence, B. D. (2008) Exercise training-induced lowering of inflammatory (CD14+CD16+) monocytes: a role in the anti-inflammatory influence of exercise? *Leukocyte Biology* 84: 1271–8.

13 Exercise, infection risk, immune function and inflammation in special populations

Nicolette C. Bishop

LEARNING OBJECTIVES

- understand the differences in immunity and immune response to exercise between males and females;
- recognise the importance of the relationship between exercise, immune function and infection risk in populations who may be immune-compromised;
- identify the effects of moderate intensity training programmes on immunity and risk of upper respiratory tract infection (URTI) in older people;
- understand the current view of the relationship between of acute and regular exercise and the effect on disease progression in people with human immunodeficiency virus (HIV);
- appreciate the relationship between exercise, immune function and inflammation in individuals with chronic conditions such as diabetes, chronic kidney disease, certain cancers and spinal cord injury;
- appreciate the potential clinical applications of exercise immunology and key future directions in exercise immunology.

INTRODUCTION

Much of the published exercise immunology research has focused on the effect of exercise on risk of URTI and immune function in athletic populations or in individuals who are involved in regular habitual exercise. In the majority of cases, the participants in these studies have been relatively young and free from long-term illness. However, the field of exercise immunology has applications in a far wider setting, particularly to those who may be immune compromised owing to disease, poor health or the effects of ageing. Furthermore, as we shall see in the next section, males and females display noticeable differences in immunity and in the immune response to exercise stress. It is important that we acknowledge sex differences in immunity particularly when exercise is employed as a non-pharmacological intervention in clinical settings.

SEX DIFFERENCES IN IMMUNITY AND THE IMMUNE RESPONSE TO EXERCISE

It is probably true to say that there is an anecdotal view among many women that some men are guilty of exaggerating symptoms of infections and illness. In all seriousness, differences between the sexes in immunity do suggest that men are indeed more susceptible to certain illnesses. Sex-based differences in immunity exist in both the innate and acquired arms of the immune system and these contribute to differences in the pathogenesis of infectious diseases in males and females (Pennell *et al.* 2012). Females tend to suffer fewer bacterial, viral and parasitic infections, at least until the menopause, but have a higher incidence of autoimmune diseases, including rheumatoid arthritis and multiple sclerosis (Pennell *et al.* 2012).

Sex differences in immunity

At this stage it is probably worth clarifying the term 'sex differences' as opposed to 'gender differences'. In the medical field, sex differences are defined as biologically conditioned dissimilarities between males and females, whereas gender differences take into account psychosocial, cultural and economic factors (Holdcroft 2007). In the context of this chapter, we focus on the basic differences between males and females in immune functions and, as such, these are 'sex differences'.

Generally, females respond to pathogens with a stronger innate and acquired immune response; this results in faster recognition and destruction of pathogens but also contributes to the greater prevalence of autoimmune diseases in females compared with males. The reasons for these differences, as with most biological differences, appear to be largely related to both hormonal and genetic influences. Broadly speaking, the female steroid hormone estrogen exerts profound effects via estrogen receptors present on macrophages, natural killer (NK) cells and T and B lymphocytes. For example, elevations in estrogen regulate T helper lymphocyte (Th)1 and Th2 responses in a bi-phasic manner during the menstrual cycle, with Th1 responses heightened during menstruation and the luteal phase when oestrogen levels are low and Th2 responses heightened during the follicular phase when estrogen levels are elevated (Pennell *et al.* 2012). Numbers of circulating T-regulatory (Treg) cells also fluctuate with the menstrual cycle, tending to be higher in the follicular phase (when estrogen levels are high) and lower in the luteal phase (Arruvtio *et al.* 2007). Estrogen also increases B cell immunoglobulin (Ig) production (Oertelt-Prigione 2012). In contrast, progesterone generally appears to decrease immune function, although it may enhance neutrophil chemotaxis (which is inhibited by estrogen) (Miyagi *et al.* 1992). The male sex hormone testosterone appears to either have little effect, or decreases immune function. In particular, testosterone inhibits B cell IgG and IgM production via inhibition of interleukin (IL)-6 production by monocytes (Oertelt-Prigione 2012).

The presence of the additional X chromosome in females is a further important influencing factor in the sex differences in immune function. The X chromosome has approximately 1,000 genes, many of which are responsible for immune function (Fish 2008). However, it is only relatively recently that investigations in this area have started and many of the polymorphisms found to date relate to autoimmune diseases. Given that most genes relevant to immune responses are present on the autosomes (i.e. the other 22 pairs of chromosomes), sexual dimorphisms here also need to be determined.

Sex differences and the immune response to exercise

Studies comparing the responses of various aspects of immune function in human males and females in response to acute exercise are limited in number. However, most suggest that the response is similar between the sexes (as reviewed in Gillum *et al.* 2011). Importantly however, very few of these have controlled for menstrual phase and oral contraceptive use. When these factors are taken into account, marked differences in the immune response to acute exercise stress are suggested. For example, circulating cytokine levels and stimulated whole-blood cytokine production did not differ between men and women after intensive exercise (Nieman *et al.* 2001a; Moyna *et al.* 1996a) when menstrual phase was not controlled for. In contrast, when controlling for menstrual phase and oral contraceptive use, a one-hour run at greater than 90% of the individual's anaerobic threshold was associated with differences in expression of pro- and anti-inflammatory genes between menstrual phases and between the sexes. In particular, expression of IL-6 at the transcriptional level was lower in women in the luteal phase and higher in the follicular phase (Northoff *et al.* 2008). The leukocytosis of exercise also appears to be influenced by menstrual phase and oral contraceptive use. After 90 minutes cycling at 65% of maximal aerobic power, numbers of circulating neutrophils, monocytes and lymphocytes were higher during the luteal phase than the follicular phase in those using oral contraceptives and also greater than the responses in men (Timmons *et al.* 2005; Figure 13.1).

Information on any sex differences in immune variables and infection incidence in the athletic population is scarce. However, a study of 80 endurance athletes found lower saliva flow rates, salivary secretory immunoglobulin A (SIgA) concentration, SIgA secretion rates, B cell and NK cell numbers in the female compared with the male athletes (Gleeson *et al.* 2011c). Female athletes also tended to have higher Toll-like receptor (TLR)-4 expression. These differences had no effect on infection incidence, duration and symptom severity, which was similar between the sexes. There were also no differences in plasma levels of IgA, IgG and IgM, total numbers of leukocytes, neutrophil, monocyte and lymphocytes and whole blood stimulated cytokine production in response to multi-antigen stimulation between the sexes. The lower IgA responses are in contrast to the usual sex associated differences in immune function, particularly as estrogen is known to enhance B cell immunoglobulin production. However, lower SIgA levels have been previously reported in elite female swimmers compared with their male counterparts (Gleeson *et al.* 1999a). The findings may suggest a greater effect of training on humoral immune functions (B cells and immunoglobulin production) in women than men although further research

Figure 13.1 Change in immune cell counts immediately after exercise in men and women during two phases of the menstrual cycle; OC = oral contraceptive, NOC = no oral contraceptive, Lut = luteal phase, Fol = follicular phase; * significantly different from all others ($P < 0.05$), ** significantly different from OC, Fol and men ($P < 0.05$) (data from Timmons *et al.* 2005)

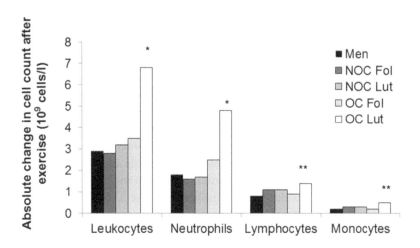

is needed to confirm this. Although menstrual phase and oral contraceptive use was not determined here, previous data suggest that menstrual cycle phase has little effect on resting SIgA responses in endurance trained female athletes (Burrows *et al.* 2002).

Summary of the sex differences in immune function

There are marked differences in immune function between men and women, with women demonstrating heightened innate and acquired immune responses that reduced their susceptibility to infections but may also increase their risk of autoimmune diseases. The literature relating to sex differences and the immune response to exercise is limited, largely because very few studies have controlled for the menstrual cycle and oral contraceptive use. Where these factors have been taken into account some quite marked differences in immune responses across the menstrual cycle and between the sexes have been reported.

EXERCISE, IMMUNE FUNCTION AND THE ELDERLY

Ageing is accompanied by a progressive decline in the functional integrity of the immune system resulting in the increased susceptibility of older people to infections and poorer responses to infection (Simpson *et al.* 2012). This state of 'immunosenescence' appears to be related to several factors over a lifetime, including accumulated exposure to external pathogens, persistent viral infections, neuroen-docrine factors and increased free radical production (Simpson *et al.* 2012; Woods *et al.* 2002). Some researchers also refer to the state of the ageing immune system as 'dysregulated', rather than simply reduced or depressed, as a reference to the view that although most aspects of immune function decline with ageing, some aspects are maintained and some aspects increase (Woods *et al.*, 2002).

Innate immune responses that decline with ageing include NK cell cytotoxicity (although the proportion of NK cells in the circulation increases (Brunsgaard and Pedersen 2000)), neutrophil phagocytosis and chemotaxis and monocyte activation, particularly in relation to TLR expression and signalling (Simpson *et al.* 2012). The decline in function of several components of acquired immunity has been found to predict future mortality; together these are termed the 'immune risk profile' and are considered to be prognostic immunological biomarkers in humans (Simpson *et al.* 2012). Markers of the immune risk profile include an inverted CD4+ : CD8+ ratio, impaired T-cell proliferative responses to antigens and the production of, and respon-siveness to, IL-2, a decline in numbers of naïve T cells (related to the atrophied thymus) and an increase in the number of memory T cells; these latter two factors inhibit immune responses to novel pathogens, increasing the risk of infectious diseases. This is particularly important when you consider that the viruses which cause common respiratory infections, such as rhinovirus, respiratory syncytial virus and influenza, constantly evolve. This means they are less likely to be recognised by an immune system with a substantially limited T-cell repertoire, leading to an increased mortality rate from these infections and associated complications in older people.

Participation in physical activity is encouraged in older people because it is associated with improved muscle function and with the prevention of such age-associated diseases as type 2 diabetes, osteoporosis, atherosclerosis, peripheral vascular disease and hypertension (Bruunsgaard and Pedersen 2000). Given the decline in many aspects of immune-cell function with ageing, it might be expected that the magnitude of any changes in immune measures following acute exercise is different between older and younger people. Furthermore, regular participation in moderate intensity exercise is associated with a lower than average risk of upper respiratory tract infections (as described in Chapter 1) and may enhance some aspects of immune function. Therefore, it is possible that that regular participation in moderate exercise training programmes may positively influence immune function in older people.

Acute exercise and immune function in older people

Few studies have investigated the effect of an acute bout of exercise on immune function in elderly people and these studies have largely concentrated on graded exercise to volitional exhaustion. For example, Ceddia *et al.* (1999) found that a bout of incremental treadmill exercise to fatigue resulted in a significant leukocytosis in previously sedentary older (mean age of 65 years) and younger (mean age of 22 years) subjects, although the magnitude of the leukocytosis was smaller and persisted for longer in the older subjects. Elevations in numbers of circulating neutrophils were observed after exercise in both the older and younger subjects but the magnitude of these changes was again much smaller in the older group. Similar responses were observed for both monocytes and total lymphocytes. Of course, the time to fatigue and absolute work rate at fatigue were markedly lower in the older subjects, which may in part account for the smaller leukocytosis. However, the number of T lymphocytes increased by approximately 50% following exercise in both the older and younger subjects and there was no significant difference between the groups in terms of the number of CD4+ and CD8+ cells recruited into the circulation at this time. Similar findings were reported by Brunsgaard *et al.* (1999), following a bout of maximal cycling exercise in a group of elderly (76–80 years) and younger (19–31 years) subjects; the elderly group demonstrated a leukocytosis of smaller magnitude than the younger group but recruited similar numbers of T lymphocytes. This relationship also persists at more moderate exercise intensities; Mazzeo *et al.* (1998) found that 20 minutes of cycling at 50% of peak work capacity was associated with a 15% increase in number of total leukocytes in a group of older men (mean age of 69 years) compared with a 33% increase in a group of younger men (mean age of 26 years) with increases of similar magnitude in numbers of CD4+ and CD8+ cells in both groups. These studies suggest that the ability to recruit T lymphocytes into the circulation in response to exercise is maintained with ageing, although neutrophil and monocyte mobilisation may be blunted in older subjects.

In the study of Mazzeo *et al.* (1998), resting T-cell proliferative responses following stimulation with the mitogen phytohemagglutinin (PHA) were significantly lower in the old compared with the younger subjects. Following the moderate exercise protocol, there was a significant increase (55%) in T-cell responsiveness compared with pre-exercise in the younger subjects but values did not significantly change in the elderly subjects. Similar findings are reported in response to graded exercise to exhaustion (Ceddia *et al.* 1999). These findings suggest that, in older individuals, the effects of exercise intensity on lymphocyte proliferation are attenuated, perhaps owing to the age-related decline in resting T-cell responsiveness.

The recruitment and function of NK cells in response to acute bouts of exercise appears to be maintained with ageing. Fiatarone *et al.* (1989) found that graded cycle exercise to volitional fatigue in older (mean age of 71 years) and younger (mean age of 30 years) women resulted in similar increases in NK-cell numbers and in NK-cell cytotoxic activity between the two groups. Resting numbers of NK cells and function were also similar between the older and younger women. In agreement with this, Mazzeo *et al.* (1998) reported similar numbers of NK cells at rest and following 20 minutes of cycling at 50% of peak work capacity between younger and older subjects.

These studies provide information on the response of an aging immune system to an acute stressor, namely a single bout of exercise. However, they do not provide information regarding the influence of regular exercise on immune function in older people. This is perhaps of greater relevance to the longer-term health and wellbeing of our ageing population.

Exercise training and immune function in older people

The effect of exercise training on immune function in older people has been investigated in both cross-sectional (a comparison of active older people with sedentary older people) and longitudinal (a period of exercise training in previously sedentary older people) studies.

Immune function differences between older active and older sedentary individuals

Early work by Nieman *et al.* (1993a) compared resting T-cell proliferative responses to mitogen and resting NK-cell activity in a group of 12 highly active older women, aged between 65 and 84 years, with a group of 32 sedentary older women of similar age. Resting NK and T cell numbers were similar between the two groups but NK cell activity and T cell proliferative responses to PHA were 54% and 56% higher, respectively, in the active older women compared with their sedentary counterparts (Figure 13.2). Shinkai *et al.* (1995) also report higher (44%) T-cell proliferative responses to PHA in a group of active older men (with an average age of 63 years) compared with that of similarly aged sedentary men, despite similar numbers of lymphocytes and lymphocyte subsets between the groups. However, in contrast to Nieman *et al.* (1993a), NK-cell activity was similar between the older conditioned men and their sedentary counterparts. Sex differences in NK cell cytoxicity and/or intensity of the regular training in which the conditioned groups participated may be reasons for the discrepancy between these two studies. In the study of Shinkai *et al.* (1995), the men were recreational runners who exercised on average for just under one hour, five days a week for around 17 years, compared with the women in the study of Nieman *et al.* (1993a), who reported exercising on average for 1.6 hours every day for the previous 11 years.

Figure 13.2 Comparison of natural killer (NK) cell activity and phytohaemagglutinin-stimulated lymphocyte proliferative responses in highly conditioned and sedentary older women; * $P < 0.01$ between the highly conditioned older women and the sedentary women (data from Nieman *et al.* 1993)

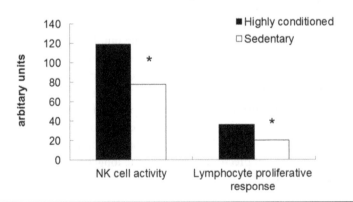

The decrease in numbers of naïve T cells with ageing is a crucial factor in reduced pathogen recognition and subsequent infection. However, this effect of ageing may be attenuated in fitter individuals. Spielmann *et al.* (2011) grouped 102 healthy men aged 18–61 years into tertiles according to their age-adjusted maximal oxygen uptake and found that aerobic fitness was positively related to the proportion of circulating naïve CD8+ T cells and negatively related to the proportion of 'exhausted' or senescent CD4+ and CD8+ T cells (i.e. T cells that have undergone many cycles of proliferation in response to antigen and are less able to respond). This relationship was apparent even after adjusting for body mass index, percentage body fat and latent herpes infections, such as cytomegalovirus and Epstein-Barr virus. These common viruses are thought to advance immunosenescence, owing to the chronic antigenic load in places on the T-cell compartment (Simpson *et al.* 2012).

Fewer studies have focused on differences in neutrophil function between sedentary and trained older people. Yan *et al.* (2001) compared recreationally active older men (with an average age of 65 years) with a group of age-matched sedentary males. The active men had exercised at least twice a week for a minimum of one hour for more than three years. Resting neutrophil counts were similar between the sedentary and active older men, yet neutrophil phagocytic activity was significantly lower in the sedentary group. Furthermore, when compared with a group of younger men (aged between 20 and 39 years) neutrophil phagocytic activity was lower in the older sedentary men, yet was similar between the older active men and their younger active and inactive counterparts, perhaps suggesting that long-term activity may help to maintain neutrophil function with advancing age (Figure 13.3). This effect of exercise could have particularly important applications for bacterial infections and also wound healing, where neutrophil migration plays a key role as part of the inflammatory response to tissue injury.

Figure 13.3 Neutrophil antibacterial activity in young compared with older active and sedentary men; * significantly lower than all other groups, $P < 0.05$ (data from Yan *et al.* 2001)

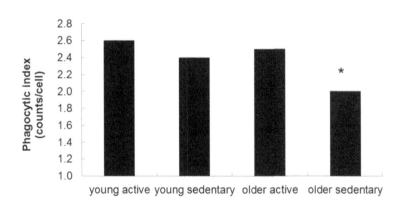

It is important to acknowledge that, unless controlled for, other lifestyle factors may influence the results of cross-sectional studies, particularly since it has been shown that many decreases in immune cell function that were previously attributed to the ageing process are actually linked to other factors such as poor nutritional status or an ongoing disease that is not clinically apparent (Lesourd *et al.* 2002). Individuals who have been active for a number of years are perhaps more likely to have followed a round 'healthier' lifestyle, yet simple cross-sectional comparisons cannot separate the specific impact that exercise training may exert on immune function from that of nutritional habits, smoking habits, genetics, psychological well-being and socio-economic status.

Regular exercise and immune function in older people

One method that can be employed to determine whether exercise training itself can impact on immune function is to look at immune function before and after a period of training in previously sedentary individuals (longitudinal studies). In this way, some of the lifestyle factors that may potentially influence immunosenescence can be controlled for, for example by recruiting non-smoking subjects who are free from chronic illness and collecting data concerning nutritional habits and psychosocial factors. On the other hand, we may be selecting the healthiest participants who may or may not be those who would benefit most from regular activity.

Following the cross-sectional comparison of older active and sedentary women, Nieman *et al.* (1993a) also looked at the effect of a supervised 12-week training programme on immune measures in 30 of the sedentary women. The women were divided into two further groups; each group exercised for 30–40 minutes, five days per week, with one group walking at 60% of heart rate reserve and the other group participating in sessions of callisthenics (light exercise involving muscular strength and flexibility work) over the same period. At the end of the training programme, $\dot{V}O_2$max increased by almost 13% in the walking group but was unchanged in the callisthenics group. However, NK-cell activity and PHA-stimulated lymphocyte proliferation did not differ between the groups at the end of the training period, suggesting that 12 weeks of moderate-intensity aerobic training was not sufficient stimulus to improve immune function in this group (Figure 13.4). Interestingly, despite the lack of differences in immune cell function between the training groups, the incidence of symptoms suggesting URTI over the 12 weeks was lower in the walking group (occurring in three of the 14 women) compared with the callisthenics group (occurring in eight of the 16 women) and only one of the highly conditioned older women experienced symptoms of URTI during the same period.

Woods *et al.* (1999) determined the effect of exercising for 40 minutes at 60–65% $\dot{V}O_2$max, three times per week over a period of six months in a group of older men and women with an average age of 65 years. A comparison group of age-matched subjects performed flexibility/toning exercise for the same duration and frequency. At the end of the training period, there were no differences in total and differential leukocyte counts or in lymphocyte subpopulations between groups. In agreement

Figure 13.4 Natural killer cell cytotoxic activity (NKCA) (A) and phytohaemagglutinin-stimulated lymphocyte proliferative responses (B) in sedentary older women before and after participation in a 12-week training programme of either moderate intensity walking or callisthenics. Dashed lines indicate corresponding levels in a group of women of similar age who had been highly active for a period of years (data from Nieman *et al.* 1993a)

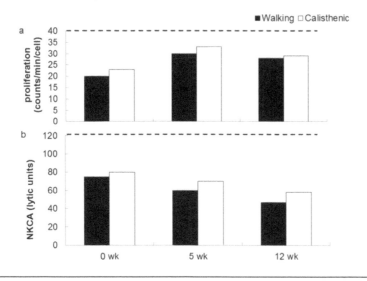

with Nieman *et al.* (1993a), no significant changes in NK-cell activity were reported, although the exercise group tended to show an increased proliferative response to stimulation with the mitogen concanavalin A (Con A). Taken together, these findings suggest that short-term moderate intensity aerobic training does not result in major changes in immune function in previously sedentary older people.

Fahlman *et al.* (2000) suggested that, rather than enhancing immune function, short-term exercise may simply help to prevent seasonal falls in immune cell measures. A ten-week training programme in which active (but not specifically trained) elderly women with an average age of 76 years walked for 50 minutes, three days each week at 70% heart rate reserve had no effect on resting NK-cell activity. However, at the end of the training period, resting NK-cell activity was decreased in a group of age-matched active but non-exercising women compared with pre-study values. The study was carried out over the winter months and this fall is in accordance with seasonal variations in cellular immune function. Therefore, these findings may suggest that rather than enhancing NK-cell function, endurance training in older people might help to maintain levels of NK-cell function. However, although a seasonal decline in NK-cell activity was also observed in the study of Nieman *et al.* (1993a), the magnitude of the decline was similar between the walking and callisthenics groups. Perhaps this again suggests that exercise intensity is a critical factor in determining any impact on immune function in older people since the elderly women in Nieman *et al.*'s (1993a) study trained at 60% heart rate reserve compared with 70% heart rate reserve in the study of Fahlman *et al.* (2000).

In addition to aerobic exercise, strength training is also advocated in the older population to prevent osteoporosis and increase ability to perform daily tasks (such as getting up from a chair) and increase capacity for independent living. However, this resistance training programmes also appears to have negligible effect on measures of immune function. Flynn *et al.* (1999) examined the effects of lower body resistance training performed three times per week over a ten-week period in women aged 67–84 years, compared with a group of similarly aged women who did not perform the resistance exercise. Training increased muscle strength but did not affect phenotypes of circulating lymphocytes, Con A-stimulated lymphocyte proliferation and NK-cell cytotoxicity. A longer duration of resistance training gave similar results; a 12-month programme in 42 clinically healthy 60–77 years olds increased strength compared with the controls, with little effect on circulating immune cell phenotypes, T-cell proliferation and NK-cell cytotoxicity (Raso *et al.* 2007). One study does report increases in response to a combined resistance and endurance training programme in 28 men and women aged 61–76 years (Shimizu *et al.* 2008). After completing five sessions per week of resistance exercise and 30 minutes of moderate-vigorous endurance exercise over six months, both numbers and proportions of anti-viral (interferon-γ+) CD4+ cells compared with age-matched non-exercising controls.

Exercise training and vaccine efficacy in older adults

The antibody response to vaccination can essentially be viewed as the 'end point' of the immune response to antigenic challenge. In this way, it may be a better reflection of the capacity of the whole immune system to respond to a challenge than specific *in vitro* measures. Importantly for the older population, the efficacy of the antibody response to vaccination decreases with age, most likely because of age-related declines in immune function. For example, it is estimated that current vaccines are 70–90% effective in young adults, but only 17–53% effective in older adults (Goodwin *et al.* 2006). This is of particular relevance when you consider that influenza is one of the major causes of death in the over-65 age group and annual vaccination against the current strain is most effective means of protecting against infection in the older population (Simpson *et al.* 2012).

A number of researchers have made attempts to improve the antibody response to influenza vaccine, for example using nutritional supplementation and, more recently, moderate exercise (Kohut *et al.* 2002, 2004; Woods *et al.* 2009). In a cross-sectional study, Kohut *et al.* (2002) found a positive association between self-reported physical activity levels and the antibody response to influenza vaccine in older adults. Those who reported participating in at least 20 minutes of vigorous exercise three or more times per week had higher responses than less active and sedentary older adults. However, it may be that those who chose to exercise regularly were in better health and as such may have had a more robust immune system, which would have influenced the findings. To address this Kohut *et al.* (2004) investigated the effect of a ten-month moderate intensity exercise training programme in 14 adults aged 64 years and over. The training programme involved exercising at 65–75% of heart rate reserve for 25–30 minutes on three days each week and responses were compared with an aged-matched group of non-exercising controls. All subjects were vaccinated with the trivalent (three strains) influenza vaccine before and after the exercise training. At the end of the training period, the exercise group significantly improved their performance in a six-minute walking distance test whereas performance in the control group was unchanged. Importantly, the magnitude of the antibody response to influenza vaccine (adjusted to take gender and differences in diet into account) was greater in the exercise group. Since the exercise intensity used in this study was 65–75% of heart rate reserve, these findings also lend support to the suggestion that exercise training needs to be of a higher intensity (greater than 60% heart-rate reserve) for any benefit on immune function to be detectable. This relationship was not apparent when the antibody response to the pre-training influenza vaccination was determined after the first eight weeks of exercise. This may suggest that exercise training programmes need to be performed for a period of several months before any benefit for immune function is evident.

To establish whether exercise can influence influenza vaccine efficiency over a period of several months (i.e. to reflect the need for protection across the whole autumn and winter season) Woods *et al.* (2009) assigned 144 inactive elderly women with an average age of 70 to a ten-month cardiovascular or flexibility exercise training programme. The women were vaccinated against influenza after four months of training and then continued exercising for the next six months. The proportion of women who had levels of antibody above the threshold for protection after six months was higher in the cardiovascular group than the flexibility group (Figure 13.5). These findings suggest that cardiovascular training can help to increase the duration of protection against influenza.

Summary of effects of ageing on immune responses to exercise

Ageing is associated with immunosenescence; a progressive decline of immune function. This is related to the increased morbidity and mortality from infectious causes in the older population. Exercise is advocated in the prevention of a number of cardiovascular and metabolic diseases associated with ageing but it is known that exercise can exert profound effects on immune function and as such exercise needs to be carefully prescribed in older people to avoid any negative impact on an already compromised immune system. In response to acute exercise, older people demonstrate a smaller leukocytosis than younger people that mainly reflects an attenuation of neutrophil mobilisation since recruitment of lymphocyte subpopulations is similar between older and younger subjects. In response to acute exercise of both moderate and maximal intensity, mitogen-stimulated lymphocyte proliferative responses are attenuated in older subjects, whereas NK-cell function appears to be preserved with ageing. Regular participation in exercise training over a period of several years is associated with enhanced measures of several innate and acquired immune functions compared with that of sedentary older people. However, shorter-term (up to one year) moderate intensity exercise training (both aerobic and

Figure 13.5 Regular exercise and long-lasting vaccine efficiency in older women. The proportion of women who had levels of antibody above the threshold for protection 24 weeks after vaccination with H1N1 and H3N3 variants of influenza virus was higher in the cardiovascular group (CARDIO) than the flexibility group (FLEX); * significant difference between groups, $P < 0.05$ (data from Woods *et al.* 2009)

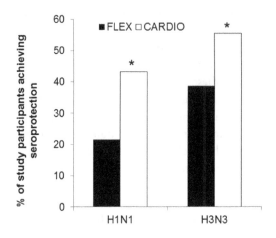

resistance) in previously sedentary clinically healthy older people does not result in a restoration of resting immune measures to the levels observed in highly conditioned older people, although it is associated with increased vaccine efficacy. However, it should be acknowledged that exclusion criteria for these studies may mean that participants are those with the most robust immune systems and greatest benefits of exercise may be more apparent in older people who are more immune compromised or who are considered to have the immune risk profile.

EXERCISE, IMMUNE FUNCTION AND HIV-SEROPOSITIVE INDIVIDUALS

HIV is a retrovirus that preferentially targets CD4+ cell surface molecules and accordingly leaves T helper cells as the major target for infection. Macrophages and microglia also express low densities of CD4 which making these cells an additional target for HIV. Transmission of HIV is usually through blood or semen containing HIV-1 or the related virus HIV-2. HIV is a type of virus known as a 'retrovirus', which has a nucleic acid core of RNA rather than DNA. Retroviruses contain an enzyme 'reverse transcriptase' that allows the virus's RNA to be transcribed into DNA and integrated into the target cell's genetic material, where it may remain dormant for long periods. Stimulation of infected cells activates HIV replication within the cell, killing the cell directly and also indirectly via the body's normal immune response to attack. The continual killing of large numbers of T helper cells by the rapidly replicating HIV virus is matched by the formation of new cells for a number of years after infection. As a result, the number of T helper cells remains normal (approximately

1,000 cells/μL blood) and individual remains free from symptoms and often unaware of that they are infected. Nevertheless, the CD4+ count can fall if the effects of the virus outweigh the body's capacity to produce new cells and given the pivotal role of T helper cells in orchestrating the acquired immune response, as described in Chapter 2, it is not surprising that as numbers of T helper cells fall, cytotoxic T cells and B cells will no longer function properly. When CD4+ T cell numbers fall to below 200 cells/μL the individual is considered to have the acquired immune deficiency syndrome (AIDS) and the risk of death from pulmonary infections and cancers that would ordinarily be handled by a healthy immune system is high.

However, HIV infection is no longer considered to be a necessarily life-threatening illness. Increased availability and efficacy of antiretroviral medicines has turned HIV into a chronic and manageable disease for many (O'Brien *et al.* 2010). Anti-retroviral therapy involves treatment of the HIV infection with drugs that act to inhibit the action of reverse transcriptase and act to prevent the assembly of new HIV. This therapy aims to slow down the progression of the infection by reducing the number of virus copies within the body (viral load). While antiretroviral therapy has significant benefits in terms of disease stability, it also is associated with the development of several metabolic complications including increased central adiposity, diabetes, dyslipidaemia and osteoporosis. The transition of HIV infection from life-threatening to manageable chronicity (and therefore life expectancy) has therefore been followed by an increased prevalence of health-related issues related to HIV infection (e.g. muscle weakness and wasting, anxiety and depression) and the metabolic side-effects of its treatment.

Aerobic and resistance exercise training programmes have been used to treat physiological symptoms associated with HIV infection, such as muscle weakness and wasting. Exercise has also been successfully used to treat anxiety and depression in HIV-infected individuals (O'Brien *et al.* 2010). However, HIV is a disease of the immune system and, given the relationship between exercise and immune function, there is concern that these exercise programmes, while enhancing cardiovascular fitness and psychological well-being, could also have an adverse effect on an already compromised immune system.

Acute exercise, immune function and HIV

Few studies have investigated the effect of acute exercise on immune function in HIV-infected individuals. Ullum *et al.* (1994b) compared measures of immune function in eight asymptomatic males with HIV with those of eight healthy control subjects of the same gender and age following one hour of cycle ergometry at 75% $\dot{V}O_2$max. The healthy individuals had significantly higher CD4+ counts at rest and in response to the exercise compared with the males with HIV. However, the magnitude of the change in CD4+ count elicited by the exercise was similar in both the patients and the controls, suggesting that mobilisation of T cells is not affected by HIV infection. In contrast, the post-exercise increases in numbers of circulating neutrophils, NK cells and NK-cell responsiveness following stimulation observed in the healthy subjects were suppressed in the HIV-infected individuals. This perhaps suggests some additional impairment of the ability of the innate immune system ('the first line of defence') to respond to a challenge following acute strenuous dynamic exercise in those with HIV.

Exercise training, immune function and HIV

Participation in regular moderate intensity exercise training programmes is suggested as a non-pharmacological therapy for treating the complications of HIV infection and the side effects of anti-retroviral therapy, as it has been shown to be beneficial for increasing lean muscle mass, decreasing fat mass and improving muscular strength (O'Brien *et al.* 2010). Furthermore, regular participation in physical activity also improves mental health, particularly reducing anxiety and depression, in HIV-infected individuals. For example, LaPerriere *et al.* (1990) studied 50 asymptomatic males who were at high risk of HIV infection but who were unaware of whether they were infected with the disease at the start of the study. The men were assigned to either an exercise or no-exercise control group. The exercisers participated in a five-week training programme that involved cycling on a stationary ergometer for 45 minutes at 80% of age-predicted maximum heart rate. After five weeks of training, cardiovascular, psychological and immunological data were collected from both the exercise group and non-exercising control group. Three days after this, the men received notification of whether or not they were infected with HIV. One week after notification, psychological and immunological data were collected for a final time. Following notification, men in the control group who were found to be infected with the disease (HIV+) showed significant decreases in numbers of NK cells (these cells are important in viral defence and are described in Chapter 2) and, as would be expected at such a time, significant increases in measures of anxiety and depression. However, at this time NK-cell numbers were maintained in the men in the exercising group that were found to be HIV+ and psychological measures resembled those of the men in the exercise and control groups that were found to be free from infection. Cardiovascular fitness (as measured by $\dot{V}O_2$max) improved in both HIV+ and HIV– men in the exercise group, suggesting that moderate aerobic exercise training programmes may be of benefit in the management of HIV.

Stringer *et al.* (1998) also examined the effect of moderate aerobic exercise training on both immune and psychological measures in 34 people with HIV, of who all but two were on anti-retroviral therapy. Individuals were assigned to three groups; a control group that did not perform any exercise training and two exercise groups that performed either moderate (around 45% $\dot{V}O_2$max) or heavy exercise (around 75% $\dot{V}O_2$max) for one hour, three times a week for six weeks. Training session duration was shortened in the heavy exercise group to ensure that the total amount of work performed per session was equivalent between the moderate and heavy exercise groups. Training significantly increased in the heavy exercise group only. The average CD4+ count at the beginning of the study was around 270 cells/μL with a range of 100–500 cells/μL (recall that the average count in a healthy individual is approximately 1,000 cells/µL). Exercise training did not affect resting CD4+ counts, which remained similar to pre-training values at the end of the study in each group and in the non-exercising controls. Similarly, the number of plasma HIV RNA copies did not change significantly in response to the exercise-training programme in either group or in the controls. However, when the authors tested the *in vivo* cell-mediated immune response by introducing a fixed amount of the yeast (*Candida albicans*) just below the skin and measuring the area of resulting swelling, a significantly enhanced response compared with the control group was found in the moderate exercise group only (Figure 13.6). Measures of quality of life also improved in both exercise groups during the study relative to the non-exercising control group. The results of this study and others (O'Brien *et al.* 2010) lend further weight to the idea that exercise training is safe and effective in individuals with HIV+ and that exercise programmes should be promoted as an additional treatment for individuals with HIV+ in the intermediate stages of the disease.

Figure 13.6 *In vivo* skin-test response to *Candida albicans* to assess cell-mediated immunity in HIV patients who undertook a 6-week training programme of either moderate or heavy aerobic exercise or were assigned to the no-exercise control group; * $P < 0.05$ compared with the control group (data from Stringer *et al.* 1998)

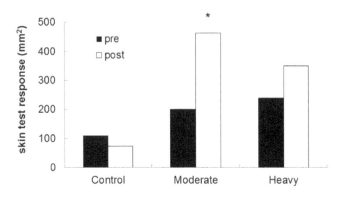

While moderate intensity exercise training was shown in this study to result in the greatest improvements in the immune response to antigen skin testing, neither moderate nor heavy exercise training affected resting CD4+ counts. This contrasts with the study of LaPerriere *et al.* (1991) that found that five weeks of interval training on a cycle ergometer at 70–80% of age predicted maximum heart rate was associated with increases in CD4+ cell count in individuals who had just found out they were infected with HIV and in a group of high-risk but healthy individuals compared with non-exercising controls. This may suggest that any benefits of exercise interventions for CD4+ cell numbers may be only apparent in those at an early stage of infection (and therefore with higher CD4+ counts).

This idea is supported by the finding that a 12-week training programme of one hour of aerobic and resistance work three days per week increased strength and exercise performance but did not affect CD4+ cell counts in HIV+ men who had resting counts of less than 200 cells/μL at the start of the study (Rigsby *et al.* 1992). CD4+ counts were also unchanged in a group of non-exercising but counselled men of similar disease status. Importantly, while this study did not find any positive effect of exercise training on numbers of CD4+ cells, it did not find any negative effect, suggesting that at this stage of disease progression, exercise can be used to enhance muscular strength and aerobic fitness without any adverse effects on the number of CD4+ cells.

A further possible reason for discrepancies between studies may be patient compliance to the exercise programme and dropout rate. In the study of Stringer *et al.* (1998) the dropout rate was 23%. This issue was investigated further by Perna *et al.* (1999); 28 early symptomatic HIV infected men and women participated in the study and the average resting CD4+ cell count for the cohort was approximately 450 cells/μL. Eighteen of the men and women participated in a 12-week interval training programme on a stationary cycle ergometer at 70–80% of age-predicted maximum heart rate for 45 minutes, three times each week. The remaining ten men and women acted as non-exercising controls. Approximately 60% of the exercise group completed the 12-week training programme but cardiovascular and immunological measures were still taken from those patients who did not complete more than 50% of the sessions (non-compliant group) for comparison with the compliant exercise group and the controls. There were significant increases in $\dot{V}O_2$ peak and resting CD4+ cell count at the end of the 12-week training period in the compliant exercise group only. Moreover, there was a significant fall in the resting CD4+ cell count in the non-compliant exercise group (Figure 13.7), with values unchanged in the control group. It is important to acknowledge that there may be other factors relating to their illness that caused them to leave the study and these, rather than the absence of exercise, could also account for the lower CD4+ counts in this group.

Further support for an increase in CD4+ cell count in patients at the earlier stages of the disease who are involved in regular exercise comes from a longitudinal study of 156 HIV+ males (Mustafa *et al.* 1999). Individuals with an initial CD4+ cell count of between 600–800 cells/μL who said that they exercised at least three or four times per week had increased CD4+ cell counts after one year compared with those with similar initial counts who did not exercise as regularly. No such relationship was found between healthy exercisers and non-exercisers over the same time. Interestingly, participation in regular exercise by HIV-infected patients also appeared to slow the progression of the disease to AIDS, with exercising three or four times per week having a more protective effect compared with exercising daily.

Progressive resistance training is also advocated in the exercise treatment in those with HIV to help alleviate symptoms of muscle wasting and loss of strength. It may also be that resistance training can also be beneficial to CD4+ counts: in a small cohort study, a group of 11 older (62–71 years) men and women who had been HIV+ for an average of nine years attended twice weekly resistance training sessions

Figure 13.7 CD4+ cell counts before and after a 12-week period of training at 70–80% of age predicted maximum heart rate for 45 minutes, 3 times each week in a group of HIV-infected men and women compared with a group of no-exercise controls. The exercise group was sub-divided into compliant and non-compliant exercisers (attended 50% of sessions or fewer); * $P < 0.05$ and ** $P < 0.01$ compared with pre-training values within group (data from Perna *et al.* 1999)

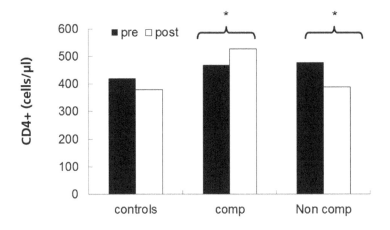

over one year (Souza *et al.* 2008). Compliance was 77%. In addition to the substantial strength increases experienced by all patients, small increases in CD4+ counts were also reported. It should be noted that the study would have been strengthed by the inclusion of a non-exercising control group.

Summary of exercise and immune function in HIV

Anecdotal reports from patients infected with HIV and clinicians associate long-term survival with maintained physical fitness and mental health. Despite the limitations of small sample sizes and high dropout rates, the evidence available supports this viewpoint; participating in regular moderate aerobic and resistance exercise is associated with maintenance of lean body mass, increases in muscular strength and cardiovascular fitness and in psychological measures of wellbeing and quality of life. There is some limited evidence to suggest that moderate exercise training programmes are associated with some increase in the numbers of CD4+ cells at rest, although this potential benefit appears to depend upon disease progression/initial CD4+ count and compliance to the activity. Nevertheless, in those patients in the later stages of the disease, regular moderate exercise training programmes do not appear to have harmful effects on resting CD4+ counts (and may even maintain numbers of CD4+ cells) and still result in improvements in muscular strength, cardiovascular fitness and psychological well-being.

EXERCISE AND IMMUNE FUNCTION AND OTHER CHRONIC LONG-TERM CONDITIONS

In the previous sections, we have seen how the influence of exercise on immune functions could potentially impact on immunity and infection risk in those who already have a weakened immune system. Just as exercise is advocated for physiological, metabolic and psychological benefits in the elderly and in those who are HIV seropositive there many other long-term conditions where exercise is recommended to restrict illness development and alleviate symptoms in those who are, by virtue of their condition and/or treatment, immune-compromised. This is often evidenced by increased susceptibility to infections and poor wound healing. Research attention is now beginning to be paid to the influence of exercise on immune function in some these conditions. Examples of these will be briefly explored in this section.

Long-term inflammatory conditions

Chronic long-term inflammation, as indicated by elevated levels of circulating inflammation markers such as IL-6 and C-reactive protein has been established as a predictor of risk for several of long-term conditions, including cardiovascular disease, diabetes, chronic obstructive pulmonary disease, chronic kidney disease, stroke, multiple sclerosis, rheumatoid arthritis and Alzheimer's disease (Gleeson *et al.* 2011a). These inflammatory conditions are also characterised by an accumulation of proinflammatory macrophages and T cells in adipose tissue, high numbers of circulating proinflammatory monocytes and low levels of the anti-inflammatory regulatory T cells. The anti-inflammatory effects of exercise are addressed in detail in Chapter 12 and include a phenotypic switch from pro- to anti-inflammatory tissue macrophages, reduced numbers of circulating proinflammatory monocytes and increased numbers of Tregs (Gleeson *et al.* 2011a).

In addition to the exacerbated inflammatory properties of immune cells in these conditions, defence mechanisms are also markedly impaired resulting in an increased incidence of infections. For example, patients with diabetes mellitus (types 1 and 2) often experience more severe and prolonged bacterial infections compared with healthy individuals. One reason for this may be impaired neutrophil function, with abnormalities in neutrophil chemotaxis, adherence, oxidative burst activity and phagocytosis all reported in diabetic patients (DiPenta *et al.* 2007). In addition, poor glucose control is associated with impaired monocyte antigen presentation and oxidative burst activity in patients with type-2 diabetes (DiPenta *et al.* 2007). Chronic kidney disease, which is linked to diabetes in some patients, is also associated with an impairment of these neutrophil functions (Cohen *et al.* 1997) in addition to defects in T-cell proliferation, reduced production of type-1 T cell cytokines and altered type-1/type-2 T-helper cell balance (Stenvinkel *et al.* 2005; Eleftheriadis *et al.* 2007). In fact, there is little aspect of the immune system that is not defective in chronic kidney disease; therefore, it is not surprising that patients with renal disease demonstrate increased rates of infection by all types of infective agent (bacterial and viral) and impaired wound healing. This, together with exposure of the blood to dialysis membranes and non-physiological fluids leads to chronic over-activation of inflammatory immune cells and pathways leading to increased risks of both infection and of inflammatory conditions.

Research regarding the effect of exercise on anti-infective immune functions in chronic inflammatory conditions is negligible compared with that of the potential benefits of exercise to inflammatory immune functions, yet the two are inevitably related. Furthermore, increased rates of infection and exacerbated inflammatory conditions have significant impact on quality of life, morbidity and mortality. One study investigating the benefits of a 12-week course of moderate tai chi exercise to T-cell function in patients with type 2 diabetes reported a reduction in HbA1c levels and enhanced type 1 (anti-viral) CD4+ cell function in patients with type 2 diabetes, in addition to enhanced expression of the Treg transcription factor FoxP3, compared with age-matched non-diabetic controls (Yeh *et al.* 2009). With regard to chronic kidney disease, a six-month programme of regular brisk walking was associated with a down-regulation of T-cell and monocyte activation, which was associated with an improvement in the ratio of pro-inflammatory IL-6 to anti-inflammatory IL-10 cytokine levels compared with chronic kidney disease patients who did not exercise (Viana *et al.* 2011). Regular exercise had no effect on circulating immune cell numbers and neutrophil degranulation responses.

Cancer

An independent protective effect of physical activity has been identified for the risk of colon (bowel) cancer and postmenopausal breast cancer, with increasing evidence suggesting a role of exercise in reducing the risk of cancers of the endometrium, lung and pancreas (Walsh *et al.* 2011a). However, the role of the immune system in the biological mechanisms relating to exercise and cancer is not well understood (Goh *et al.* 2012). Chronic inflammation has a role in the aetiology of colon and breast cancers, yet data linking a reduction in biomarkers of chronic inflammation via regular exercise and cancer risk have yet to be clearly demonstrated. Likewise, it has been hypothesised that the mobilisation of anti-tumour immune cells, such as NK cells and macrophages, with exercise increases anti-tumour surveillance, recognition and destruction. However, issues such as the nature of the anti-tumour defence mechanisms affected by exercise and the optimal exercise intensity, duration and frequency needed to maximise any anti-tumour (and anti-inflammatory) effects still need to be resolved (Walsh *et al.* 2011a; Goh *et al.* 2012).

Spinal cord injury

Individuals with spinal cord injury experience autonomic dysfunction to a degree that depends on the level and severity of the damage to the spinal cord. Given the role of the autonomic nervous system on immune cell mobilisation and functions it is not surprising that many immune cell functions are known to be depressed in spinal cord injured individuals including NK cell numbers and cytotoxicity, T-cell function and activation and macrophage phagocytosis (Nash 2000). The decline in immune function occurs rapidly after injury; for example NK-cell functions fell to 21% of that in non-injured age-matched controls two weeks after injury in a group of 49 paraplegic and tetraplegic individuals. T-cell functions fell to 40% of that of the controls by three months post-injury (Kliesch *et al.* 1999). Infections of the skin, respiratory and urinary tracts are the most common causes of morbidity in individuals with SCI (DeVivo 1999) while long-term inflammatory conditions are more common than in non-injured individuals of the same age, most likely the result of inactivity and poor diet (Nash *et al.* 2000).

Well-designed investigations of any effects of exercise on immune functions in individuals with spinal cord injury are limited to a few studies of NK cell numbers and cytotoxicity and salivary SIgA. For example, NK-cell cytotoxicity decreased immediately after two hours arm-crank exercise at 60% $\dot{V}O_2$ peak in paraplegic individuals with injuries to the spinal cord at the level of the thoracic and lumber vertebrae (levels T11–L4) but increased at the same time in a group of non-injured control participants (Ueta *et al.* 2008). In contrast, the cytotoxic activity of NK cells was impaired in tetraplegic individuals (injury at the level of the sixth and seventh cervical vertebrae; C6–C7) in response to 20 minutes of arm-cranking exercise at a similar intensity, compared with non-injured controls (Yamanaka *et al.* 2010; Figure 13.8).

Figure 13.8 Attenuated natural killer (NK) cell cytotoxic activity in response to 20 minutes arm-cranking exercise at 60% $\dot{V}O_2$ max in tetraplegic athletes (SCI) and non-injured controls (Non SCI); * significantly lower than controls, $P < 0.001$ (data from Yamanaka *et al.* 2010)

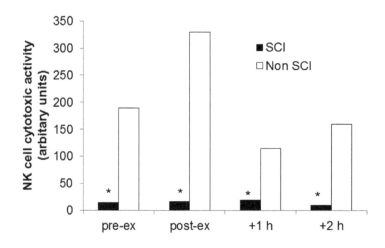

With regard to salivary SIgA, tetraplegic athletes (injury at C6–C7 cervical vertebrae) were able to increase SIgA secretion rate similarly to paraplegic (injury at T6–T12) and ambulant wheelchair athletes in response to both 60 minutes of moderate continuous and 60 minutes of intensive intermittent wheelchair propulsive exercise, although the magnitude of the increase was greater for the tetraplegic athletes (Leicht *et al.* 2011). This was despite the level of their injury resulting in disrupted sympathetic innervation of salivary glands and most likely reflects greater contribution of parasympathetic inputs and/or sympathetic reflex activity. The contribution of such compensatory mechanisms was further highlighted by the observation that during an intense training session tetraplegic wheelchair athletes showed responses thought to be governed by the sympathetic nervous system, such as reductions of saliva flow rate as a result of strenuous exercise (Leicht *et al.* 2012a). Similarly, a period of heavy training was associated with a decrease in resting levels of SIgA in elite tetraplegic athletes (Leicht *et al.* 2012b), just as has been commonly reported in the able-bodied population.

Circulating levels of inflammatory markers are also greater in those with spinal cord injury than in controls of similar age (Wang *et al.* 2007). There is little information on the potential of exercise to exert anti-inflammatory effects of exercise in those with spinal cord injury but some early data suggests an impaired cytokine response to wheelchair propulsive exercise in tetraplegics compared with paraplegics and non-injured controls (Paulson *et al.* 2013), which may suggest a that the anti-inflammatory effects of voluntary exercise are limited in these individuals.

Application of genomics and proteomics to exercise immunology research

We have seen in this chapter that the potential clinical applications of exercise immunology research are wide ranging. However, to translate research findings into effective exercise prescription there is a pressing need to better understand the mechanisms underlying the relationship between exercise and immune function in both healthy and clinical populations. Application of genomics and proteomics to the relationship between exercise and immune function is one method that exercise immunologists hope will help to more easily identify mechanistic pathways and reliable clinical biomarkers in the near future. These methods use high-throughput/high-sensitivity laboratory methods and complex statistical analysis to essentially scan an entire biological field, or part of it, without hypothesis (Walsh *et al.* 2011a). As you can imagine, such methods generate vast amounts of detailed data. While this increases the chances of finding unexpected biological relationships and indeed has revealed numerous pathways and candidates for biomarkers, given the great redundancy inherent in the immune system it should be acknowledged that each relationship found may not necessarily be of equal biological importance. That said, genomics and proteomics have revealed that gene expression in peripheral blood mononuclear cells are rapidly activated and deactivated even after short bouts of exercise (Connolly *et al.* 2004), gene expression is dependent on workload (Büttner *et al.* 2007) and is influenced by age and menstrual cycle (Northoff *et al.* 2008; Thalacker-Mercer *et al.* 2010); all factors that go some way to explaining some of the effects of exercise on immune function. Furthermore, the expression of micro-RNAs, a class of post-transcriptional regulators that are capable of altering gene expression by targeting mRNAs usually resulting in their silencing, has been reported to alter in response to brief heavy exercise (Radom-Aisik *et al.* 2012). Specifically, exercise was associated with changes microRNA profiles in monocytes and lymphocytes, many of which are related to inflammatory processes.

While these techniques will undoubtedly enhance our mechanistic understanding, their practical application is currently limited. This is because, to use genomic and proteomic data to make reliable predictions of individual risk of infection or illness, it is necessary to standardise genomic and proteomic analytical procedures between laboratories; this is something that is almost impossible to do at the present time (Walsh *et al.* 2011a). As such, a widespread practical application of these techniques is not yet viable but given the pace of new technologies and innovations, can't be too far away.

Summary

One of the key aims of the American College of Sports Medicine's 'Exercise is Medicine' initiative launched in 2007 is to foster implementation of exercise counselling into clinical practice and promote collaboration between healthcare providers and exercise professionals. In this regard, the potential clinical applications of exercise immunology are vast. Exercise is recommended to restrict the development and alleviate symptoms of long-term conditions in those who are, by virtue of their condition and/or treatment, immune-compromised. Research regarding the effect of exercise on anti-infective immune functions in chronic inflammatory conditions is limited compared with that of the potential benefits of exercise in inflammatory immune functions, yet the two are inevitably related. Furthermore, inflammatory events are an important part of wound healing, which is impaired in ageing and many clinical conditions, often leading to chronic ulcers and pressure sores. Therefore, the clinical applications of the immune response to exercise are a key area for future research to enable healthcare and exercise professionals to be able to prescribe optimal exercise programmes to maximise the benefits of exercise to immune function, inflammation and infection risk.

KEY POINTS

- Much of the exercise immunology literature has focused on the effects of exercise in healthy, relatively young individuals who are highly conditioned or, at the very least, recreationally active. However, field of exercise immunology has potential applications in a far wider setting.
- Males and females exhibit marked differences in immunity, with females naturally more resistant to infections but more prone to autoimmune conditions.

- Limited information from well-controlled studies suggests that leukocyte mobilisation, as well as inflammatory cytokine responses, may be influenced by menstrual phase and oral contraceptive use.
- Ageing is associated with immunosenescence; a progressive decline of immune function which is related to the increased morbidity and mortality from infectious causes in the older population.
- Long-term active older people demonstrate enhanced measures of several innate and acquired immune functions exercise. Shorter-term moderate intensity exercise training in previously sedentary older people does not result in a restoration of resting immune measures to the levels observed in highly conditioned older people but is associated with increased vaccine efficacy.
- Participation in regular moderate aerobic exercise is advocated as a non-pharmacological therapy for the management of HIV infection, since it is associated with physiological and psychological benefits without any adverse effects on immune function; it may even help to maintain or increase numbers of CD4+ cells in adherent exercisers.
- Exercise is recommended to restrict the development and alleviate symptoms of long-term conditions in those who are, by virtue of their condition and/or treatment, immune-compromised.
- Research regarding the effect of exercise on anti-infective immune functions in chronic inflammatory conditions is limited compared with that of the potential benefits of exercise to inflammatory immune functions, yet the two are inevitably related.
- It has been hypothesised that the mobilisation of anti-tumour immune cells, such as NK cells and macrophages, with exercise increases anti-tumour surveillance, recognition and destruction, although this remains to be conclusively shown.
- Spinal cord injury is associated with impaired immune function, most probably related to the injury-related disruption to the autonomic nervous system. Well-designed investigations of the effects of exercise on immune functions in individuals with spinal chord injury suggest impairment of altered NK-cell responses yet a maintenance of the salivary SIgA response compared with non-injured individuals.
- The potential clinical applications of the immune response to exercise are extensive but to translate research findings into effective exercise prescription, there is a pressing need for better mechanistic understanding. This will no doubt involve the wider application of genomics and proteomics to exercise immunology research.

FURTHER READING

Gillum, T. L., Kuennen, M. R., Schneider, S. and Mosely, P. (2011) A review of sex differences in immune function after aerobic exercise. *Exercise Immunology Review* 17: 104–21.

O'Brien, K., Nixon, S., Tynan, A. M. and Glazier, R. (2010) Aerobic exercise interventions for adults living with HIV/AIDS. *Cochrane Database of Systematic Reviews* 4: CD001796. [Pages 17–22 relate specifically to immunological outcomes.]

Simpson, R. J., Lowder, T. W., Speilmann, G., Bigley, A., LaVoy, E. C. and Kunz, H. (2012) Exercise and the ageing immune system. *Ageing Research Reviews* 11: 404–20.

Walsh, N. P., Gleeson, M., Shephard, R. J., Gleeson, M., Woods, J. A., Bishop, N. C., Fleshner, M., Green, C., Pedersen, B. K., Hoffman-Goetz, L., Rogers, C. J., Northoff, H., Abbasi, A. and Simon, P. (2011) Position statement. Part one: Immune function and exercise. *Exercise Immunology Review* 17: 6–63. [Pages 36–9 relate specifically to exercise and cancer and pages 39–43 relate to genomics and proteomics in exercise immunology.]

Woods, J. A., Lowder, T. W. and Keylock, K. T. (2002) Can exercise training improve immune function in the aged? *Annals of the New York Academy of Science* 959: 117–27.

Glossary

AA (amino acid) the chief structural molecule of protein, consisting of an amino group (NH_2) and a carboxylic acid group (CO_2H) plus another so-called R-group that determines the amino acid's properties; 20 different amino acids can be used to make proteins

α-amylase (or amylase) a digestive enzyme found in saliva that begins the digestion of starches in the mouth (also called ptyalin); it also has an antibacterial action

acclimatisation adaptation of the body to an environmental extreme (e.g. heat, cold, and altitude)

acidosis a disturbance of the normal acid-base balance in which excess acids accumulate causing a fall in pH (e.g. when lactic acid accumulates in muscle and blood during high-intensity exercise)

acquired immune response immunity mediated by lymphocytes and characterised by antigen specificity and memory

ACSM American College of Sports Medicine

ACTH (adrenocorticotrophic hormone) hormone secreted from anterior pituitary gland, which stimulates release of cortisol from adrenal glands

active transport movement or transport across cell membranes by membrane carriers; an expenditure of energy (ATP) is required

acute phase proteins several proteins released from liver (e.g. C-reactive protein) and leukocytes that aid body's response to injury or infection; rapid change in circulating concentration of acute phase proteins occurs following the initiation of an inflammatory response

adaptogen name used for substances that help the body to adapt to stress situations

adipocyte adipose tissue cell whose main function is to store triacylglycerol (fat)

adipose tissue white fatty tissue that stores triacylglycerol

ADMR (average daily metabolic rate) the average energy expenditure over 24 hours

adrenaline hormone secreted by the adrenal gland; a stimulant that prepares the body for 'fight or flight' and an important activator of fat and carbohydrate breakdown during exercise (also known as epinephrine)

aerobic occurring in the presence of free oxygen

AI (adequate intake) recommended dietary intake comparable to the RNI or RDA but based on less scientific evidence

AIDS   acquired immune deficiency syndrome

allergen   antigen that causes an allergy

allergy   abnormally high sensitivity to certain substances, such as pollens, foods or microorganisms

alpha-tocopherol   the most biologically active alcohol in vitamin E

ammonia   (NH_3) metabolic by-product of the oxidation of amino acids. It may be transformed into urea for excretion from the body.

AMP   antimicrobial protein

AMPK   adenosine monophosphate-activated protein kinase

AMS   acute mountain sickness

anaemia   a condition defined by an abnormally low blood haemoglobin content resulting in a lowered oxygen carrying capacity

anaerobic   occurring in the absence of free oxygen

anaphylaxis   an acute, potentially life-threatening hypersensitivity reaction, involving the release of mediators from mast cells, basophils and recruited inflammatory cells

anorexia athletica   a form of anorexia nervosa observed in athletes who show significant symptoms of eating disorders but who do not meet the criteria of the Diagnostic and Statistical Manual of Mental Disorders (American Psychiatric Association 1987) for anorexia or bulimia nervosa

anorexia nervosa   an eating disorder characterised by an abnormally small food intake and a refusal to maintain a normal body weight (according to what is expected for gender, age and height), a distorted view of body image, an intense fear of being fat or overweight and gaining weight or 'feeling fat' when clearly the individual is below normal weight, and the absence of at least three successive menstrual cycles in females (amenorrhoea)

ANOVA   analysis of variance

anthropometry   use of body girths and diameters to evaluate body composition

antibody   soluble protein produced by B lymphocytes with antimicrobial effects; also known as immunoglobulin

antigen   usually a molecule foreign to the body but can be any molecule capable of being recognised by an antibody or T-cell receptor

antioxidant   molecules that can prevent or limit the actions of free radicals usually by removing their unpaired electron and thus converting them into something far less reactive

APC   antigen-presenting cell

apoptosis   an internal programme that allows damaged or obsolete cells to commit suicide

AQUA   Allergy Questionnaire for Athletes

arteriosclerosis   hardening of the arteries (*see also* atherosclerosis)

ascorbic acid   vitamin C; major role is as a water-soluble antioxidant

atherosclerosis   a specific form of arteriosclerosis characterised by the formation of fatty plaques on the luminal walls of arteries

atopy   a genetic predisposition toward the development of immediate hypersensitivity reactions against common environmental antigens

ATP   (adenosine triphosphate) a high-energy compound that is the immediate source for muscular contraction and other energy requiring processes in the cell

atrophy   wasting away, a diminution in the size of a cell, tissue, organ, or part

AV   (arteriovenous) refers to comparison of arterial and venous blood composition

AV differences   difference between arterial and venous concentration of a substance, indicating net uptake or release of that substance

B cells   bursa of Fabricius-derived cells

bacterium   single-celled microscopic organism larger than a virus and lacking a nucleus and other organised cell structures

base   substance that tends to donate an electron pair or coordinate an electron

BASES   British Association of Sport and Exercise Sciences

basophil   type of granulocyte found in the blood

BCAA   (branched-chain amino acid) three essential amino acids that can be oxidised by muscle; includes leucine, isoleucine and valine

β-carotene   precursor for vitamin A found in plants; also called provitamin A

bioavailability   in relation to nutrients in food, the amount that may be absorbed into the body

biopsy   a small sample of tissue taken for analysis

b.m.   body mass in kilograms

BMI   (body mass index) body mass in kilograms divided by height in square metres (kg/m^2); an index used as a measure of obesity

BMR   (basal metabolic rate) energy expenditure under basal, post-absorptive conditions representing the energy needed to maintain life under these basal conditions

bronchoconstriction   narrowing of air passages of the lungs from smooth muscle contraction, as in asthma

caffeine   stimulant drug found in many food products, such as coffee, tea and cola drinks; stimulates the central nervous system and used as an ergogenic aid

calorie (cal)   traditional unit of energy; 1 calorie expresses the quantity of energy (heat) needed to raise the temperature of 1 g (1 ml) of water 1°C (from 14.5°C to 15.5°C)

CAM   cell adhesion molecule

cAMP   (cyclic adenosine monophosphate) an important intracellular messenger in the action of hormones

capillary   the smallest vessel in the cardiovascular system; capillary walls are only one cell thick; all exchanges of molecules between the blood and tissue fluid occur across the capillary walls

carcinogen   cancer-inducing substance

catabolism   destructive metabolism whereby complex chemical compounds in the body are degraded to simpler ones (e.g. glycogen to glucose; proteins to amino acids)

catalyst   substance that accelerates a chemical reaction, usually by temporarily combining with the substrates and lowering the activation energy, and is recovered unchanged at the end of the reaction (e.g. an enzyme)

CBSM cognitive behavioural stress management

CCR chemokine receptor

CD (clusters of differentiation or cluster designators) proteins expressed on cell surface of leukocytes (white blood cells) that can be used to identify different types of leukocyte or subsets of lymphocytes

cell smallest discrete living unit of the body

cell-mediated immunity refers to T cell-mediated immune responses; killing of infected host cells by T-cytotoxic lymphocytes

cellulose major component of plant cell walls and the most abundant non-starch polysaccharide; cannot be digested by human digestive enzymes

CFS chronic fatigue syndrome

CHD (coronary heart disease) narrowing of the arteries supplying the heart muscle that can cause heart attacks

chemokines cytokines that selectively induce chemotaxis and activation of leukocytes

chemotaxis movement of cells up a concentration gradient of attractant chemical factors

CHO (carbohydrate) compound composed of carbon, hydrogen and oxygen in ratio of $1 : 2 : 1$ (CH_2O); carbohydrates include sugars, starches and dietary fibres

CK (creatine kinase) enzyme that catalyses the transfer of phosphate from phospho-creatine to ADP to form ATP; also known as creatine phosphokinase

clone identical cells derived from a single progenitor

CMV cytomegalovirus

coenzyme small molecules that are essential in stoichiometric amounts for the activity of some enzymes; examples include nicotinamide adenine dinucleotide, flavin adenine dinucleotide, pyridoxal phosphate, thiamine pyrophosphate and biotin

colon the large intestine; this part of the intestine is mainly responsible for forming, storing and expelling faeces

colony-stimulating factor cytokine that stimulates increased production and release of leukocytes (white blood cells) from the bone marrow

complement soluble proteins found in body fluids and produced by liver; once activated, they exert several antimicrobial effects

complex carbohydrates foods containing starch and other polysaccharides as found in bread, pasta, cereals, fruits and vegetables, in contrast to simple carbohydrates such as glucose, milk sugar, and table sugar

Con A (concanavalin A) a T-cell mitogen

concentration gradient difference in concentration of a substance on either side of a membrane

condensation reaction involving the union of two or more molecules with the elimination of a simpler group such as H_2O

conformation shape of molecules determined by rotation about single bonds, especially in polypeptide chains about carbon-carbon links

COOH   carboxylic acid group

cortisol   steroid hormone secreted from the adrenal glands

covalent bond   chemical bond in which two or more atoms are held together by the interaction of their outer electrons

C-reactive protein   acute phase protein that is able to bind to the surface of micro-organisms and stimulates complement activation and phagocytosis by neutrophils and macrophages

CSFE   carboxyfluorescein succinamidyl ester; a fluorescent molecule used in flow cytometry to track the proliferation of CD4+ and CD8+ T-lymphocyte subsets

Cu   copper

CXCR4   chemokine receptor type 4 (also called fusin or CD184)

cytokine   protein released from cells that acts as a chemical messenger by binding to receptors on other cells; cytokines include interleukins, tumour necrosis factors, colony-stimulating factors and interferons

cytotoxic   ability to kill other cells (e.g. those infected with a virus)

DALDA   daily analyses of life demands in athletes questionnaire

degranulation   release of granule contents (e.g. digestive enzymes form neutrophils)

demargination   release into the circulation of leukocytes that were bound to endothelial cells of blood vessel walls

dendritic cell   specialised antigen presenting cell found in the tissues

DHA   docosahexaenoic acid

diabetes mellitus   disorder of carbohydrate metabolism caused by disturbances in production or utilisation of insulin; causes high blood-glucose levels and loss of sugar in the urine

diarrhoea   frequent passage of a watery faecal discharge because of a gastrointestinal disturbance or infection

diffusion   movement of molecules from a region of high concentration to one of low concentration, brought about by their kinetic energy

digestion   process of breaking down food to its smallest components so that it can be absorbed in the intestine

disaccharide   sugars that yield two monosaccharides on hydrolysis; sucrose is the most common and is composed of glucose and fructose

diuretics   drugs that act on the kidney to promote urine formation

dl   (decilitre) one tenth of a litre

dm   (dry matter or dry material) usually refers to tissue weight after removal of water

DNA   (deoxyribonucleic acid) compound that forms genes (i.e. the genetic material)

DPCP   diphenylcyclopropenone

DTH   (delayed type hypersensitivity) cell-mediated immune reaction to a recognised antigen occurring within 24–72 hours

EBV   (Epstein-Barr virus) virus responsible for infectious mononucleosis

eccentric exercise   types of exercise that involve lengthening of the muscle during activation, which can cause damage to some of the myofibres; types of exercise that have a significant eccentric component include downhill running, bench stepping and lowering of weights

ECF (extracellular fluid) body fluid that is located outside the cells, including the blood plasma, interstitial fluid, cerebrospinal fluid, synovial fluid and ocular fluid

EDTA (ethylene diamine tetra acetate) anticoagulant that prevents blood from clotting by binding to and removing free calcium ions

EE (energy expenditure) energy expended per unit of time to produce power

EEA (energy expenditure for activity) energy cost associated with physical activity (exercise)

EGCG epigallocatechin 3-gallate

EHI exertional heat illness

EHS exertional heat stroke

EIAn exercise-induced anaphylaxis

EIB exercise-induced bronchospasm

eicosanoids derivatives of fatty acids in the body that act as cell-cell signalling molecules; they include prostaglandins, thromboxanes and leukotrienes

electrolyte substance that, when dissolved in water, conducts an electric current; include acids, bases, and salts, and usually dissociate into ions carrying either a positive charge (cation) or a negative charge (anion)

ELISA (enzyme-linked immunosorbent assay) a type of assay used to measure the concentration of soluble cytokines, hormones, antibodies, etc.

ELISPOT sensitive type of assay used to quantify cytokine-secreting cells

EMRA CD45RA+ effector memory cells, sometimes referred to as senescent or terminally differentiated cells

endocrine ductless glands that secrete hormones into the blood

endogenous from within the body

energy ability to perform work; exists in various forms, including mechanical, heat and chemical

energy balance balance between energy intake and energy expenditure

enzyme protein with specific catalytic activity; designated by the suffix '-ase' and frequently attached to the type of reaction catalysed; virtually all metabolic reactions in the body are dependent upon and controlled by enzymes

eosinophil type of blood granulocyte; increased numbers in the circulation are found in allergic conditions

EPA eicosapentaenoic acid

epinephrine *see* adrenaline

epitope part of an antigen recognised by an antibody or T-cell receptor

ergogenic aids substances that improve exercise performance and are used in attempts to increase athletic or physical performance capacity

ergolytic performance impairing

erythrocyte red blood cell that contains haemoglobin and transports oxygen

essential amino acids amino acids that must be obtained in the diet and cannot be synthesised in the body; also known as indispensable amino acids

essential fatty acids   unsaturated fatty acids that cannot be synthesised in the body and must be obtained in the diet (e.g. linoleic acid and linolenic acid)

euhydration   normal state of body hydration (water content)

eumenorrhoea   occurrence of normal menstrual cycles

excretion   removal of metabolic wastes

exogenous   from outside the body

FACS   fluorescence-activated cell sorter

FAD   flavin adenine dinucleotide (*see also* coenzyme)

faeces   excrement discharged from the intestines, consisting of bacteria, cells from the intestines, secretions and a small amount of food residue

fat   fat molecules contain the same structural elements as carbohydrates but with little oxygen relative to carbon and hydrogen and poorly soluble in water; also known as lipids (derived from the Greek word *lipos*); a general name for oils, fats, waxes and related compounds; oils are liquid at room temperature, whereas fats are solid

fatty acid   type of fat having a carboxylic acid group at one end of the molecule and a methyl (CH_3) group at the other end, separated by a hydrocarbon chain that can vary in length; a typical structure of a fatty acid is $CH_3(CH_2)_{14}COOH$ (palmitic acid or palmitate)

Fc   crystallisable, non-antigen-binding fragment of an immunoglobulin molecule

Fc receptor   cell-surface receptor that binds to the Fc part of immunoglobulin molecules

FcεRI   high-affinity IgE receptor, also known as Fc epsilon RI; is a receptor for the Fc region of IgE, an antibody subclass involved in allergy disorders and immunity against parasites. FcεRI is found on epidermal Langerhans cells, eosinophils, mast cells and basophils. Crosslinking of the FcεRI via IgE–antigen complexes leads to degranulation of mast cells or basophils and release of inflammatory mediators, most notably histamine

FDEIA   food-dependent exercise-induced anaphylaxis

female athlete triad   syndrome that is characterised by the three conditions that are prevalent in female athletes: amenorrhoea, disordered eating and osteoporosis

ferritin   protein used to store iron; mostly found in the liver, spleen and bone marrow; soluble ferritin is released from cells into the blood plasma in direct proportion to cellular ferritin content; hence, the serum ferritin concentration can be used to indicate the status of the body's iron stores

fibre   indigestible carbohydrates

fish oil   oils high in unsaturated fats extracted from the bodies of fish or fish parts, especially the livers; used as a dietary supplement

FITC   fluorescein isothiocyanate; a fluorescent marker used in flow cytometry

flux   rate of flow through a metabolic pathway

fMLP   (formyl-methionyl-leucyl-phenylalanine) a bacterial cell-wall peptide that is a chemical stimulant of phagocytes

folic acid or folate   water-soluble vitamin required in the synthesis of nucleic acids; it appears to be essential in preventing certain types of anaemia

free radical   atom or molecule that possesses at least one unpaired electron in its outer orbit. The free radicals the superoxide ($\cdot O_2^-$), hydroxyl ($\cdot OH$), and nitric oxide ($NO\cdot$) radicals; highly reactive and may cause damage to lipid membranes causing membrane instability and increased permeability; can also cause oxidative damage to proteins, including enzymes, and damage to DNA

FSH   (follicle stimulating hormone) a gonadotrophin secreted from the anterior pituitary gland

g   gram

gamma delta (γδ) T cell   subset of T lymphocyte that recognises lipid and other non-peptide antigens; potent cytotoxic cells that aid the host in bacterial elimination, wound repair and delayed-type hypersensitivity reactions

gastrointestinal tract   gastrointestinal system or alimentary tract; the main sites in the body used for digestion and absorption of nutrients, consisting of the mouth, oesophagus, stomach, small intestine (ileum) and large intestine (colon)

gene   specific sequence in DNA that codes for a particular protein; genes are located on the chromosomes; each gene is found in a definite position (locus)

genotype   genetic composition or assortment of genes that, together with environmental influences, determines the appearance or phenotype of an individual

germ line   genetic material transmitted from parents to offspring through the gametes (sperm and ova)

ginseng   root found in Asia and the USA, although the Asian variety is more easily obtainable; a popular nutritional supplement and medication in Asia

g/L   grams per litre

gluconeogenesis   synthesis of glucose from non-carbohydrate precursors such as glycerol, ketoacids or amino acids

GLUT4   glucose transporter type 4

glutamine   one of the 20 amino acids commonly found in proteins; the most abundant free amino acid in the blood plasma; considered to be an important energy source for leukocytes

glycaemic index   increase in blood glucose and insulin response to a meal; the glycaemic index of a food is expressed against a reference food, usually glucose

glycogen   polymer of glucose used as storage form of carbohydrate in the liver and muscles

glycogenolysis   breakdown of glycogen into glucose-1-phosphate by the action of phosphorylase

glycolysis   sequence of reactions that converts glucose (or glycogen) to pyruvate

glycoprotein   protein that is attached to one or more sugar molecules

glycosidic bond   chemical bond in which the oxygen atom is the common link between a carbon of one sugar molecule and the carbon of another; glycogen, the glucose polymer, is a branched-chain polysaccharide consisting of glucose molecules linked by glycosidic bonds

GM-CSF   granulocyte-monocyte colony stimulating factor

GMFI   (geometric mean fluorescence intensity) a quantitative measure of the staining intensity of a fluorescent marker used in flow cytometry

gonadotrophic hormones   hormones released from the anterior pituitary gland that promote sex steroid hormone synthesis by the ovaries in females and the testes in males

GP   general practitioner

H+   hydrogen ion or proton

H₂O₂   hydrogen peroxide

haem   molecular ring structure that is incorporated in the haemoglobin molecule, enabling this protein to carry oxygen

haematocrit   proportion of the blood volume that is occupied by the cellular elements (red cells, white cells, and platelets); also known as the packed-cell volume

haematopoiesis   production of erythrocytes and leukocytes in the bone marrow

haematuria   red blood cells or haemoglobin in the urine

haemodilution   thinning of the blood caused by an expansion of the plasma volume without an equivalent rise in red blood cells

haemoglobin   red, iron-containing respiratory pigment found in red blood cells; important in the transport of respiratory gases and in the regulation of blood pH

haemolysis   destruction of red blood cells within the circulation

haemorrhage   damage to blood-vessel walls resulting in bleeding

half-life   time in which half the quantity or concentration of a substance is eliminated or removed

HCl   (hydrochloric acid) part of gastric digestive juices

HClO   (hydrochlorous acid) produced by phagocytes

HCO₃-   bicarbonate ion, the principal extracellular buffer

HDL   (high-density lipoprotein) protein–lipid complex in the blood plasma that facilitates the transport of triacylglycerols, cholesterol and phospholipids

hepatic glucose output   liver glucose output; the glucose that is released from the liver as a result of glycogenolysis or gluconeogenesis

HIV   human immunodeficiency virus

HLA   human leukocyte antigen

hormone   organic chemical produced in cells of one part of the body (usually an endocrine gland) that diffuses or is transported by the blood circulation to cells in other parts of the body, where it regulates and coordinates their activities

HPA axis   hypothalamic-pituitary-adrenal axis

HPLC   high-pressure liquid chromatography

hROS   highly reactive oxygen species

humoral   fluid-borne

hydrogen bond   weak intermolecular or intramolecular attraction resulting from the interaction of a hydrogen atom and an electronegative atom possessing a lone pair of electrons (e.g. oxygen or nitrogen); hydrogen bonding is important in DNA and RNA and is responsible for much of the tertiary structure of proteins

hydrolysis   reaction in which an organic compound is split by interaction with water into simpler compounds

hyperthermia   elevated body temperature (> 37°C or 98.6°F)

hypertonic   having a higher concentration of dissolved particles (osmolality) than that of another solution with which it is being compared (usually blood plasma, which has an osmolality of 290 mOsm/kg)

hyperventilation   state in which an increased amount of air enters the pulmonary alveoli (increased alveolar ventilation), resulting in reduction of carbon dioxide tension and eventually leading to alkalosis

hyponatraemia   below normal serum sodium concentration (< 140 mmol/L)

hypothalamus   region at base of brain responsible for integration of sensory input and effector responses in regulation of body temperature; also contains centres for control of hunger, appetite and thirst

hypothermia   lower than normal body temperature

hypotonic   having a lower concentration of dissolved particles (osmolality) than that of another solution with which it is being compared (usually blood plasma, which has an osmolality of 290 mOsm/kg).

hypovolaemia   reduced blood volume

ICAM   intercellular adhesion molecule

IFN   (interferon) type of cytokine; some interferons inhibit viral replication in infected cells

Ig   (immunoglobulin) same as antibody

IGF   insulin-like growth factor

IL   (interleukin) type of cytokine produced by leukocytes and some other tissues; acts as a chemical messenger, rather like a hormone but usually with localised effects

IL-1ra   interleukin-1 receptor antagonist

immunodepression   lowered functional activity of the immune system

in vitro   within a glass, observable in a test tube, in an artificial environment; can also be referred to as *ex vivo* (outside the living body)

in vivo   within the living body

indispensable amino acids   *see* essential amino acids

inflammation   body's response to injury, which includes redness (increased blood flow) and swelling (oedema) caused by increased capillary permeability

innate immunity   immunity that is not dependent on prior contact with antigen

insulin   hormone secreted by the pancreas involved in carbohydrate metabolism and, in particular, the control of the blood glucose concentration

interferon   type of cytokine; inhibits viral replication

interstitial   fluid-filled spaces that lie between cells

IOC   International Olympic Committee

ion   any atom or molecule that has an electrical charge owing to loss or gain of valency (outer shell) electrons; may carry a positive charge (cation) or a negative charge (anion)

ionic bond   bond in which valence electrons are either lost or gained and atoms that are oppositely charged are held together by electrostatic forces

ischaemia   reduced blood supply to a tissue or organ

isoform   chemically distinct forms of a enzyme with identical activities usually coded by different genes; also called isoenzyme

isomer one of two or more substances that have an identical molecular composition and relative molecular mass but different structure because of a different arrangement of atoms within the molecule

isotonicity having the same concentration of dissolved particles (osmolality) than that of another solution with which it is being compared (usually blood plasma, which has an osmolality of 290 mOsm/kg)

isotope one of a set of chemically identical species of atom that have the same atomic number but different mass numbers (e.g. 12-isotopes,13-isotopes and 14-isotopes of carbon whose atomic number is 12)

iu international units

J (joule) unit of energy according to the International System of Units. 1 joule is the amount of energy needed to move a mass of 1 g at a velocity of 1 m/s

kcal (kilocalorie) 1,000 calories; 1 kcal = 1 Calorie = 1,000 calories

kD kilodalton

ketone bodies acidic organic compounds produced during the incomplete oxidation of fatty acids in the liver; contain a carboxyl group ($-COOH$) and a ketone group ($-C=O$); examples include acetoacetate and 3-hydroxybutyrate

kinase enzyme that regulates a phosphorylation-dephosphorylation reaction (i.e. the addition or removal of a phosphate group); this process is one important way in which enzyme activity can be regulated

kJ (kilojoule) unit of energy (1 kJ = 10^3 J)

KLH keyhole limpet haemocyanin; a protein antigen that is unlikely to have been encountered previously and which elicits a thymus-dependent antibody response

KLR killer lectin-like receptor

L litre

lactic acid metabolic end product of anaerobic glycolysis

lactoferrin antimicrobial protein found in plasma and saliva that chelates iron (essential for bacterial proliferation) and has antiviral properties

LAK (lymphokine-activated killer cells) types of lymphocyte similar to natural killer cells that are activated by interleukin-2

LBM (lean body mass) all parts of the body, excluding fat

LDL (low-density lipoproteins) protein–lipid complex in the blood plasma that facilitates the transport of triacylglycerols, cholesterol and phospholipids

lecithin common name for phosphatidyl choline, the most abundant phospholipid found in cell membranes

lectins proteins, mostly from plants, that bind specific sugars on glycoproteins and glycolipids; several lectins are mitogenic (e.g. Con-A; PHA)

legume high-protein fruit or pod of vegetables, including beans, peas and lentils

leptin regulatory hormone produced by adipocytes (fat cells); when released into the circulation, it influences the hypothalamus to control appetite

leucine essential amino acid that is alleged to slow the breakdown of muscle protein during strenuous exercise and to improve gains in muscle mass with strength training

leukocyte white blood cell; important in inflammation and immune defence

leukocytosis   increased number of leukocytes in the circulation

leukotrienes   metabolic products of the polyunsaturated fatty acid arachidonic acid which promote inflammatory responses; mostly produced by macrophages, mast cells and basophils

LGG   *L. rhamnosus* GG

LH   (luteinising hormone) a gonadotrophin secreted from the anterior pituitary gland

ligand   any molecule that is recognised by a binding structure such as a receptor

linoleic acid   an essential fatty acid

linolenic acid   an essential fatty acid

lipid   compound composed of carbon, hydrogen and oxygen and sometimes other elements; lipids dissolve in organic solvents but not in water and include triacylglycerol, cholesterol and phospholipids; commonly called fats

lipid peroxidation   oxidation of fatty acids in lipid structures (e.g. membranes) caused by the actions of free radicals

lipolysis   breakdown of triacylglycerols into fatty acids and glycerol

LPS   (lipopolysaccharide) endotoxin derived from Gram-positive bacterial cell walls that has inflammatory and mitogenic actions

LTB-B4   (leukotriene-B4) metabolic product of the polyunsaturated fatty acid arachidonic acid, which promotes inflammatory responses; mostly produced by macrophages

lymph   tissue fluid which drains into and from the lymphatic system

lymphocyte   type of white blood cell important in the acquired immune response; includes both T cells and B cells, the latter producing antibodies

lymphokines   cytokines produced by lymphocytes

lysis   process of disintegration of a cell

lysosome   membranous vesicle found in the cell cytoplasm; lysosomes contain digestive enzymes capable of autodigesting the cell

lysozyme   enzyme that breaks down proteins and proteoglycans in bacterial cell walls; produced by macrophages and found in tears and saliva

M   (molar) unit of concentration (nM: nanomolar = 10^{-9}M; μM: micromolar = 10^{-6}M; mM: millimolar = 10^{-3}M).

macromineral   dietary elements essential to life processes that each constitute at least 0.01% of total body mass; the seven macrominerals are potassium, sodium, chloride, calcium, magnesium, phosphorus, and sulphur

macronutrients   nutrients ingested in relatively large amounts (carbohydrate, fat, protein, and water)

macrophage   phagocyte and antigen-presenting cell found in the tissues; precursor is the blood monocyte; initiates the acquired immune response

maltodextrin   glucose polymer (commonly containing 6–12 glucose molecules) that exerts lesser osmotic effects compared with glucose and is used in a variety of sports drinks as the main source of carbohydrate

maltose   disaccharide that yields two molecules of glucose upon hydrolysis

margination   adherence of leukocytes to the endothelial wall of blood vessels

mast cell   cell found in the tissues that resembles a blood basophil; both cell types are activated by IgE-antigen complexes resulting in degranulation and release of inflammatory mediators including histamine and leukotrienes

MCP   monocyte chemotactic protein

mDC   myeloid dendritic cell

megadose   excessive amount of a substance in comparison to a normal dose (such as the RDA); usually used to refer to vitamin supplements

memory cells   clonally expanded T and B lymphocytes that are primed to respond faster on exposure to a previously encountered antigen

meta-analysis   an analytical technique which takes a bird's-eye perspective by comparing and summarising the effects of a large number of studies

metabolic acidosis   metabolic derangement of acid–base balance where the blood pH is abnormally low

metabolite   product of a metabolic reaction

metalloenzyme   enzyme that needs a mineral component (e.g. copper, iron, magnesium, and zinc) to function effectively

METS   (metabolic equivalents) measurement of energy expenditure expressed as multiples of the resting metabolic rate; 1 MET equals approximately an oxygen uptake rate of 3.5 ml O_2/kg b.m./minute

MFI   (mean fluorescence intensity) used to quantify expression of molecules

μg   (microgram) one millionth of a gram

MHC   (major histocompatibility complex) molecules involved in antigen presentation to T cells; class I MHC proteins are present on virtually all nucleated cells, whereas class II MHC proteins are expressed on antigen presenting cells (primarily macrophages and dendritic cells)

micromineral   those dietary elements essential to life processes that each comprise less than 0.001% of total body mass and are needed in quantities of less than 100 mg a day; among the 14 trace elements are iron, zinc, copper, chromium and selenium; also known as trace elements

micronutrients   organic vitamins and inorganic minerals that must be consumed in relatively small amounts in the diet to maintain health

mineral   inorganic element found in nature, although the term is usually reserved for those elements that are solid; in nutrition, the term is usually used to classify those dietary elements essential to life processes; examples are calcium and iron

minute   unit of time; 60 seconds

MIP   macrophage inflammatory protein

mitochondrion   oval or spherical organelle containing the enzymes of the tricarboxylic acid cycle and electron transport chain; site of oxidative phosphorylation (re-synthesis of ATP involving the use of oxygen)

mitogen   chemical that can stimulate lymphocytes to proliferate (undergo rapid cell divisions)

mitosis   type of cell division in which each of the two daughter cells receives exactly the same number of chromosomes present in the nucleus of the parent cell

MJ   (megajoule) 10^6 joules

mL   millilitre

mM   millimole (10^{-3}M)

µM   micromole (10^{-6}M) one millionth of a mole; a mole is the molecular weight in grams

Mn   magnesium

mole   amount of a chemical compound whose mass in grams is equivalent to its molecular weight, the sum of the atomic weights of its constituent atoms

molecule   aggregation of at least two atoms of the same or different elements held together by special forces (covalent bonds) and having a precise chemical formula (e.g. O_2, $C_6H_6O_6$)

monoclonal antibody   specific antibody derived from a single B-cell clone

monocyte   type of white blood cell that can ingest and destroy foreign material and initiate the acquired immune response; precursor of tissue macrophage

monosaccharide   simple sugar that cannot be hydrolysed to smaller units (e.g. glucose, fructose and galactose)

mOsm/kg   milliosmoles per kilogram

mRNA   messenger ribonucleic acid

m/s   metres per second

MTT   3-(4,5-dimethlythiazol-2-yl)-2,5-diphenyltetrazolium bromide; a yellow compound used in assays of lymphocyte proliferation

mucosa   layer of cells lining the mouth, nasal passages, airways and gut that presents a barrier to pathogen entry into the body

myoglobin   protein that functions as an intracellular respiratory pigment that is capable of binding oxygen and only releasing it at very low partial pressures

NAD   nicotinamide adenine dinucleotide (*see also* coenzyme)

NADPH   (nicotinamide adenine dinucleotide phosphate-oxidase) a membrane-bound enzyme complex

NETs   (neutrophil extracellular traps) a web of fibres composed of chromatin and serine proteases that trap and kill microbes extracellularly; NETs provide a high local concentration of antimicrobial components and bind, disarm and kill microbes independent of phagocytic uptake

neurotransmitters   endogenous signalling molecules that transfer information from one nerve ending to the next

neutrophil   type of white blood cell that can ingest and destroy foreign material; very important as a first line of defence against bacteria

NH₂   amino group

NH₃   ammonia

NH₄⁺   ammonium ion

nitrogen balance   dietary state in which the input and output of nitrogen is balanced so that the body neither gains nor loses tissue protein

NK   (natural killer) cell; type of lymphocyte important in eliminating viral infections and preventing cancer

NKCA   (natural killer cell cytotoxic activity) ability of NK cells to destroy virally infected cells and tumour cells

NKT (natural killer T cells) these cells are almost entirely CD3+ and CD8+ (so are a type of T lymphocyte) but also express the 'NK-cell markers' CD56 and CD161 and respond to glycolipids presented by CD1d

N/L ratio ratio of neutrophils to lymphocytes in the blood

nM nanomolar (10^{-9}M)

NO nitric oxide

NO· nitric oxide radical

NOD receptors (nucleotide-binding oligomerisation domain) receptors; a group of intracellular surveillance proteins that can detect bacterial peptidoglycan, signalling the presence of bacteria in the host cell

non-essential amino acids amino acids that can be synthesised in the body

noradrenaline catecholamine hormone and the neurotransmitter of most of the sympathetic nervous system (of so-called adrenergic neurons); also known as norepinephrine

norepinephrine *see* noradrenaline

nutraceutical nutrient that may function as a pharmaceutical (drug) when taken in certain quantities

nutrient substance found in food that provides energy or promote growth and repair of tissues

nutrition total of the processes of ingestion, digestion, absorption and metabolism of food and the subsequent assimilation of nutrient materials into the tissues

O_2 oxygen molecule

·O_2^- (superoxide radical) a highly reactive free radical

obesity excessive accumulation of body fat; usually reserved for those individuals who are 20% or more above the average weight for their size

OH hydroxyl group

·OH (hydroxyl radical) a highly reactive free radical

opsonin molecule that enhances phagocytosis by promoting adhesion of the antigen to the phagocyte

osmosis diffusion of water molecules from the lesser to the greater concentration of solute (dissolved substance) when two solutions are separated by a membrane that selectively prevents the passage of solute molecules but is permeable to water molecules

OTS overtraining syndrome

oxidative burst increased oxygen consumption and production of reactive oxygen species by phagocytes following their activation; also known as respiratory burst

PAMP (pathogen associated molecular pattern) molecules that are commonly expressed by micro-organisms that are not expressed by host cells

pathogen micro-organism that can cause symptoms of disease

PBMC peripheral blood mononuclear cells which includes all lymphocytes and monocytes but excludes granulocytes

PBS phosphate-buffered saline

pDC plasmacytoid dendritic cell

PE R-phycoerythrin; a fluorescent marker used in flow cytometry

PEM (protein energy malnutrition) inadequate intake of dietary protein and energy

peptide small compound formed by the bonding of two or more amino acids; larger chains of linked amino acids are called polypeptides or proteins

PerCP (peridinin chlorophyll) a fluorescent marker used in flow cytometry

perforin molecule produced by natural killer cells and cytotoxic T cells that forms a pore in the membrane of target cells leading to lysis and cell death

PGE$_2$ prostaglandin E$_2$

pH measure of acidity/alkalinity; pH = $-\log_{10}[H^+]$

PHA (phytohaemagglutinin) plant lectin that acts as a T cell mitogen

phagocyte leukocyte capable of ingesting and digesting microorganisms

phagocytosis process of ingestion of bacteria, virus or cell debris by cells such as neutrophils and macrophages (*phago* = eat; *cyte* = cell)

phenotype appearance or physiological characteristic of an individual that results from the interaction of the genotype and the environment

phospholipids fats containing a phosphate group that on hydrolysis yield fatty acids, glycerol and a nitrogenous compound; lecithin is an example; phospholipids are important components of membranes

PIgR (polyimmunoglobulin receptor) receptor molecule that specifically binds dimeric secretory IgA and transports it across the mucosal epithelial cells

plasma liquid portion of the blood in which the blood cells are suspended; typically accounts for 55–60% of total blood volume; differs from serum in that it contains fibrinogen, the clot-forming protein

plasma cell terminally differentiated B lymphocyte that secretes large amounts of antibody

PLP pyridoxal phosphate (*see also* coenzyme)

PMBC peripheral blood mononuclear cell

PMA (phorbol myristate acetate) mitogen that directly stimulates protein kinase C

PMN (polymorphonuclear) cells, which principally refers to neutrophils

PMT photomultiplier tube

polypeptide peptide that, upon hydrolysis, yields more than two amino acids

polyphenols large class of naturally occurring compounds that include the flavonoids, flavonols, flavonones, and anthocyanidins; these compounds contain a number of phenolic hydroxyl (–OH) groups attached to ring structures, which confers them with powerful antioxidant activity

polysaccharide polymers of (arbitrarily) more than about ten monosaccharide residues linked glycosidically in branched or unbranched chains; examples include starch and glycogen

POMS profile of mood state questionnaire

post-absorptive state period after a meal has been absorbed from the gastrointestinal tract

power work performed per unit of time

precursor substance from which another, usually more active or mature substance, is formed

prohormones   protein hormone before processing to remove parts of its sequence and thus make it active

prostaglandins   lipids derived from the polyunsaturated fatty acid arachidonic acid that increase vascular permeability, sensitise pain receptors, initiate fever and stimulate or inhibit immune responses

prosthetic group   coenzyme that is tightly bound to an enzyme

protease   enzyme that catalyses the digestion or cleavage of proteins

protein   biological macromolecules composed of a chain of covalently linked amino acids; may have structural or functional roles

PRR   (pattern recognition receptors) receptors on APCs and phagocytes that recognise PAMPs

PUFA   (polyunsaturated fatty acid) fatty acid that contains more than one carbon-carbon double bond

PWM   (pokeweed mitogen) plant lectin that is a T-cell dependent B cell mitogen

pyrogen   substance that causes body temperature to elevated, as in fever, and be regulated at a higher set point

Ra   (rate of appearance) usually refers to the rate at which a substance enters the blood circulation

RAST test   radioallergosorbent test (*see* Technique box 11.1)

RBC   (red blood cell) erythrocyte

Rd   (rate of disappearance) usually refers to the rate at which a substance leaves the blood circulation

RDA   (recommended daily allowance) recommended intake of a particular nutrient that meets the needs of nearly all (97%) healthy individuals of similar age and gender; established by the Food and Nutrition Boards of the National Academy of Sciences

respiratory burst   *see* oxidative burst

reperfusion   restoration of the blood supply to a tissue or organ

rhIL-6   recombinant human interleukin-6

RIA   radioimmunoassay

ribosome   very small organelle composed of protein and RNA that is either free in the cytoplasm or attached to the membranes of the endoplasmic reticulum of a cell; site of protein synthesis

RNA   ribonucleic acid

RNI   (recommended nutrient intake) defined as the level of intake required to meet the known nutritional needs of more than 97.5% of healthy persons; In the UK, the RNI is very similar to the original RDA

ROS   (reactive oxygen species) collective name for free radicals and other highly reactive molecules derived from molecular oxygen; ROS include superoxide radical ($^{\bullet}O_2^-$), hydroxyl radical ($^{\bullet}OH$), hydrogen peroxide (H_2O_2) and perchlorous acid (HOCl)

s   (second) a unit of time

SAM   sympatheticoadrenal–medullary axis

sarcolemma   cell membrane of a muscle fibre

sarcomere   smallest contractile unit or segment of a muscle fibre and is defined as the region between two Z lines

sarcoplasm   cytoplasm or intracellular fluid within a muscle fibre

sarcoplasmic reticulum   elaborate bag-like membranous structure found within a muscle cell; its interconnecting membranous tubules lie in the narrow spaces between the myofibrils, surrounding and running parallel to them

SD   (standard deviation) measure of variability about the mean; 68% of the population is within 1 standard deviation above and below the mean, and about 95% of the population is within 2 standard deviations of the mean

SE   (standard error) measure of variability about the mean

sensitivity   a measure of how often a test will correctly identify a positive

serum   fluid left after blood has clotted

s-IgA   salivary immunoglobulin A

SI units   (Système Internationale d'unités) the International System of Units, a worldwide agreed uniform system of units of measurement

SIRS   systemic inflammatory response syndrome

SOCS   suppressor of cytokine signalling

SOD   superoxide dismutase

solute   substance dissolved in a solvent liquid such as water

solvent   liquid medium in which particles can dissolve

specificity   a measure of how accurate a test is against false positives

stable isotope   isotope is a specific form of a chemical element; it differs from atoms of other forms (isotopes) of the same element in the number of neutrons in its nucleus; 'stable' refers to the fact that the isotope is not radioactive, in contrast to some other types of isotopes

starch   carbohydrate made of multiple units of glucose attached together by bonds that can be broken down by human digestion processes (*see also* complex carbohydrates)

steroid   complex molecule derived from the lipid cholesterol containing four interlocking carbon rings

stimulation index   lymphocyte proliferation expressed as ratio of mitogen-stimulated proliferation rate to unstimulated proliferation rate

T cells   lymphocytes processed in the thymus glands

TBARS   (thiobarbituric acid-reactive substances) stable compounds produced as a consequence of free radical actions on lipid structures; commonly used as a measure of oxidative stress

Tc   (T-cytotoxic lymphocyte) effector cell of cell-mediated immunity

TCR   (T cell receptor) antigen receptor present on surface of T lymphocytes that recognises fragments of antigenic peptides presented by MHC class II proteins on APCs

testosterone   male sex hormone responsible for male secondary sex characteristics at puberty; it has anabolic and androgenic effects

TGF   (transforming growth factor) an inhibitory cytokine produced by T regulatory cells

Th   T-helper lymphocyte

thymus   lymphoid gland located in the chest where lymphocytes differentiate into immunocompetent T cells

tissue   organised association of similar cells that perform a common function (e.g. muscle tissue)

TLR   (Toll-like receptor) family of evolutionary conserved pattern recognition receptors present on APCs and phagocytes that detect PAMPs and initiate the acquired immune response to pathogens

TNF   (tumour necrosis factor) cytokine that promotes inflammation

TPP   thiamine pyrophosphate (*see also* coenzyme)

trace element   *see* micromineral

trafficking (of leukocytes)   movements of leukocytes into or out of the circulation

transcription   process by which RNA polymerase produces single-stranded RNA complementary to one strand of the DNA

translation   process by which ribosomes and tRNA decipher the genetic code in mRNA to synthesise a specific polypeptide or protein

Treg   T-regulatory lymphocyte, a major producer of the anti-inflammatory cytokine, interleukin-10

UK   United Kingdom

UPS   unexplained underperformance syndrome (also known as overtraining syndrome)

urea   end product of protein metabolism; chemical formula $CO(NH_2)_2$

URI   upper respiratory illness

uric acid   breakdown product of nucleic acids; present in small quantity in the plasma and urine of man and most mammals

urine   fluid produced in the kidney and excreted from the body; contains urea, ammonia and other metabolic wastes

URTI   (upper respiratory tract infections) increasingly used to describe symptoms of illness affecting the upper respiratory tract where an infectious cause of symptoms cannot be confirmed and other causes (e.g. airway inflammation) may be responsible

URTS   upper respiratory tract (infection-type) symptoms

USA   United States of America

vegan   vegetarian who eats no animal products

vegetarian   one whose food is of vegetable or plant origin

virus   microscopic organism that cannot replicate or express its genes without a host living cell; viruses invade living cells and use the nucleic acid material they contain to replicate themselves

vitamin   organic substance necessary in small amounts for the normal metabolic functioning of the body; must be present in the diet because the body cannot synthesise it (or cannot synthesise an adequate amount of it)

vitamin B$_1$ thiamine

vitamin B$_2$ riboflavin

vitamin B$_6$ pyridoxine

vitamin B$_{12}$ cyanocobalamin

vitamin C   ascorbic acid

vitamin D   cholecalciferol; the product of irradiation of 7-dehydrocholesterol found in the skin

vitamin E   alpha-tocopherol

vitamin K   menoquinone

V_{max} maximal velocity of an enzymatic reaction when substrate concentration is not limiting

$\dot{V}O_2$ Rate of oxygen uptake

$\dot{V}O_2$ **max**   maximal oxygen uptake; the highest rate of oxygen consumption by the body that can be determined in an incremental exercise test to exhaustion. $\dot{V}O_2$ max is confirmed by the observation of plateau in oxygen uptake despite an increase in exercise intensity

$\dot{V}O_2$ **peak**   peak oxygen uptake; the highest rate of oxygen consumption by the body observed in an incremental exercise test to exhaustion but not necessarily confirmed as the true maximum value. For good athletes $\dot{V}O_2$ max can often be measured but, for less fit individuals, children and the elderly, usually only $\dot{V}O_2$ peak can be measured because they cannot sustain high-intensity exercise long enough to reach a plateau in oxygen uptake

W   (watt) unit of power or work rate (J/s)

water   universal solvent of life (H_2O); the body is composed of 60% water

white blood cells   leukocytes; important cells of the immune system that defend the body against invading micro-organisms

WHO   World Health Organization

w.w.   wet weight

Bibliography

Abbott, R. D., White, L. R., Ross, G. W., Masaki, K. H., Curb, J. D. and Petrovitch, H. (2004) Walking and dementia in physically capable elderly men. *Journal of the American Medical Association* 292:1447–53.

Agrawal, A., Sridharan, A., Prakash, S. and Agrawal, H. (2012) Dendritic cells and aging: consequences for autoimmunity. *Expert Reviews in Clinical Immunology* 8: 73–80.

Akbar, A. N., Terry, L., Timms, A., Beverley, P. C. and Janossy, G. (1988) Loss of CD45R and gain of UCHL1 reactivity is a feature of primed T cells. *Journal of Immunology* 140: 2171–8.

Akimoto, T., Kumai, Y., Akama, T., Hayashi, E., Murakami, H., Soma, R., Kuno, S. and Kono, I. (2003) Effects of 12 months of exercise training on salivary secretory IgA levels in elderly subjects. *British Journal of Sports Medicine* 37: 76–9.

Akira, S., Taga, T. and Kishimoto, T. (1993) Interleukin-6 in biology and medicine. *Advances in Immunology* 54: 1–78.

Al Hegelan, M., Tighe, R. M., Castillo, C. and Hollingsworth, J.W. (2011) Ambient ozone and pulmonary innate immunity. *Immunology Research* 49: 173–91.

Alaranta, A., Alaranta, H., Heliovaara, M., Alha, P., Palmu, P. and Helenius, I. (2005) Allergic rhinitis and pharmacological management in elite athletes. *Medicine and Science in Sports and Exercise* 37: 707–11.

Albers, R., Antoine, J. M., Bourdet-Sicard, R., Calder, P. C., Gleeson, M., Lesourd, B., Samartin, S., Sanderson, I. R., Van Loo, J., Vas Dias, F. W. and Watzl, B. (2005) Markers to measure immunomodulation in human nutrition intervention studies. *British Journal of Nutrition* 94: 452–81.

Allgrove, J. E., Gomes, E., Hough, J. and Gleeson, M. (2008) Effects of exercise intensity on salivary antimicrobial proteins and markers of stress in active men. *Journal of Sports Sciences* 26: 653–61.

Allsop, P., Peters, A. M., Arnot, R. N., Stuttle, A. W., Deenmamode, M., Gwilliam, M. E., Myers, M. J. and Hall, G. M. (1992) Intrasplenic blood cell kinetics in man before and after brief maximal exercise. *Clinical Sciences (London)* 83: 47–54.

Alm, J. S., Swartz, J., Lilja, G., Scheynius, A. and Pershagen, G. (1999) Atopy in children of families with an anthroposophic lifestyle. *The Lancet* 353: 1485–8.

Aloe, L., Simone, M. D. and Properzi, F. (1999) Nerve growth factor: a neurotrophin with activity on cells of the immune system. *Microscopy Research and Technique* 45: 285–91.

Alonso, J. M., Tscholl, P. M., Engebretsen, L., Mountjoy, M., Dvorak, J. and Junge, A. (2010) Occurrence of injuries and illnesses during the 2009 IAAF World Athletics Championships. *British Journal of Sports Medicine* 44: 1100–5.

Alonso, J. M., Edouard, P., Fischetto, G., Adams, B., Depiesse, F. and Mountjoy, M. (2012) Determination of future prevention strategies in elite track and field: analysis of Daegu 2011 IAAF Championships injuries and illnesses surveillance. *British Journal of Sports Medicine* 46: 505–14.

Anane, L. H., Edwards, K. M., Burns, V. E., Drayson, M. T., Riddell, N. E., van Zanten, J. J., Wallace, G. R., Mills, P. J. and Bosch, J. A. (2009) Mobilization of gammadelta T lymphocytes in response to psychological stress, exercise, and beta-agonist infusion. *Brain, Behavior, and Immunity* 23: 823–9.

Anderson, S. D. and Kippelen, P. (2005) Exercise-induced bronchoconstriction: pathogenesis. *Current Allergy and Asthma Reports* 5: 116–22.

Andrewes, C. H. (1950) Adventures among viruses; the puzzle of the common cold. *New England Journal of Medicine* 242: 235–240.

Ansley, L., Kippelen, P., Dickinson, J. and Hull, J. H. (2012) Misdiagnosis of exercise-induced bronchoconstriction in professional soccer players. *Allergy* 67: 390–5.

Antoni, M. H., Lutgendorf, S. K., Cole, S.W., Dhabhar, F. S., Sephton, S. E., McDonald, P. G., Stefanek, M. and Sood, A. K. (2006) The influence of biobehavioural factors on tumour biology: pathways and mechanisms. *Nature Reviews Cancer* 6: 240–8.

Appay, V., van Lier, R. A., Sallusto, F. and Roederer, M. (2008) Phenotype and function of human T lymphocyte subsets: consensus and issues. *Cytometry A* 73: 975–83.

Armstrong, L. E., Pumerantz, A. C., Fiala, K. A., Roti, M. W., Kavouras, S. A., Casa, D. J. and Maresh, C. M. (2010) Human hydration indices: acute and longitudinal reference values. *International Journal of Sport Nutrition and Exercise Metabolism* 20: 145–53.

Arnold, M. C., Papanicolaou, D. A., O'Grady, J. A., Lotsikas, A., Dale, J. K., Straus, S. E. and Grafman, J. (2002) Using an interleukin-6 challenge to evaluate neuropsychological performance in chronic fatigue syndrome. *Psychological Medicine* 32: 1075–89.

Arruvtio, L., Sanz, M., Banham, A. H., Fainboim L (2007) Expansion of CD4+CD25+ and FoxP3+ regulatory T cells during the follicular phase of the menstrual cycle: implications for human reproduction. *Journal of Immunology* 178: 2572–8.

Atanackovic, D., Schnee, B., Schuch, G., Faltz, C., Schulze, J., Weber, C. S., Schafhausen, P., Bartels, K., Bokemeyer, C., Brunner-Weinzierl, M. C. and Deter, H.C. (2006) Acute psychological stress alerts the adaptive immune response: stress-induced mobilization of effector T cells. *Journal of Neuroimmunology* 176: 141–52.

Athens, J. W., Haab, O. P., Raab, S. O., Mauer, A. M., Ashenbrucker, H., Cartwright, G. E. and Wintrobe, M. M. (1961) Leukokinetic studies. IV. The total blood, circulating and marginal granulocyte pools and the granulocyte turnover rate in normal subjects. *Journal of Clinical Investigation* 40: 989–95.

Baeten, D., Boots, A. M., Steenbakkers, P. G., Elewaut, D., Bos, E., Verheijden, G. F., Berheijden, G., Miltenburg, A. M., Rijnders, A. W., Veys, E. M. and De Keyser, F. (2000) Human cartilage gp39+,CD16+ monocytes in peripheral blood and synovium: correlation with joint destruction in rheumatoid arthritis. *Arthritis & Rheumatism* 43: 1233–43.

Bailey, D. M., Davies, B., Castell, L. M., Collier, D. J., Milledge, J. S., Hullin, D. A., Seddon, P. S. and Young, I. S. (2003) Symptoms of infection and acute mountain sickness; associated metabolic sequelae and problems in differential diagnosis. *High Altitude Medicine & Biology* 4: 319–31.

Bailey, D. M., Davies, B., Romer, L., Castell, L., Newsholme, E. and Gandy, G. (1998) Implications of moderate altitude training for sea-level endurance in elite distance runners. *European Journal of Applied Physiology and Occupational Physiology* 78: 360–8.

Bain, B. J., Phillips, D., Thomson, K., Richardson, D. and Gabriel, I. (2000) Investigation of the effect of marathon running on leucocyte counts of subjects of different ethnic origins: relevance to the aetiology of ethnic neutropenia. *British Journal of Haematology* 108: 483–7.

Baj, Z., Kantorski, J., Majewska, E., Zeman, K., Pokoca, L., Fornalczyk, E., Tchorzewski, H., Sulowska, Z. and Lewicki, R. (1994) Immunological status of competitive cyclists before and after the training season. *International Journal of Sports Medicine* 15: 319–24.

Balducci, S., Zanuso, S., Nicolucci, A., De Feo, P., Cavallo, S., Cardelli, P., Fallucca, S., Alessi, E., Fallucca, F. and Pugliese, G. (2010) Effect of an intensive exercise intervention strategy on modifiable cardiovascular risk factors in subjects with type 2 diabetes mellitus: a randomized controlled trial: the Italian Diabetes and Exercise Study (IDES). *Archives of Internal Medicine* 170: 1794–803.

Barrett, B. (2003) Medicinal properties of Echinacea: critical review. *Phytomedicine* 10: 66–86.

Barrett, B. P., Brown, R. L., Locken, K., Maberry, R., Bobula, J. A. and D'Alessio, D. (2002) Treatment of the common cold with unrefined echinacea. A randomized, double-blind, placebo-controlled trial. *Annals of Internal Medicine* 137: 939–46.

Bassit, R. A., Sawada, L. A., Bacurau, R. F., Navarro, F., Martins, E., Jr, Santos, R. V., Caperuto, E. C., Rogeri, P. and Costa Rosa, L. F. (2002) Branched-chain amino acid supplementation and the immune response of long-distance athletes. *Nutrition* 18: 376–9.

Bate, S. L., Dollard, S. C. and Cannon, M. J. (2010) Cytomegalovirus seroprevalence in the United States: the national health and nutrition examination surveys, 1988–2004. *Clinical Infectious Diseases* 50: 1439–47.

Baum, M., Geitner, T. and Liesen, H. (1996) The role of the spleen in the leucocytosis of exercise: consequences for physiology and pathophysiology. *International Journal of Sports Medicine* 17: 604–7.

Baumert, M., Brechtel, L., Lock, J., Hermsdorf, M., Wolff, R., Baier, V. and Voss, A. (2006) Heart rate variability, blood pressure variability, and baroreflex sensitivity in overtrained athletes. *Clinical Journal of Sports Medicine* 16: 412–417.

Bays, H. E. (2009) 'Sick fat', metabolic disease, and atherosclerosis. *American Journal of Medicine* 122: S26–37.

Beals, K. A. and Manore, M. M. (1994) The prevalence and consequences of subclinical eating disorders in female athletes. *International Journal of Sports Nutrition* 4: 175–95.

Beeley, J. M., Smith, D. J. and Oakley, E. H. (1993) Environmental hazards and health. *British Medical Bulletin* 49: 305–25.

Beery, T. A. (2003) Sex differences in infection and sepsis. *Critical Care Nursing Clinics of North America* 15: 55–62.

Beilin, B., Shavit, Y., Razumovsky, J., Wolloch, Y., Zeidel, A. and Bessler, H. (1998) Effects of mild perioperative hypothermia on cellular immune responses. *Anesthesiology* 89: 1133–40.

Belge, K. U., Dayyani, F., Horelt, A., Siedlar, M., Frankenberger, M., Frankenberger, B., Espevik, T. and Ziegler-Heitbrock, L. (2002) The proinflammatory CD14+CD16+DR++ monocytes are a major source of TNF. *Journal of Immunology* 168: 3536–42.

Berg, A., Northoff, H. and Konig, D. (1998) Influence of Echinacin (E31) treatment on the exercise-induced immune response in athletes. *Journal of Clinical Research* 1: 367–80.

Berglund, B. and Hemmingson, P. (1990) Infectious disease in elite cross-country skiers: A one-year incidence study. *Clinical Journal of Sports Medicine* 2: 19–23.

Bergmann, M., Gornikiewicz, A., Sautner, T., Waldmann, E., Weber, T., Mittlböck, M.,

Roth, E. and Függer, R. (1999) Attenuation of catecholamine-induced immunosuppression in whole blood from patients with sepsis. *Shock* 12: 421–7.

Berkow, R. L. and Dodson, R. W. (1987) Functional analysis of the marginating pool of human polymorphonuclear leukocytes. *American Journal of Hematology* 24: 47–54.

Bermon, S. (2007) Airway inflammation and upper respiratory tract infection in athletes: is there a link? *Exercise Immunology Review* 13: 6–14.

Besedovsky, L., Lange, T. and Born, J. (2012) Sleep and immune function. *European Journal of Physiology* 463: 121–37.

Beutler, B. and Rietschel, E. T. (2003) Innate immune sensing and its roots: the story of endotoxin. *Nature Reviews Immunology* 3: 169–76.

Beziat, V., Descours, B., Parizot, C., Debre, P. and Vieillard, V. (2010) NK cell terminal differentiation: correlated stepwise decrease of NKG2A and acquisition of KIRs. *PLoS One* 5: e11966.

Bieger, W. P., Weiss, M., Michel, G. and Weicker, H. (1980) Exercise-induced monocytosis and modulation of monocyte function. *International Journal of Sports Medicine* 1: 30–6.

Bigley, A. B., Lowder, T. W., Spielmann, G., Rector, J. L., Pircher, H., Woods, J. A. and Simpson, R. J. (2012) NK-cells have an impaired response to acute exercise and a lower expression of the inhibitory receptors KLRG1 and CD158a in humans with latent cytomegalovirus infection. *Brain, Behavior and Immunity* 26: 177–86.

Biselli, R., Le Moli, S., Matricardi, P. M., Farrace, S., Fattorossi, A., Nisini, R. and D'Amelio, R. (1991) The effects of hypobaric hypoxia on specific B cell responses following immunization in mice and humans. *Aviation, Space, and Environmental Medicine* 62: 870–4.

Bishop, N. C. (2012) Overcoming microbial hurdles: keeping the Olympics infection-free. *Future Microbiology* 7: 913–15.

Bishop, N. C. and Gleeson, M. (2009) Acute and chronic effects of exercise on markers of mucosal immunity. *Frontiers in Bioscience* 14: 4444–56.

Bishop, N. C., Blannin, A. K., Robson, P. J., Walsh, N. P. and Gleeson, M. (1999a) The effects of carbohydrate supplementation on immune responses to a soccer-specific exercise protocol. *Journal of Sports Sciences* 17: 787–96.

Bishop, N. C., Blannin, A. K., Walsh, N. P., Robson, P. J. and Gleeson, M. (1999b) Nutritional aspects of immunosuppression in athletes. *Sports Medicine* 28: 151–76.

Bishop, N. C., Blannin, A. K., Armstrong, E., Rickman, M. and Gleeson, M. (2000a) Carbohydrate and fluid intake affect the saliva flow rate and IgA response to cycling. *Medicine and Science in Sports and Exercise* 32: 2046–51.

Bishop, N. C., Blannin, A. K., Rand, R., Johnson, R. and Gleeson, M. (2000b) Effects of carbohydrate supplementation on the blood neutrophil degranulation responses to prolonged cycling. *International Journal of Sport Medicine* 21(Suppl 1): S73.

Bishop, N. C., Blannin, A. K., Walsh, N. P. and Gleeson, M. (2001a) Carbohydrate beverage ingestion and neutrophil degranulation responses following cycling to fatigue at 75% $\dot{V}O_2$ max. *International Journal of Sport Medicine* 22: 226–31.

Bishop, N. C., Walsh, N. P., Haines, D. L., Richards, E. E. and Gleeson, M. (2001b) Pre-exercise carbohydrate status and immune responses to prolonged cycling: II. Effect on plasma cytokine concentration. *International Journal of Sports Nutrition* 11: 503–12.

Bishop, N. C., Gleeson, M., Nicholas, C. W. and Ali, A. (2002) Influence of carbohydrate supplementation on plasma cytokine and neutrophil degranulation responses to high intensity intermittent exercise. *International Journal of Sport Nutrition and Exercise Metabolism* 12: 145–56.

Bishop, N.C., Walsh, N.P. and Scanlon, G.A. (2003) Effect of prolonged exercise and carbohydrate on total neutrophil elastase content. *Medicine and Science in Sports and Exercise* 35: 1326–1332.

Bishop, N. C., Scanlon, G. A., Walsh, N. P., McCallum, L. J. and Walker, G. J. (2004) No effect of fluid intake on neutrophil responses to prolonged cycling. *Journal of Sports Sciences* 22: 1091–8.

Bishop, N. C., Fitzgerald, C., Porter, P. J., Scanlon, G. A. and Smith, A. C. (2005a) Effect of caffeine ingestion on lymphocyte counts and subset activation in vivo following strenuous cycling. *European Journal of Applied Physiology* 93: 606–13.

Bishop, N. C., Walker, G. J., Bowley, L. A., Evans, K. F., Molyneux, K., Wallace, F. A. and Smith, A. C. (2005b) Lymphocyte responses to influenza and tetanus toxoid in vitro following intensive exercise and carbohydrate ingestion on consecutive days. *Journal of Applied Physiology* 99: 1327–35.

Bishop, N. C., Walker, G. J., Scanlon, G. A., Richards, S. and Rogers, E. (2006) Salivary IgA responses to prolonged intensive exercise following caffeine ingestion. *Medicine and Science in Sports and Exercise* 38: 513–19.

Bishop, N. C., Walker, G. J., Gleeson, M., Wallace, F. A. and Hewitt, C. R. A. (2009) Human T lymphocyte migration towards the supernatants of human rhinovirus infected airway epithelial cells: influence of exercise and carbohydrate intake. *Exercise Immunology Review* 15: 42–59.

Blannin, A.K., Chatwin, L.J., Cave, R. and Gleeson, M. (1996a) Effects of submaximal cycling and endurance training on neutrophil phagocytic activity in middle–aged men. *British Journal of Sports Medicine* 39: 125–9.

Blannin, A. K., Gleeson, M., Brooks, S. and Cave, R. (1996b) Acute effect of exercise on human neutrophil degranulation. *Journal of Physiology* 495: 140P.

Blannin, A. K., Gleeson, M., Cobbold, M., Brooks, S. and Cave, R. (1997) Elastase release from neutrophils in relation to total cellular elastase content. *Journal of Sports Sciences* 15: 37–8.

Blannin, A. K., Robson, P. J., Walsh, N. P., Clark, A. M., Glennon, L. and Gleeson, M. (1998) The effect of exercising to exhaustion at different intensities on saliva immunoglobulin A, protein and electrolyte secretion. *International Journal of Sport Medicine* 19: 547–52.

Bonini, M., Braido, F., Baiardini, I., Del, G. S., Gramiccioni, C., Manara, M., Tagliapietra, G., Scardigno, A., Sargentini, V., Brozzi, M., Rasi, G. and Bonini, S. (2009) AQUA: Allergy Questionnaire for Athletes. Development and validation. *Medicine and Science in Sports and Exercise* 41: 1034–41.

Boonstra, A., Asselin-Paturel, C., Gilliet, M., Crain, C., Trinchieri, G., Liu, Y. J. and O'Garra, A. (2003) Flexibility of mouse classical and plasmacytoid-derived DCs in directing T helper type 1 and 2 cell development: dependency on antigen dose and differential toll-like receptor ligation. *Journal of Experimental Medicine* 197: 101–9.

Booth, C. K., Coad, R. A., Forbes-Ewan, C. H., Thomson, G. F. and Niro, P. J. (2003) The physiological and psychological effects of combat ration feeding during a 12-day training exercise in the tropics. *Military Medicine* 168: 63–70.

Booth, S., Florida-James, G. D., McFarlin, B. K., Spielmann, G., O'Connor, D. P. and Simpson, R. J. (2010) The impact of acute strenuous exercise on TLR2, TLR4 and HLA.DR expression on human blood monocytes induced by autologous serum. *European Journal of Applied Physiology* 110: 1259–68.

Borchers, A. T., Selmi, C., Meyers, F. J., Keen, C. L. and Gershwin, M. E. (2009) Probiotics and immunity. *Journal of Gastroenterology* 44: 26–46.

Bosanská, L., Michalský, D., Lacinová, Z., Dostálová, I., Bártlová, M., Haluzíková, D., Matoulek, M., Kasalický, M. and Haluzík, M. (2010) The influence of obesity and different fat depots on adipose tissue gene expression and protein levels of cell adhesion molecules. *Physiological Research* 59: 79–88.

Bosch, J. A., Berntson, G. G., Cacioppo, J. T., Dhabhar, F. S. and Marucha, P. T. (2003) Acute stress evokes selective mobilization of T cells that differ in chemokine receptor expression: a potential pathway linking immunologic reactivity to cardiovascular disease. *Brain, Behavior and Immunity* 17: 251–9.

Bosch, J. A., Berntson, G. G., Cacioppo, J. T. and Marucha, P. T. (2005) Differential mobilization of functionally distinct natural killer subsets during acute psychologic stress. *Psychosomatic Medicine* 67: 366–75.

Bosch, J. A., Ring, C., De Geus, E. J. C., Veerman, E. C. I. and Nieuw Amerongen, A. V. (2002) Stress and secretory immunity. *International Review of Neurobiology* 52: 213–53.

Bosenberg, A. T., Brock-Utne, J. G., Gaffin, S. L., Wells, M. T. and Blake, G. T. (1988) Strenuous exercise causes systemic endotoxemia. *Journal of Applied Physiology* 65: 106–8.

Bouchama, A., Parhar, R. S., el-Yazigi, A., Sheth, K. and al-Sedairy, S. (1991) Endotoxemia and release of tumor necrosis factor and interleukin 1 alpha in acute heatstroke. *Journal of Applied Physiology* 70: 2640–4.

Bousquet, J., Van, C. P. and Khaltaev, N. (2001) Allergic rhinitis and its impact on asthma. *Journal of Allergy and Clinical Immunology* 108(Suppl 5): S147–S334.

Bousquet, J., Khaltaev, N., Cruz, A. A., Denburg, J., Fokkens, W. J., Togias, A., Zuberbier, T., Baena-Cagnani, C. E., Canonica, G. W., van Weel, C., Agache, I., Aït-Khaled, N., Bachert, C., Blaiss, M. S., Bonini, S., Boulet, L. P., Bousquet, P. J., Camargos, P., Carlsen, K. H., Chen, Y., Custovic, A., Dahl, R., Demoly, P., Douagui, H., Durham, S. R., van Wijk, R. G., Kalayci, O., Kaliner, M. A., Kim, Y. Y., Kowalski, M. L., Kuna, P., Le, L. T., Lemiere, C., Li, J., Lockey, R. F., Mavale-Manuel, S., Meltzer, E. O., Mohammad, Y., Mullol, J., Naclerio, R., O'Hehir, R. E., Ohta, K., Ouedraogo, S., Palkonen, S., Papadopoulos, N., Passalacqua, G., Pawankar, R., Popov, T. A., Rabe, K. F., Rosado-Pinto, J., Scadding, G. K., Simons, F. E., Toskala, E., Valovirta, E., van Cauwenberge, P., Wang, D. Y., Wickman, M., Yawn, B. P., Yorgancioglu, A., Yusuf, O. M., Zar, H., Annesi-Maesano, I., Bateman, E. D., Ben Kheder, A., Boakye, D. A., Bouchard, J., Burney, P., Busse, W.W., Chan-Yeung, M., Chavannes, N. H., Chuchalin, A., Dolen, W. K., Emuzyte, R., Grouse, L., Humbert, M., Jackson, C., Johnston, S. L., Keith, P. K., Kemp, J. P., Klossek, J. M., Larenas-Linnemann, D., Lipworth, B., Malo, J. L., Marshall, G. D., Naspitz, C., Nekam, K., Niggemann, B., Nizankowska-Mogilnicka, E., Okamoto, Y., Orru, M. P., Potter, P., Price, D., Stoloff, S. W., Vandenplas, O., Viegi, G., Williams, D.; World Health Organization; GA(2)LEN; AllerGen. (2008) Allergic Rhinitis and its Impact on Asthma (ARIA) 2008 update (in collaboration with the World Health Organization, GA(2)LEN and AllerGen). *Allergy* 63(Suppl 86): 8–160.

Brandtzaeg, P. (1996) History of oral tolerance and mucosal immunity. *Annals of the New York Academy of Sciences* 778: 1–27.

Brannigan, D., Rogers, I. R., Jacobs, I., Montgomery, A., Williams, A. and Khangure, N. (2009) Hypothermia is a significant medical risk of mass participation long-distance open water swimming. *Wilderness and Environmental Medicine* 20: 14–18.

Brenner, I. K., Castellani, J. W., Gabaree, C., Young, A. J., Zamecnik, J., Shephard, R. J. and Shek, P. N. (1999) Immune changes in humans during cold exposure: effects of prior heating and exercise. *Journal of Applied Physiology* 87: 699–710.

Bridge, C. A. and Jones, M. A. (2006) The effect of caffeine ingestion on 8 km run performance in a field setting. *Journal of Sports Sciences* 24: 433–9.

Brown, G. D. and Gordon, S. (2003) Fungal beta-glucans and mammalian immunity. *Immunity* 19: 311–15.

Brunekreef, B., Hoek, G., Breugelmans, O. and Leentvaar, M. (1994) Respiratory effects of low–level photochemical air pollution in amateur cyclists. *American Journal of Respiratory and Critical Care Medicine* 150: 962–6.

Bruun, J. M., Lihn, A. S., Pedersen, S. B. and Richelsen, B. (2005) Monocyte chemoat-tractant protein-1 release is higher in visceral than subcutaneous human adipose tissue (AT): implication of macrophages resident in the AT. *The Journal of Clinical Endocrinology and Metabolism* 90: 2282–9.

Bruunsgaard H and Pedersen BK (2000) Special feature for the Olympics: effects of exercise on the immune system in the elderly population. *Immunology and Cell Biology* 78: 523–31.

Bruunsgaard, H., Galbo, H., Halkjaer-Kristensen, J., Johansen, T. L., MacLean, D. A. and Pedersen, B. K. (1997a) Exercise-induced increase in serum interleukin-6 in humans is related to muscle damage. *Journal of Physiology* 499: 833–41.

Bruunsgaard, H., Hartkopp, A., Mohr, T., Konradsen, H., Heron, I., Mordhorst, C. H. and Pedersen, B. K. (1997b) In vivo cell-mediated immunity and vaccination response following prolonged, intense exercise. *Medicine and Science in Sports and Exercise* 29: 1176–81.

Bruunsgaard, H., Jensen, M. S., Scheling, P., Halkjaer-Kristensen, J., Ogawa, K., Skinhoj, P. and Pedersen, B. K. (1999) Exercise induces recruitment of lymphocytes with an activated phenotype and short telomeres in young and elderly humans. *Life Sciences* 35: 2623–33.

Budgett, R. (1990) Overtraining syndrome. *British Journal of Sports Medicine* 24: 231–6.

Budgett, R., Newsholme, E., Lehmann, M., Sharp, C., Jones, D., Peto, T., Collins, D., Nerurkar, R. and White, P. (2000) Redefining the overtraining syndrome as the unexplained underperformance syndrome. *British Journal of Sports Medicine* 34: 67–8.

Bulati, M., Buffa, S., Candore, G., Caruso, C., Dunn-Walters, D. K., Pellicano, M., Wu, Y. C. and Colonna Romano, G. (2011) B cells and immunosenescence: a focus on IgG+IgD–CD27– (DN) B cells in aged humans. *Ageing Research Reviews* 10: 274–84.

Burke, L. M., Hawley, J. A., Wong, S. H. and Jeukendrup, A. E. (2011) Carbohydrates for training and competition. *Journal of Sports Sciences* 29: S17–S27.

Burns, V. E. Using vaccinations to assess in vivo immune function in psychoneuroim-munology. *Methods in Molecular Biology* 934: 371–81.

Burrows, M., Bird, S. R. and Bishop, N. C. (2002) The menstrual cycle and its effect on the immune status of female endurance runners. *Journal of Sports Science* 20: 339–44.

Bury, T., Marechal, R., Mahieu, P. and Pirnay, F. (1998) Immunological status of competitive football players during the training season. *International Journal of Sports Medicine* 19: 364–8.

Butcher, S.K., Chahal, H., Nayak, L., Sinclair, A., Henriquez, N. V., Sapey, E., O'Mahony, D. and Lord, J. M. (2001) Senescence in innate immune responses: reduced neutrophil phagocytic capacity and CD16 expression in elderly humans. *Journal of Leukocyte Biology* 70: 881–6.

Butler, J., O'Brien, M., O'Malley, K. and Kelly, J. G. (1982) Relationship of beta-adrenore-ceptor density to fitness in athletes. *Nature* 298: 60–2.

Büttner, P., Mosig, S., Lechtermann, A., Funke, H. and Mooren, F. C. (2007) Exercise affects the gene expression profiles of human white blood cells. *Journal of Applied Physiology* 102: 26–36.

Byrne, C., Lee, J. K., Chew, S. A., Lim, C. L. and Tan, E. Y. (2006) Continuous thermoregulatory responses to mass participation distance running in heat. *Medicine and Science in Sports and Exercise* 38: 803–10.

Calabria, C. W., Dietrich, J. and Hagan, L. (2009) Comparison of serum-specific IgE (ImmunoCAP) and skin-prick test results for 53 inhalant allergens in patients with chronic rhinitis, *Allergy and asthma proceedings* 30: 386–96.

Calder, P. C. (2011) Fatty acids and inflammation: the cutting edge between food and pharma. *European Journal of Pharmacology* 668: S50–8.

Calder, P. C. and Kew, S. (2002) The immune system: a target for functional foods? *British Journal of Nutrition* 88(Suppl 2): S165–77.

Campbell, J. P., Guy, K., Cosgrove, C., Florida-James, G. D. and Simpson, R. J. (2008) Total lymphocyte CD8 expression is not a reliable marker of cytotoxic T-cell populations in human peripheral blood following an acute bout of high-intensity exercise. *Brain, Behavior and Immunity* 22: 375–80.

Campbell, J. P., Riddell, N. E., Burns, V. E., Turner, M., van Zanten, J. J., Drayson, M. T. and Bosch, J. A. (2009) Acute exercise mobilises CD8+ T lymphocytes exhibiting an effector-memory phenotype. *Brain, Behavior and Immunity* 23: 767–75.

Campbell, P. T., Wener, M. H., Sorensen, B., Wood, B., Chen-Levy, Z., Potter, J. D., McTiernan, A. and Ulrich, C. M. (2008) Effect of exercise on in vitro immune function: a 12-month randomized, controlled trial among postmenopausal women. *Journal of Applied Physiology* 104: 1648–55.

Camus, G., Pincemail, J., Ledent, M., Juchmès-Ferir, A., Lamy, M., Deby-Dupont, G. and Deby, C. (1992) Plasma levels of polymorphonuclear elastase and myeloperoxidase after uphill walking and downhill running at similar energy cost. *International Journal of Sports Medicine* 13: 443–6.

Camus, G., Duchateau, J., Deby-Dupont, G., Pincemail, J., Deby, C., Juchmès-Ferir, A., Feron, F. and Lamy, M. (1994) Anaphylatoxin C5a production during short-term submaximal dynamic exercise in man. *International Journal of Sports Medicine* 15: 32–35.

Cannon, J. G., Fiatarone, M. A., Fielding, R. A. and Evans, W. J. (1994) Aging and stress-induced changes in complement activation and neutrophil mobilization. *Journal of Applied Physiology* 76: 2616–20.

Capuron, L. and Miller, A. H. (2011) Immune system to brain signaling: neuropsychopharmacological implications. *Pharmacological Therapy* 130: 226–38.

Carins, J. and Booth, C. (2002) Salivary immunoglobulin-A as a marker of stress during strenuous physical training. *Aviation, Space and Environmental Medicine* 73: 1203–7.

Carlisle, A. J. and Sharp, N. C. (2001) Exercise and outdoor ambient air pollution. *British Journal of Sports Medicine* 35: 214–22.

Carpenter, G. H., Proctor, G. B., Ebersole, L. E. and Garrett, J. R. (2004) Secretion of IgA by rat parotid and submandibular cells in response to autonomimetic stimulation in vitro. *International Immunopharmacology* 4: 1005–14.

Castell, L. M. and Newsholme, E. A. (1998) Glutamine and the effects of exhaustive exercise upon the immune response. *Canadian Journal of Physiology and Pharmacology* 76: 524–32.

Castell, L. M., Poortmans, J. R. and Newsholme, E. A. (1996) Does glutamine have a role in reducing infections in athletes? *European Journal of Applied Physiology* 73: 488–90.

Castellani, J. W., Young, A. J., Ducharme, M. B., Giesbrecht, G. G., Glickman, E. and Sallis,

R. E. (2006) American College of Sports Medicine position stand: prevention of cold injuries during exercise. *Medicine and Science in Sports and Exercise* 38: 2012–29.

Ceddia, M. A. and Woods, J. A. (1999) Exercise suppresses macrophage antigen presentation. *Journal of Applied Physiology* 87: 2253–8.

Ceddia, M. A., Price, E. A., Kohlmeier, C. K., Evans, J. K., Lu, Q., McAuley, E. and Woods, J. A. (1999) Differential leukocytosis and lymphocyte mitogenic response to acute maximal exercise in the young and old. *Medicine and Science in Sports and Exercise* 31: 829–36.

Ceddia, M. A., Voss, E. W. Jr., and Woods, J. A. (2000) Intracellular mechanisms responsible for exercise-induced suppression of macrophage antigen presentation. *Journal of Applied Physiology* 88: 804–10.

Cerwenka, A. and Lanier, L. L. (2001) Natural killer cells, viruses and cancer. *Nature Reviews Immunology* 1: 41–9.

Chan, M. H. S., Carey, A. L., Watt, M. J. and Febbraio, M. A. (2004) Cytokine gene expression in human skeletal muscle during concentric contraction: evidence that IL-8, like IL-6, is influenced by glycogen availability. *American Journal of Physiology: Regulatory, Integrative and Comparative Physiology* 287: R322–7.

Chandra, R. K. (1984) Excessive intake of zinc impairs immune responses. *Journal of the American Medical Association* 252: 1443–6.

Chen, K. and Cherutti, C. (2011) The function and regulation of immunoglobulin D. *Current Opinion in Immunology* 23: 1–8.

Chiang, L. M., Chen, Y. J., Chiang, J., Lai, L. Y., Chen, Y. Y. and Liao, H. F. (2007) Modulation of dendritic cells by endurance training. *International Journal of Sports Medicine* 28: 798–803.

Chikanza, I. C. (1999) Prolactin and neuroimmunomodulation: in vitro and in vivo observations. *Annals of the New York Academy of Sciences* 876: 119–30.

Chinda, D., Nakaji, S., Umeda, T., Shimoyama, T., Kurakake, S., Okamura, N., Kumae, T. and Sugawara, K. (2003) A competitive marathon race decreases neutrophil functions in athletes. *Luminescence* 18: 324–9.

Chiu, W. T., Kao, T. Y. and Lin, M. T. (1996) Increased survival in experimental rat heatstroke by continuous perfusion of interleukin-1 receptor antagonist. *Neuroscience Research* 24: 159–63.

Chouker, A., Demetz, F., Martignoni, A., Smith, L., Setzer, F., Bauer, A., Holzl, J. Peter, K., Christ, F. and Thiel, M. (2005) Strenuous physical exercise inhibits granulocyte activation induced by high altitude. *Journal of Applied Physiology* 98: 640–7.

Chow, F. Y., Nikolic-Paterson, D. J., Ozols, E., Atkins, R. C. and Tesch, G. H. (2005) Intercellular adhesion molecule-1 deficiency is protective against nephropathy in type 2 diabetic db/db mice. *Journal of the American Society of Nephrology* 16: 1711–22.

Christ, F. and Thiel, M. (2005) Strenuous physical exercise inhibits granulocyte activation induced by high altitude. *Journal of Applied Physiology* 98: 640–7.

Chubak, J., McTiernan, A., Sorensen, B., Wener, M. H., Yasui, Y., Velasquez, M., Wood, B., Rajan, K. B., Wetmore, C. M., Potter, J. D. and Ulrich, C. M. (2006) Moderate-intensity exercise reduces the incidence of colds among postmenopausal women. *American Journal of Medicine* 119: 937–42.

Clancy, R. L., Gleeson, M., Cox, A., Callister, R., Dorrington, M., D'Este, C., Pang, G., Pyne, D., Fricker, P. and Henriksson, A. (2006) Reversal in fatigued athletes of a defect in interferon gamma secretion after administration of Lactobacillus acidophilus. *British Journal of Sports Medicine* 40: 351–4.

Cohen, G., HaagWeber, M. and Hörl, W. H. (1997) Immune dysfunction in uremia. *Kidney International* Suppl 62: S79–S82.

Cohen, S. (2005) Keynote Presentation at the Eight International Congress of Behavioral Medicine: the Pittsburgh common cold studies: psychosocial predictors of susceptibility to respiratory infectious illness. *International Journal of Behavioral Medicine* 12: 123–31.

Cohen, S., Doyle, W. J., Alper, C. M., Janicki-Deverts, D. and Turner, R. B. (2009) Sleep habits and susceptibility to the common cold. *Archives of Internal Medicine* 169: 62–7.

Connolly, P. H., Caiozzo, V. J., Zaldivar, F., Nemet, D., Larson, J., Hung, S. P., Heck, J. D., Hatfield, G. W. and Cooper, D. M. (2004) Effects of exercise on gene expression in human peripheral blood mononuclear cells. *Journal of Applied Physiology* 97: 1461–9.

Cosgrove, C., Galloway, S. D., Neal, C., Hunter, A. M., McFarlin, B. K., Spielmann, G. and Simpson, R. J. (2012) The impact of 6-month training preparation for an Ironman triathlon on the proportions of naive, memory and senescent T cells in resting blood. *European Journal of Applied Physiology* 112: 2989–98.

Costa, R. J., Oliver, S. J., Laing, S. J., Waiters, R., Bilzon, J. L. and Walsh, N. P. (2009) Influence of timing of postexercise carbohydrate–protein ingestion on selected immune indices. *International Journal of Sport Nutrition and Exercise Metabolism* 19: 366–84.

Costa, R. J., Smith, A. H., Oliver, S. J., Walters, R., Maassen, N., Bilzon, J. L. and Walsh, N. P. (2010) The effects of two nights of sleep deprivation with or without energy restriction on immune indices at rest and in response to cold exposure. *European Journal of Applied Physiology* 109: 417–28.

Costa, R. J., Fortes, M. B., Richardson, K., Bilzon, J. L. and Walsh, N. P. (2012) The effects of postexercise feeding on saliva antimicrobial proteins. *International Journal of Sport Nutrition and Exercise Metabolism* 22: 184–91.

Cox, A. J., Gleeson, M., Pyne, D. B., Saunders, P. U., Clancy, R. . and Fricker P. A. (2004) Valtrex therapy for Epstein-Barr virus reactivation and upper respiratory symptoms in elite runners. *Medicine and Science in Sports and Exercise* 36: 1104–10.

Cox, A. J., Pyne, D. B., Saunders, P. U., Callister, R. and Gleeson, M. (2007) Cytokine responses to treadmill running in healthy and illness-prone athletes. *Medicine and Science in Sports and Exercise* 9: 1918–26.

Cox, A. J., Gleeson, M., Pyne, D. B., Callister, R., Hopkins, W. G. and Fricker, P. A. (2008) Clinical and laboratory evaluation of upper respiratory symptoms in elite athletes. *Clinical Journal of Sports Medicine* 18: 438–45.

Cox, A. J., Gleeson, M., Pyne, D. B., Callister, R., Fricker, P. A. and Scott, R. J. (2010a) Cytokine gene polymorphisms and risk for upper respiratory symptoms in highly-trained athletes. *Exercise Immunology Review* 16: 8–21.

Cox, A. J., Gleeson, M., Pyne, D. B., Saunders, P. U., Callister, R. and Fricker, P. A. (2010b) Respiratory symptoms and inflammatory responses to Difflam throat-spray intervention in half-marathon runners: a randomised controlled trial. *British Journal of Sports Medicine* 44: 127–33.

Cox, A. J., Pyne, D. B., Saunders, P. U. and Fricker, P. A. (2010c) Oral administration of the probiotic Lactobacillus fermentum VRI–003 and mucosal immunity in endurance athletes. *British Journal of Sports Medicine* 44: 222–6.

Croisier, J. L., Camus, G., Venneman, I., Deby-Dupont, G., Juchmès-Ferir, A., Lamy, M., Crielaard, J. M., Deby, C. and Duchateau, J. (1999) Effects of training on exercise-induced muscle damage and interleukin 6 production. *Muscle and Nerve* 22: 208–12.

Crooks, C. V., Wall, C. R., Cross, M. L. and Rutherfurd-Markwick, K. J. (2006) The effect of bovine colostrum supplementation on salivary IgA in distance runners. *International Journal of Sport Nutrition and Exercise Metabolism* 16: 47–64.

Cross, M. C., Radomski, M. W., VanHelder, W. P., Rhind, S. G. and Shephard, R. J. (1996) Endurance exercise with and without a thermal clamp: effects on leukocytes and leukocyte subsets. *Journal of Applied Physiology* 81: 822–9.

Crucian, B., Stowe, R., Quiriarte, H., Pierson, D. and Sams, C. (2011) Monocyte phenotype and cytokine production profiles are dysregulated by short-duration spaceflight. *Aviation, Space, and Environmental Medicine* 82: 857–62.

Crystal-Peters, J., Neslusan, C., Crown, W. H. and Torres, A. (2002) Treating allergic rhinitis in patients with comorbid asthma: the risk of asthma-related hospitalizations and emergency department visits. *Journal of Allergy and Clinical Immunology* 109: 57–62.

Cunniffe, B., Griffiths, H., Proctor, W., Davies, B., Baker, J. S. and Jones, K.P. (2011) Mucosal immunity and illness incidence in elite rugby union players across a season. *Medicine and Science in Sports and Exercise* 43: 388–97.

Cupps, T. R. and Fauci, A. S. (1982) Corticosteroid-mediated immunoregulation in man. *Immunology Review* 65: 133–55.

Curwen, M. (1997) Excess winter mortality in England and Wales with special reference to the effects of temperature and influenza. In: *The Health of Adult Britain 1841–1994*, (edited by J. Charlton and M. Murphy). London: The Stationery Office. Vol. 1, pp. 205–16.

Custovic, A., Simpson, A., Chapman, M. D. and Woodcock, A. (1998) Allergen avoidance in the treatment of asthma and atopic disorders. *Thorax* 53: 63–72.

Daly, J. M., Reynolds, J., Sigal, R. K., Shou, J. and Liberman, M. D. (1990) Effect of dietary protein and amino acids on immune function. *Critical Care Medicine* 18: S86–S93.

Dantzer, R., O'Connor, J. C., Freund, G. G., Johnson, R. W. and Kelley, K. W. (2008) From inflammation to sickness and depression: when the immune system subjugates the brain. *Nature Reviews Neuroscience* 9: 46–56.

Davis, J. M., Kohut, M. L., Colbert, L. H., Jackson, D. A., Ghaffar, A. and Mayer, E. P. (1997) Exercise, alveolar macrophage function, and susceptibility to respiratory infection. *Journal of Applied Physiology* 83: 1461–6.

Davis, J. M., Kohut, M. L., Jackson, D. A., Colbert, L. H., Mayer, E. P. and Ghaffar, A. (1998) Exercise effects on lung tumor metastases and in vitro alveolar macrophage antitumor cytotoxicity. *American Journal of Physiology* 274: R1454–9.

Davis, J. M., Murphy, E. A., Brown, A. S., Carmichael, M. D., Ghaffar, A. and Mayer, E. P. (2004) Effects of oat beta-glucan on innate immunity and infection after exercise stress. *Medicine and Science in Sports and Exercise* 36: 1321–7.

Davis, J. M., Murphy, E. A., McClellan, J. L., Carmichael, M. D. and Gangemi, J. D. (2008) Quercetin reduces susceptibility to influenza infection following stressful exercise. *American Journal of Physiology: Regulatory, Integrative and Comparative Physiology* 295: R505–9.

Davison, G. (2011) Innate immune responses to a single session of sprint interval training. *Applied Physiology, Nutrition and Metabolism* 36: 395–404.

Davison, G. and Diment, B. C. (2010) Bovine colostrum supplementation attenuates the decrease of salivary lysozyme and enhances the recovery of neutrophil function after prolonged exercise. *British Journal of Nutrition* 103: 1425–32.

Davison, G. and Gleeson, M. (2005) Influence of acute vitamin C and/or carbohydrate ingestion on hormonal, cytokine, and immune responses to prolonged exercise. *International Journal of Sport Nutrition and Exercise Metabolism* 15: 465–79.

Davison, G. and Gleeson, M. (2006) The effect of 2 weeks vitamin C supplementation on immunoendocrine responses to 2.5 h cycling exercise in man. *European Journal of Applied Physiology* 97: 454–61.

Davison, G., Gleeson, M, and Phillips, S. (2007) Antioxidant supplementation and immunoendocrine responses to prolonged exercise. *Medicine and Science in Sports and Exercise* 39: 645–52.

de Gonzalo-Calvo, D., Fernandez-Garcia, B., de Luxan-Delgado, B., Rodriguez-Gonzalez, S., Garcia-Macia, M., Suarez, F. M., Solano, J. J., Rodriguez-Colunga, M. J. and Coto-Montes, A. (2011) Long-term training induces a healthy inflammatory and endocrine emergent biomarker profile in elderly men. *Age* 34: 761–71.

Derhovanessian, E., Maier, A. B., Hahnel, K., Beck, R., de Craen, A. J., Slagboom, E. P., Westendorp, R. G. and Pawelec, G. (2011) Infection with cytomegalovirus but not herpes simplex virus induces the accumulation of late-differentiated CD4+ and CD8+ T-cells in humans. *Journal of General Virology* 92: 2746–56.

DeVivo, M. J., Krause, J. S. and Lammertse, D. P. (1999) Recent trends in mortality and causes of death among persons with spinal cord injury. *Archives of Physical and Medical Rehabilitation* 80: 1411–19.

Devlin, R. B., McDonnell, W. F., Mann, R., Becker, S., House, D. E., Schreinemachers, D. and Koren, H. S. (1991) Exposure of humans to ambient levels of ozone for 6.6 hours causes cellular and biochemical changes in the lung. *American Journal of Respiratory Cell and Molecular Biology* 4: 72–81.

Devlin, R. B., McDonnell, W. F., Becker, S., Madden, M. C., McGee, M. P., Perez, R., Hatch, G., House, D. E. and Koren, H. S. (1996) Time-dependent changes of inflammatory mediators in the lungs of humans exposed to 0.4 ppm ozone for 2 hr: a comparison of mediators found in bronchoalveolar lavage fluid 1 and 18 hr after exposure. *Toxicology and Applied Pharmacology* 138: 176–85.

Dhabhar, F. S. (2009) Enhancing versus suppressive effects of stress on immune function: implications for immunoprotection and immunopathology. *Neuroimmunomodulation* 16: 300–17.

Diehl, S. and Rincón, M. (2002) The two faces of IL-6 on Th1/Th2 differentiation. *Molecular Immunolunology* 39: 531–6.

Dienz, O. and Rincon, M. (2009) The effects of IL-6 on CD4 T cell responses. *Clinical Immunology* 130: 27–33.

Dijkstra, H. P. and Robson-Ansley, P. (2011) The prevalence and current opinion of treatment of allergic rhinitis in elite athletes. *Current Opinion in Allergy and Clinical Immunology* 11: 103–8.

Diment, B. C., Fortes, M. B., Greeves, J. P., Casey, A., Costa, R. J., Walters, R. and Walsh, N. P. (2012) Effect of daily mixed nutritional supplementation on immune indices in soldiers undertaking an 8-week arduous training programme. *European Journal of Applied Physiology* 112: 1411–18.

Dimitrov, S., Benedict, C., Heutling, D., Westermann, J., Born, J. and Lange, T. (2009) Cortisol and epinephrine control opposing circadian rhythms in T cell subsets. *Blood* 113: 5134–43.

Dimitrov, S., Lange, T. and Born, J. (2010) Selective mobilization of cytotoxic leukocytes by epinephrine. *Journal of Immunology* 184: 503–11.

DiPenta, J. M., Green-Johnson, J. M., Murphy, R. J. (2007) Type 2 diabetes mellitus, resistance training, and innate immunity: is there a common link? *Applied Physiology Nutrition and Metabolism* 32: 1025–35.

Douglas, R. M., Hemila, H., Chalker, E. and Treacy, B. (2007) Vitamin C for preventing and treating the common cold. *Cochrane Database of Systematic Reviews* CD000980.

Downing, J. F. and Taylor, M. W. (1987) The effect of in vivo hyperthermia on selected lymphokines in man. *Lymphokine Research* 6: 103–9.

Downing, J. F., Martinez-Valdez, H., Elizondo, R. S., Walker, E. B. and Taylor, M. W. (1988) Hyperthermia in humans enhances interferon-gamma synthesis and alters the peripheral lymphocyte population. *Journal of Interferon Research* 8: 143–50.

Duchmann, R., Neurath, M. F. and Meyer zum Buschenfelde, K. H. (1997) Responses to self and non-self intestinal microflora in health and inflammatory bowel disease. *Research in Immunology* 148: 589–94.

Duclos, M., Gouarne, C. and Bonnemaison, D. (2003) Acute and chronic effects of exercise on tissue sensitivity to glucocorticoids. *Journal of Applied Physiology* 94: 869–75.

Dufaux, B. and Order, U. (1989) Complement activation after prolonged exercise. *Clinica Chimica Acta* 179: 45–50.

Dufaux, B., Order, U. and Liesen, H. (1991) Effect of a short maximal physical exercise on coagulation, fibrinolysis and complement system. *International Journal of Sports Medicine* 12: S38–S42.

Dziedziak, W. (1990) The effect of incremental cycling on physiological functions of peripheral blood granulocytes. *Biology of Sport* 7: 239–47.

Eccles, R. (2002a) Acute cooling of the body surface and the common cold. *Rhinology* 40: 109–14.

Eccles, R. (2002b) An explanation for the seasonality of acute upper respiratory tract viral infections. *Acta Otolaryngology* 122: 183–91.

Edwards, A. J., Bacon, T. H., Elms, C. A., Verardi, R., Felder, M. and Knight, S. C. (1984) Changes in the populations of lymphoid cells in human peripheral blood following physical exercise. *Clinical Experimental Immunology* 58: 420–7.

Eichner, E. R. (1987) Infectious mononucleosis: Recognition and management in athletes. *Physician and Sportsmedicine* 15: 61–71.

Eichner, E. R. (1994) Overtraining: Consequences and prevention. *Journal of Sports Sciences* 13: S41–8.

Ekblom, B., Ekblom, O. and Malm, C. (2006) Infectious episodes before and after a marathon race. *Scandinavian Journal of Medicine and Science in Sports* 16: 287–93.

Eleftheriadis, T., Antoniadi, G., Liakopoulos, V., Kartsios, C. and Stefanidis, I. (2007) Disturbances of acquired immunity in hemodialysis patients. *Seminars in Dialysis* 20: 440–51.

Elenkov, I. J. and Chrousos, G. P. (2002) Stress hormones, proinflammatory and antiinflammatory cytokines, and autoimmunity. *Annals of the New York Academy of Sciences* 966: 290–303.

Eliassen, H. A., Hankinson, S. E., Rosner, B., Holmes, M. D. and Willet, W. C. (2010) Physical activity and risk of breast cancer among postmenopausal women. *Archives of Internal Medicine* 170: 1758–64.

Ely, B. R., Cheuvront, S. N., Kenefick, R. W. and Sawka, M. N. (2010) Aerobic performance is degraded, despite modest hyperthermia, in hot environments. *Medicine and Science in Sports and Exercise* 42: 135–41.

Engström, P. E., Norhagen, G., Osipova, L., Helal, A., Wiebe, V., Brusco, A., Carbonara, A. O., Lefranc, G. and Lefranc, M. P. (1996) Salivary IgG subclasses in individuals with and without homozygous IGHG gene deletions. *Immunology* 89: 178–82.

Eriksson, K. F. and Lindgärde, F. (1991) Prevention of type 2 (non-insulin-dependent) diabetes mellitus by diet and physical exercise. The 6-year Malmö feasibility study. *Diabetologia* 34: 891–8.

Evans, D. L., Charney, D. S., Lewis, L., Golden, R. N., Gorman, J. M., Krishnan, K. R., Nemeroff, C. B., Bremner, J. D., Carney, R. M., Coyne, J. C., Delong, M. R., Frasure-Smith, N., Glassman, A. H., Gold, P. W., Grant, I., Gwyther, L., Ironson, G., Johnson, R. L., Kanner, A. M., Katon, W. J., Kaufmann, P. G., Keefe, F. J., Ketter, T., Laughren, T. P., Leserman, J., Lyketsos, C. G., McDonald, W. M., McEwen, B. S., Miller, A. H., Musselman, D., O'Connor, C., Petitto, J. M., Pollock, B. G., Robinson, R. G., Roose, S. P., Rowland, J., Sheline, Y., Sheps, D. S., Simon, G., Spiegel, D., Stunkard, A., Sunderland, T., Tibbits, P. Jr. and Valvo, W. J. (2005) Mood disorders in the medically ill: scientific review and recommendations. *Biological Psychiatry* 58: 175–89.

Eyolfson, D. A., Tikuisis, P., Xu, X., Weseen, G. and Giesbrecht, G. G. (2001) Measurement and prediction of peak shivering intensity in humans. *European Journal of Applied Physiology* 84: 100–6.

Faas, M., Bouman, A., Moesa, H., Heineman, M. J., de Leij, L. and Schuiling, G. (2000) The immune response during the luteal phase of the ovarian cycle: a Th2-type response. *Fertility and Sterility* 74: 1008–13.

Fabbri, M., Smart, C. and Pardi, R. (2003) T lymphocytes. *The International Journal of Biochemistry and Cell Biology* 35: 1004–8

Facco, M., Zilli, C., Siviero, M., Ermolao, A., Travain, G., Baesso, I., Bonamico, S., Cabrelle, A., Zaccaria, M. and Agostini, C. (2005) Modulation of immune response by the acute and chronic exposure to high altitude. *Medicine and Science in Sports and Exercise* 37: 768–74.

Fahlman, M., Boardley, D., Flynn, M. G., Braun, W. A., Lambert, C. P. and Bouillon, L. E. (2000) Effects of endurance training on selected parameters of immune function in elderly women. *Gerontology* 46: 97–107.

Fahlman, M. M. and Engels, H. J. (2005) Mucosal IgA and URTI in American college football players: A year longitudinal study. *Medicine and Science in Sports and Exercise* 37: 374–80.

Fairey, A. S., Courneya, K. S., Field, C. J., Bell, G. J., Jones, L. W. and Mackey, J. R. (2005) Randomized controlled trial of exercise and blood immune function in postmenopausal breast cancer survivors. *Journal of Applied Physiology* 98: 1534–40.

Febbraio, M. A. (2001) Alterations in energy metabolism during exercise and heat stress. *Sports Medicine* 31: 47–59.

Febbraio, M. A. and Pedersen, B. K. (2002) Muscle–derived interleukin-6: mechanisms for activation and possible biological roles. *FASEB Journal* 16: 1335–47.

Febbraio, M. A., Hiscock, N., Sacchetti, M., Fischer, C. P. and Pedersen, B. K. (2004) Interleukin-6 is a novel factor mediating glucose homeostasis during skeletal muscle contraction. *Diabetes* 53: 1643–8.

Fehr, J. and Grossman, H. C. (1979) Disparity between circulating and marginated neutrophils: evidence from studies on the granulocyte alkaline phosphatase, a marker of cell maturity. *American Journal of Haematology* 7: 369–79.

Feldman, R. D., Limbird, L. E., Nadeau, J., Robertson, D. and Wood, A. J. (1984) Alterations in leukocyte beta-receptor affinity with aging. A potential explanation for altered beta-adrenergic sensitivity in the elderly. *New England Journal of Medicine* 310: 815–19.

Fernandez, M. A., Puttur, F. K., Wang, Y. M., Howden, W., Alexander, S. I. and Jones, C. A.

(2008) T regulatory cells contribute to the attenuated primary CD8+ and CD4+ T cell responses to herpes simplex virus type 2 in neonatal mice. *Journal of Immunology* 180: 1556–4.

Fiatarone, M. A., Morley, J. E., Bloom, E. T., Benton, D., Solomon, G. F. and Makinodan, T. (1989) The effect of exercise on natural killer cell activity in young and old subjects. *Journal of Gerontology* 44: M37–M45.

Field, C. J., Gougeon, R. and Marliss, E. B. (1991) Circulating mononuclear cell numbers and function during intense exercise and recovery. *Journal of Applied Physiology* 71: 1089–97.

Fingerle-Rowson, G., Angstwurm, M., Andreesen, R. and Ziegler-Heitbrock, H.W. (1998) Selective depletion of CD14+CD16+ monocytes by glucocorticoid therapy. *Clinical Experimental Immunology* 112: 501–6.

Fischer, C. P. (2006) Interleukin-6 in acute exercise and training: what is the biological relevance? *Exercise Immunology Review* 12: 6–33.

Fischer, C. P., Hiscock, N. J., Penkowa, M., Basu, S., Vessby, B., Kallner, A., Sjoberg, L. B. and Pedersen, B. K. (2004) Supplementation with vitamins C and E inhibits the release of interleukin-6 from contracting human skeletal muscle. *Journal of Physiology* 558: 633–45.

Fish, E. N. (2008) The X-files in immunity, sex-based differences pre-dispose immune responses. *Nature Reviews Immunology* 8: 737–44.

Fletcher, D. K. and Bishop, N. C. (2011) Effect of a high and low dose of caffeine on antigen-stimulated activation of human natural killer cells after prolonged cycling. *International Journal of Sport Nutrition and Exercise Metabolism* 21: 155–65.

Florida-James, G., Donaldson, K. and Stone, V. (2004) Athens 2004: the pollution climate and athletic performance. *Journal of Sports Sciences* 22: 967–80.

Flynn, M. G. and McFarlin, B. K. (2006) Toll-like receptor 4: link to the anti-inflammatory effects of exercise? *Exercise and Sport Sciences Reviews* 34: 176–81.

Flynn, M. G., Fahlman, M., Braun, W. A., Lambert, C. P., Bouillon, L. E., Brolinson, P. G. and Armstrong, C. W. (1999) Effects of resistance exercise training on selected indices of immune function in elderly women. *Journal of Applied Physiology* 86: 1905–13.

Flynn, M. G., McFarlin, B. K., Phillips, M. D., Stewart, L. K. and Timmerman, K. L. (2003) Toll-like receptor 4 and CD14 mRNA expression are lower in resistive exercise-trained elderly women. *Journal of Applied Physiology* 95: 1833–42.

Fortes, M. B., Diment, B. C., Di Felice, U., Gunn, A. E., Kendall, J. L., Esmaeelpour, M. and Walsh, N. P. (2011) Tear fluid osmolarity as a potential marker of hydration status. *Medicine and Science in Sports and Exercise* 43: 1590–7.

Fortes, M. B., Diment, B. C., Di Felice, U. and Walsh, N. P. (2012) Dehydration decreases saliva antimicrobial proteins important for mucosal immunity. *Applied Physiology, Nutrition and Metabolism* 37: 850–9.

Foster, C. and Lehmann, M. (1999) *Overtraining syndrome.* Insider (Isostar Sport Nutrition Foundation). 7: 1–5.

Foster, N. K., Martyn, J. B., Rangno, R. E., Hogg, J. C. and Pardy, R. L. (1986) Leukocytosis of exercise: role of cardiac output and catecholamines. *Journal of Applied Physiology* 61: 2218–23.

Fox, P. C., van der Ven, P. F., Sonies, B. C., Weiffenbach, J. M. and Baum, B. J. (1985) Xerostomia: evaluation of a symptom with increasing significance. *Journal of the American Dental Association* 110: 519–25.

Francis, J. L., Gleeson, M, Pyne, D. B., Callister, R. and Clancy, R. L. (2005) Variation of salivary immunoglobulins in exercising and sedentary populations. *Medicine and Science in Sports and Exercise* 37: 571–8.

Freeman, B. D. and Buchman, T. G. (2001) Interleukin-1 receptor antagonist as therapy for inflammatory disorders. *Expert Opinion on Biological Therapy* 1: 301–8.

Fricker, P. A. (2007) Incidence, etiology, and symptomatology of upper respiratory illness in elite athletes. *Medicine and Science in Sports and Exercise* 39: 577–86.

Fricker, P. A. and Pyne, D. B. (2005) Why do athletes seem prone to infection? *Medicine Today* 6: 66.

Fricker, P. A., McDonald, W. A., Gleeson, M. and Clancy, R. L. (1999) Exercise-associated hypogammaglobulinemia. *Clinical Journal of Sport Medicine* 9: 46–8.

Fricker, P. A., Gleeson, M., Flanagan, A., Pyne, D. B., McDonald, W. A. and Clancy, R. L. (2000) A clinical snapshot: do elite swimmers experience more upper respiratory illness than nonathletes? *Clinical Exercise Physiology* 2: 155–8.

Fry, R. W., Morton, A. R. and Keast, D. (1991) Overtraining in athletes: An update. *Sports Medicine* 12: 21–65.

Fry, R. W., Morton, A. R., Crawford, G. P. M. and Keast, D. (1992a) Cell numbers and in vitro responses of leucocytes and lymphocyte subpopulations following maximal exercise and interval training sessions of different intensities. *European Journal of Applied Physiology* 64: 218–27.

Fry, R. W., Morton, A. R., Garcia-Webb, P., Crawford, G. P. and Keast, D. (1992b) Biological responses to overload training in endurance sports. *European Journal of Applied Physiology and Occupational Physiology* 64: 335–44.

Gabriel, H., Urhausen, A. and Kindermann, W. (1991) Circulating leukocyte and lymphocyte subpopulations before and after intensive endurance exercise to exhaustion. *European Journal of Applied Physiology* 63: 449–57.

Gabriel, H., Schwarz, L., Steffens, G. and Kindermann, W. (1992a) Immunoregulatory hormones, circulating leukocyte and lymphocyte subpopulations before and after endurance exercise of different intensities. *International Journal of Sports Medicine* 13: 359–66.

Gabriel, H., Urhausen, A. and Kindermann, W. (1992b) Mobilisation of circulating leukocyte and lymphocyte subpopulations during and after short, anaerobic exercise. *European Journal of Applied Physiology* 65: 164–70.

Gabriel, H., Schwarz, L., Born, P. and Kindermann, W. (1992c) Differential mobilization of leucocyte and lymphocyte subpopulations into the circulation during endurance exercise. *European Journal of Applied Physiology and Occupational Physiology* 65: 529–34.

Gabriel, H., Brechtel, L., Urhausen, A. and Kindermann, W. (1994) Recruitment and recirculation of leukocytes after an ultramarathon run: preferential homing of cells expressing high levels of the adhesion molecule LFA-1. *International Journal of Sports Medicine* 15(Suppl 3): S148–53.

Gabriel, H., Müller, H. J., Urhausen, A. and Kindermann, W. (1994b) Suppressed PMA-induced oxidative burst and unimpaired phagocytosis of circulating granulocytes one week after a long endurance exercise. *International Journal of Sports Medicine* 15: 441–5.

Gabriel, H. H., Urhausen, A., Valet, G., Heidelbach, U. and Kindermann, W. (1998) Overtraining and immune system: a prospective longitudinal study in endurance athletes. *Medicine and Science in Sports and Exercise* 30 : 1151–7.

Gala, R. R. (1991) Prolactin and growth hormone in the regulation of the immune system. *Proceedings of the Society for Experimental Biology and Medicine* 198: 513–27.

Galbo, H. (1983) *Hormonal and Metabolic Adaptation to Exercise.* New York: Verlag.

Galloway, S. D. and Maughan, R. J. (1997) Effects of ambient temperature on the capacity to perform prolonged cycle exercise in man. *Medicine and Science in Sports and Exercise* 29: 1240–9.

Galluci, S. and Matzinger, P. (2001) Danger signals: SOS to the immune system. *Current Opinion in Immunology* 13: 114–19.

Gannon, G., Shek, P. N. and Shephard, R. J. (1995) Natural killer cells: modulation by intensity and duration of exercise. *Exercise Immunology Review* 1: 26–48.

Gannon, G. A., Rhind, S. G., Shek, P. N. and Shephard, R. J. (2001) Differential cell adhesion molecule expression and lymphocyte mobilisation during prolonged aerobic exercise. *European Journal of Applied Physiology* 84: 272–82.

Gathiram, P., Wells, M. T., Brock-Utne, J. G., Wessels, B. C. and Gaffin, S. L. (1987) Prevention of endotoxaemia by non-absorbable antibiotics in heat stress. *Journal of Clinical Pathology* 40: 1364–8.

Gathiram, P., Wells, M. T., Brock-Utne, J. G. and Gaffin, S. L. (1988) Prophylactic corticosteroid increases survival in experimental heat stroke in primates. *Aviation, Space, and Environmental Medicine* 59: 352–5.

Giesbrecht, G. G. (1995) The respiratory system in a cold environment. *Aviation, Space, and Environmental Medicine* 66: 890–902.

Giesbrecht, G. G. (2000) Cold stress, near drowning and accidental hypothermia: a review. *Aviation, Space, and Environmental Medicine* 71: 733–52.

Gill, J. M. R. and Cooper, A. R. (2008) Physical activity and prevention of type 2 diabetes mellitus. *Sports Medicine* 38: 807–24.

Gillum, T. L., Kuennen, M. R., Schneider, S. and Moseley, P. (2011) A review of sex differences in immune function after aerobic exercise. *Exercise Immunology Review* 17: 104–21.

Gimenez, M., Mohan-Kumar, T., Humbert, J. C., De Talance, N. and Buisine, J. (1986) Leukocyte, lymphocyte and platelet response to dynamic exercise. Duration or intensity effect? *European Journal of Applied Physiology and Occupational Physiology* 55: 465–70.

Glaser, R. and Kiecolt-Glaser, J. K. (2005) Stress–induced immune dysfunction: implications for health. *Nature Reviews Immunology* 5: 243–51.

Gleeson, M. (2000a) Interleukins and exercise. *Journal of Physiology* 529: 1.

Gleeson, M. (2000b) Mucosal immune responses and risk of respiratory illness in elite athletes. *Exercise Immunology Review* 6: 5–42.

Gleeson, M. (2005) *Immune Function in Sport and Exercise*. Edinburgh: Elsevier.

Gleeson, M. (2006a) Can nutrition limit exercise-induced immunodepression? *Nutrition Reviews* 64: 119–31.

Gleeson, M. (2006b) Immune system adaptation in elite athletes. *Current Opinion in Clinical Nutrition and Metabolic Care* 9: 659–65.

Gleeson, M. (2007) Exercise and immune function. *Journal of Applied Physiology* 103: 693–9.

Gleeson, M. and Bishop, N. C. (1999) Immunology. In R. J. Maughan (Editor) *Basic and Applied Sciences for Sports Medicine*. Oxford: Butterworth Heinemann, pp. 199–236.

Gleeson, M. and Bishop, N. C. (2005) The T cell and NK cell immune response to exercise. *Annals of Transplantation* 10: 43–8.

Gleeson, M. and Pyne, D. B. (2000) Special feature for the Olympics: effects of exercise on the immune system: exercise effects on mucosal immunity. *Immunology and Cell Biology* 78: 536–44.

Gleeson, M., Brooks, S. and Cave, R. (1993) The relationship between the serum cortisol concentration and the delayed leukocytosis of exercise in untrained humans. *Journal of Physiology* 467: 115.

Gleeson, M., Almey, J., Brooks, S., Cave, R., Lewis, A. and Griffiths, H. (1995a) Haematological and acute phase responses associated with delayed onset muscle soreness in man. *European Journal of Applied Physiology* 71: 137–42.

Gleeson, M., McDonald, W. A., Cripps, A. W., Pyne, D. B., Clancy, R. L. and Fricker, P. A. (1995b) The effect on immunity of long-term intensive training in elite swimmers. *Clinical Experimental Immunology* 102: 210–16.

Gleeson, M., Blannin, A. K., Zhu, B., Brooks, S. and Cave, R. (1995c) Cardiorespiratory, hormonal and haematological responses to submaximal cycling performed 2 days after eccentric or concentric exercise bouts. *Journal of Sports Sciences* 13: 471–9.

Gleeson, M., Blannin, A. K., Walsh, N. P., Field, C. N. and Pritchard, J. C. (1998) Effect of exercise-induced muscle damage on the blood lactate response to incremental exercise in humans. *European Journal of Applied Physiology* 77: 292–5.

Gleeson, M., McDonald, W. A., Pyne, D. B., Cripps, A. W., Francis, J. L., Fricker, P. A. and Clancy, R. L. (1999a) Salivary IgA levels and infection risk in elite swimmers. *Medicine and Science in Sports and Exercise* 31: 67–73.

Gleeson, M., Hall, S. T., McDonald, W. A., Flanagan, A. J. and Clancy, R. L. (1999b) Salivary IgA subclasses and infection risk in elite swimmers. *Immunology and Cell Biology* 77: 351–5.

Gleeson, M., Ginn, E. and Francis, J.L. (2000a) Salivary immunoglobulin monitoring in an elite kayaker. *Clinical Journal of Sport Medicine* 10: 206–8.

Gleeson, M., McDonald, W. A., Pyne, D. B., Clancy, R. L., Cripps, A. W., Francis, J. L. and Fricker, P. A. (2000b) Immune status and respiratory illness for elite swimmers during a 12-week training cycle. *International Journal of Sport Medicine* 21: 302–7.

Gleeson, M., McFarlin, B. and Flynn, M. (2006) Exercise and Toll-like receptors. *Exercise Immunology Review* 12: 34–53.

Gleeson, M., Pyne, D. B., Austin, J. P., Lynn, F. J., Clancy, R. L., McDonald, W. A. and Fricker, P. A. (2002) Epstein-Barr virus reactivation and upper-respiratory illness in elite swimmers. *Medicine and Science in Sports and Exercise* 34: 411–17.

Gleeson, M., McFarlin, B. K. and Flynn, M. G. (2006) Exercise and toll-like receptors. *Exercise Immunology Review* 12: 34–53.

Gleeson, M., Bishop, N. C., Stensel, D. J., Lindley, M. R., Mastana, S. S. and Nimmo, M. A. (2011a) The anti-inflammatory effects of exercise: mechanisms and implications for the prevention and treatment of disease. *Nature Reviews Immunology* 11: 607–15.

Gleeson, M., Bishop, N. C., Oliveira, M. and Tauler, P. (2011b) Daily probiotic's (Lactobacillus casei Shirota) reduction of infection incidence in athletes. *International Journal of Sport Nutrition and Exercise Metabolism* 21: 55–64.

Gleeson, M., Bishop, N., Oliveira, M., McCauley, T. and Tauler, P. (2011c) Sex differences in immune variables and respiratory infection incidence in an athletic population. *Exercise Immunology Review* 17: 122–35.

Gleeson, M., Bishop, N. C., Oliveira, M., McCauley, T. and Tauler, P. (2012a) Influence of training load on upper respiratory tract infection incidence and antigen-stimulated cytokine production. *Scandinavian Journal of Medicine and Science in Sports* doi: 10.1111/j.1600–0838.2011.01422.x.

Gleeson, M., Bishop, N. C., Oliveira, M., McCauley, T., Tauler, P. and Muhamad, A. S. (2012b) Respiratory infection risk in athletes: association with antigen–stimulated IL–10 production and salivary IgA secretion. *Scandinavian Journal of Medicine and Science in Sports* 22: 410–17.

Gleeson, M., Siegler, J., Burke, L. M., Stear, S. and Castell, L. M. (2012c) A to Z of nutritional supplements: dietary supplements, sports nutrition foods and ergogenic aids for health and performance – Part 31. (Probiotics). *British Journal of Sports Medicine* 46: 377–8.

Gmunder, F. K., Konstantinova, I., Cogoli, A., Lesnyak, A., Bogomolov, W. and Grachov, A. W. (1994) Cellular immunity in cosmonauts during long duration spaceflight on board the orbital MIR station. *Aviation, Space, and Environmental Medicine* 65: 419–23.

Goebel, M. U. and Mills, P. J. (2000) Acute psychological stress and exercise and changes in peripheral leukocyte adhesion molecule expression and density. *Psychosomatic Medicine* 62: 664–70.

Goh, J., Kirk, E. A., Lee, S. X. and Ladiges, W. C. (2012) Exercise, physical activity and breast cancer: the role of tumour associated macrophages. *Exercise Immunology Review* 18: 158–76.

Gomes, E. C., Stone, V. and Florida-James, G. (2011) Impact of heat and pollution on oxidative stress and CC16 secretion after 8 km run. *European Journal of Applied Physiology* 111: 2089–97.

Gomez-Merino, D., Drogou, C., Chennaoui, M., Tiollier, E., Mathieu, J. and Guezennec, C. Y. (2005) Effects of combined stress during intense training on cellular immunity, hormones and respiratory infections. *Neuroimmunomodulation* 12: 164–72.

Gonzalez-Alonso, J., Teller, C., Andersen, S. L., Jensen, F. B., Hyldig, T. and Nielsen, B. (1999) Influence of body temperature on the development of fatigue during prolonged exercise in the heat. *Journal of Applied Physiology* 86: 1032–9.

Goodman, C. (2010) Relationship between inflammatory cytokines and self-report measures of training overload. *Research in Sports Medicine* 18: 127–39.

Goodwin, K., Viboud, C. and Simonsen, L. (2006) Antibody response to influenza vaccination in the elderly: a quantitative review. *Vaccine* 24:1159–69.

Gore, C. J., Hahn, A., Rice, A., Bourdon, P., Lawrence, S., Walsh, C., Stanef, T., Barnes, P., Parisotto, R., Martin, D. and Pyne, D. (1998) Altitude training at 2690m does not increase total haemoglobin mass or sea level $\dot{V}O_2$max in world champion track cyclists. *Journal of Science and Medicine in Sport* 1: 156–70.

Grant, R. W., Mariani, R. A., Vieira, V. J., Fleshner, M., Smith, T. P., Keylock, K. T., Lowder, T. W., McAuley, E., Hu, L., Chapman-Novakofski, K. and Woods, J.A. (2008) Cardio-vascular exercise intervention improves the primary antibody response to keyhole limpet hemocyanin (KLH) in previously sedentary older adults. *Brain, Behavior and Immunity* 22: 923–32.

Green, C., Pedersen, B. K., Hoffman-Goetz, L., Rogers, C. J., Northoff, H., Abbasi, A. and Simon, P. (2011) Position Statement Part One: Immune function and exercise. *Exercise Immunology Review* 17: 6–63.

Green, K. J. and Rowbottom, D. G. (2003) Exercise–induced changes to in vitro T-lymphocyte mitogen responses using CFSE. *Journal of Applied Physiology* 95: 57–63.

Green, K. J., Rowbottom, D. G. and Mackinnon, L. T. (2002) Exercise and T-lymphocyte function: a comparison of proliferation in PBMC and NK-cell depleted PMC culture. *Journal of Applied Physiology* 92: 2390–5.

Gress, R. E. and Deeks, S. G. (2009) Reduced thymus activity and infection prematurely age the immune system. *Journal of Clinical Investigation* 119: 2884–7.

Grogan, J. B., Parks, L. C. and Minaberry, D. (1980) Polymorphonuclear leukocyte function in cancer patients treated with total body hyperthermia. *Cancer* 45: 2611–15.

Grover, R. F., Weil, J. V. and Reeves, J. T. (1986) Cardiovascular adaptation to exercise at high altitude *Exercise Immunology Review* 14: 269–302.

Groves, J. R. and Prapavessis, H. (1992) Preliminary evidence for the reliability and validity of an abbreviated Profile of Mood State questionnaire. *International Journal of Sport Psychology* 23: 93–109.

Gueguinou, N., Huin-Schohn, C., Bascove, M., Bueb, J. L., Tschirhart, E., Legrand-Frossi, C. and Frippiat, J. P. (2009) Could spaceflight-associated immune system weakening preclude the expansion of human presence beyond Earth's orbit? *Journal of Leukocyte Biology* 86: 1027–38.

Guilietti, A., van Etten, E., Overbergh, L., Stoffels, K., Bouillon, R. and Mathieu, C. (2007) Monocytes from type 2 diabetic patients have a pro-inflammatory profile. 1,25-Dihydroxyvitamin D(3) works as anti–inflammatory. *Diabetes Research and Clinical Practice* 77: 47–57.

Hack, V., Strobel, G., Rau, J. P. and Weicker, H. (1992) The effect of maximal exercise on the activity of neutrophil granulocytes in highly trained athletes in a moderate training period. *European Journal of Applied Physiology* 65: 520–4.

Hack, V., Strobel, G., Weiss, M. and Weicker, H. (1994) PMN cell counts and phagocytic activity of highly trained athletes depend on training period. *Journal of Applied Physiology* 77: 1731–5.

Haffner, S. M. (2007) Abdominal adiposity and cardiometabolic risk: do we have all the answers? *American Journal of Medicine* 120: S10–S16.

Haller Hasskamp, J., Zapas, J. L. and Elias, E. G. (2005) Dendritic cell counts in the peripheral blood of healthy adults. *American Journal of Hematology* 78: 314–15.

Hanson, L. Ä., Björkander, J. and Oxelius, V. A. (1983) Selective IgA deficiency. In: R. K. Chandra (Editor), *Primary and Secondary Immunodeficiency Disorders*. Edinburgh: Churchill Livingstone, pp. 62–4.

Hao, Q., Lu, Z., Dong, B. R., Huang, C. Q. and Wu, T. (2011) Probiotics for preventing acute upper respiratory tract infections. *Cochrane Database of Systematic Reviews* CD006895.

Hardman, A. E. and Stensel, D. J. (2009) *Physical Activity and Health: The Evidence Explained.* (2nd ed.). Abingdon: Routledge. pp. 120–1.

Harper Smith, A. D., Coakley, S. L., Ward, M. D., Macfarlane, A. W., Friedmann, P. S. and Walsh, N. P. (2011) Exercise-induced stress inhibits both the induction and elicitation phases of in vivo T-cell-mediated immune responses in humans. *Brain, Behavior and Immunity* 25: 1136–42.

Harrison, R. M. (2006) Sources of air pollution, In: M. Chan and M. Danzon (Editors), *World Health Organization Air Quality Guidelines: Global Update 2005.* Germany: Druckpartner Moser.

Hattori, N. (2009) Expression, regulation and biological actions of growth hormone (GH) and ghrelin in the immune system. *Growth Hormone and IGF Research* 19: 187–97.

Haus, E. and Smolensky, M. H. (1999) Biologic rhythms in the immune system. *Chronobiology International* 16: 581–622.

Hawkins, W. R. and Ziegelschmid, J. F. (1975) Clinical aspects of crew health: biomedical results of Apollo, NASA-SP-368. Washington, DC: National Aeronautical and Space Administration.

Hazucha, M. J., Madden, M., Pape, G., Becker, S., Devlin, R., Koren, H. S., Kehrl, H. and Bromberg, P. A. (1996) Effects of cyclo-oxygenase inhibition on ozone-induced respiratory inflammation and lung function changes. *European Journal of Applied Physiology and Occupational Physiology* 73: 17–27.

He, C. S., Tsai, M. L., Ko, M. H., Chang, C. K. and Fang, S. H. (2010) Relationships among salivary immunoglobulin A, lactoferrin and cortisol in basketball players during a basketball season. *European Journal of Applied Physiology* 110: 989–95.

Health Protection Agency (2005) *Health Protection in the 21st Century: Understanding the Burden of Disease.* London: HPA.

Helenius, I. and Haahtela, T. (2000) Allergy and asthma in elite summer sport athletes. *Journal of Allergy and Clinical Immunology* 106: 444–52.

Helenius, I., Lumme, A. and Haahtela, T. (2005) Asthma, airway inflammation and treatment in elite athletes. *Sports Medicine* 35: 565–74.

Helenius, I. J., Tikkanen, H. O., Sarna, S. and Haahtela, T. (1998) Asthma and increased bronchial responsiveness in elite athletes: atopy and sport event as risk factors. *Journal of Allergy and Clinical Immunology* 101: 646–52.

Hemila, H. (2011) Zinc lozenges may shorten the duration of colds: a systematic review. *Open Respiratory Medicine Journal J* 5: 51–8.

Henson, D. A., Nieman, D. C., Parker, J. C., Rainwater, M. K., Butterworth, D. E., Warren, B. J., Utter, A., Davis, J. M., Fagoaga, O. R. and Nehlsen-Cannarella, S. L. (1998) Carbohydrate supplementation and the lymphocyte proliferative response to long endurance running. *International Journal of Sports Medicine* 19: 574–80.

Henson, D. A., Nieman, D. C., Blodgett, A. D., Butterworth, D. E., Utter, A. C., Davis, J. M., Sonnefeld, G., Morton, S. D., Fagoaga, O. R. and Nehlsen-Cannarella, S. L. (1999) Influence of exercise mode and carbohydrate on the immune response to prolonged exercise. *International Journal of Sports Nutrition* 9: 213–28.

Hill, L. and Clemen, M. (1929) *Common Colds, Causes and Preventive Measures.* London: William Heinemann.

Hiscock, N. and Pedersen, B. K. (2002) Exercise-induced immunodepression – plasma glutamine is not the link. *Journal of Applied Physiology* 93: 813–22.

Hiscock, N., Chan, M. H., Bisucci, T., Darby, I. A. and Febbraio, M. A. (2004) Skeletal muscle myocytes are a source of interleukin-6 mRNA expression and protein release during contraction: evidence of fiber type specificity. *FASEB Journal* 18: 992–4.

Hitomi, Y., Miyamura, M., Mori, S., Suzuki, K., Kizaki, T., Itoh, C., Murakami, K., Haga, S. and Ohno, H. (2003) Intermittent hypobaric hypoxia increases the ability of neutrophils to generate superoxide anion in humans. *Clinical and Experimental Pharmacology and Physiology* 30: 659–64.

Ho, C. S., Lopez, J. A., Vuckovic, S., Pyke, C. M., Hockey, R. L. and Hart, D. N. (2001) Surgical and physical stress increases circulating blood dendritic cell counts independently of monocyte counts. *Blood* 98: 140–5.

Hoffman-Goetz, L. and Pedersen, B. K. (1994) Exercise and the immune system: a model of the stress response? *Immunology Today* 15: 382–7.

Hoffman-Goetz, L., Simpson, J. R., Cipp, N., Arumugam, Y. and Houston, M. E. (1990) Lymphocyte subset responses to repeated submaximal exercise in men. *Journal of Applied Physiology* 68: 1069–74.

Hogg, J. C. and Doerschuk, C. M. (1995) Leukocyte traffic in the lung. *Annual Review of Physiology* 57: 97–114.

Holdcroft, A. (2007) Integrating the dimensions of sex and gender into basic life sciences research: methodologic and ethical issues. *Gender Medicine* 4(Suppl B): S64–S74.

Holgate, S. T., Church, M. and Lichtenstein, L. M. (2006) *Allergy* (3rd ed.), Philadelphia, PA: Mosby Elsevier.

Holgate, S. T., Arshad, H. S., Roberts, G. C., Howarth, P. H., Thurner, P. and Davies, D. E. (2009) A new look at the pathogenesis of asthma. *Clinical Science (London)* 118: 439–50.

Holger, G., Urhausen, A., Valet, G., Heidelbach, U. and Kindermann, W. (1998) Overtraining and immune system: a prospective longitudinal study in endurance athletes. *Medicine and Science in Sports and Exercise* 30: 1151–7.

Holz, O., Jorres, R. A., Timm, P., Mucke, M., Richter, K., Koschyk, S. and Magnussen, H. (1999) Ozone-induced airway inflammatory changes differ between individuals and are reproducible. *American Journal of Respiratory and Critical Care Medicine* 159: 776–84.

Hong, E. G., Ko, H. J., Cho, Y. R., Kim, H. J., Ma, Z., Yu, T. Y., Friedline, R. H., Kurt-Jones, E., Finberg, R., Fischer, M. A., Granger, E. L., Norbury, C. C., Hauschka, S. D., Philbrick, W. M., Lee, C. G., Elias, J. A. and Kim, J. K. (2009) Interleukin-10 prevents diet-induced insulin resistance by attenuating macrophage and cytokine response in skeletal muscle. *Diabetes* 58: 2525–35.

Hong, S. and Mills, P. J. (2008) Effects of an exercise challenge on mobilization and surface marker expression of monocyte subsets in individuals with normal vs. elevated blood pressure. *Brain, Behavior and Immunity* 22: 590–9.

Hong, S., Farag, N. H., Nelesen, R. A., Ziegler, M. G. and Mills, P. J. (2004) Effects of regular exercise on lymphocyte subsets and CD62L after psychological vs. physical stress. *Journal of Psychosomatic Research* 56: 363–70.

Horn, P. L., Pyne, D. B., Hopkins, W. G. and Barnes, C. J. (2010) Lower white blood cell counts in elite athletes training for highly aerobic sports. *European Journal of Applied Physiology* 110: 925–32.

Horvath, S. M., Raven, P. B., Dahms, T. E. and Gray, D. J. (1975) Maximal aerobic capacity at different levels of carboxyhemoglobin. *Journal of Applied Physiology* 38: 300–3.

Howren, M. B., Lamkin, D. M. and Suls, J. (2009) Associations of depression with C-reactive protein, IL-1, and IL-6: a meta-analysis. *Psychosomatic Medicine* 71: 171–86.

Hull, J. H., Hull, P. J., Parsons, J. P., Dickinson, J. W. and Ansley, L. (2009) Approach to the diagnosis and management of suspected exercise–induced bronchoconstriction by primary care physicians. *BMC Pulmonary Medicine* 9: 29.

Ibfelt, T., Petersen, E. W., Bruunsgaard, H., Sandmand, M. and Pedersen, B. K. (2002) Exercise-induced change in type 1 cytokine-producing CD8+ T cells is related to a decrease in memory T cells. *Journal of Applied Physiology* 93: 645–8.

Imai, K., Matsuyama, S., Miyake, S., Suga, K. and Nakachi, K. (2000) Natural cytotoxic activity of peripheral-blood lymphocytes and cancer incidence: an 11-year follow-up study of a general population. *The Lancet* 356: 1795–9.

Jackson, G. G., Dowling, H. F., Spiesman, I. G. and Boano, A. V. (1958) Transmission of the common cold to volunteers under controlled conditions. *Archives in Internal Medicine* 101: 267–78.

Jacobs, L., Nawrot, T. S., de Geus, B., Meeusen, R., Degraeuwe, B., Bernard, A., Sughis, M., Nemery, B. and Panis, L. I. (2010) Subclinical responses in healthy cyclists briefly exposed to traffic-related air pollution: an intervention study. *Environmental Health* 9: 64–71.

Janeway, C. A. Jr, Travers, P., Walport, M. and Shlomchik, M. (2001) The distribution and functions of immunoglobulin isotypes. In: C. A. Janeway, Jr., P. Travers, M. Walport and M. J. Shlomchik (Editors), *Immunobiology: The Immune System in Health and Disease* (5th ed.) New York: Garland Science. Chapter 9, The humoral immune response.

Jemmot, J. B. 3rd, Borysenko, J. Z., Borysenko, M., McClelland, D. C., Chapman, R., Meyer, D. and Benson, H. (1983) Academic stress, power motivation, and decrease in secretion rate of salivary secretory Immunoglobulin A. *The Lancet* 1: 1400–2.

Jeukendrup, A. E., Hesselink, M. K. C., Snyder, A. C., Kuipers, H. and Keizer, H. A. (1992) Physiological changes in male competitive cyclists after two weeks of intensified training. *International Journal of Sports Medicine* 13: 534–41.

Jiao, P., Chen, Q., Shah, S., Du, J., Tao, B., Tzameli, I., Yan, W. and Xu, H. (2009) Obesity-related upregulation of monocyte chemotactic factors in adipocytes: involvement of nuclear factor-kappaB and c-Jun NH2-terminal kinase pathways. *Diabetes* 58: 104–15.

Johannsen, N. M., Priest, E. L., Dixit, V. D., Earnest, C. P., Blair, S. N. and Church, T. S. (2010) Association of white blood cell subfraction concentration with fitness and fatness. *British Journal of Sports Medicine* 44: 588–93.

Johannsen, N. M., Swift, D. L., Johnson, W. D., Dixit, V. D., Earnest, C. P., Blair, S. N. and Church, T. S. (2012) Effect of different doses of aerobic exercise on total white blood cell (WBC) and WBC subfraction number in postmenopausal women: results from DREW. *PLoS One* 7: e31319.

Johnson, C. and Eccles, R. (2005) Acute cooling of the feet and the onset of common cold symptoms. *Family Practice* 22: 608–13.

Jonsdottir, I. H. (2000) Special feature for the Olympics: effects of exercise on the immune system: neuropeptides and their interaction with exercise and immune function. *Immunology and Cell Biology* 78: 562–70.

Jonsdottir, I. H., Hellstrand, K., Thoren, P. and Hoffmann, P. (2000) Enhancement of natural immunity seen after voluntary exercise in rats. Role of central opioid receptors. *Life Sciences* 66: 1231–9.

Kaisho, T. and Akira, S. (2006) Toll-like receptor function and signalling. *Journal of Allergy and Clinical Immunology* 117: 979–87.

Kamen, D. L. and Tangpricha, V. (2010) Vitamin D and molecular actions on the immune system: modulation of innate and autoimmunity. *Journal of Molecular Medicine* 88: 441–50.

Kanda, H., Tateya, S., Tamori, Y., Kotani, K., Hiasa, K., Kitazawa, R., Kitazawa, S., Miyachi, H., Maeda, S., Egashira, K. and Kasuga, M. (2006) MCP-1 contributes to macrophage infiltration into adipose tissue, insulin resistance, and hepatic steatosis in obesity. *Journal of Clinical Investigation* 116: 1494–505.

Kantamala, D., Vongsakul, M. and Satayavivad, J. (1990) The in vivo and in vitro effects of caffeine on rat immune cells activities: B, T and NK cells. *Asian Pacific Journal of Allergy and Immunology* 8: 77–82.

Kapasi, Z. F., Ouslander, J. G., Schnelle, J. F., Kutner, M. and Fahey, J. L. (2003) Effects of an exercise intervention on immunologic parameters in frail elderly nursing home residents. *The Journals of Gerontology Series A: Biological Sciences and Medical Sciences* 58: 636–43.

Kappel, M., Stadeager, C., Tvede, N., Galbo, H. and Pedersen, B. K. (1991) Effects of in vivo hyperthermia on natural killer cell activity, in vitro proliferative responses and blood mononuclear cell subpopulations. *Clinical Experimental Immunology* 84: 175–80.

Kappel, M., Tvede, N., Galbo, H., Haahr, P. M., Kjaer, M., Linstow, M., Klarlund, K. and Pedersen, B. K. (1991) Evidence that the effect of physical exercise on NK cell activity is mediated by epinephrine. *Journal of Applied Physiology* 70: 2530–4.

Kappel, M., Poulsen, T. D., Hansen, M. B., Galbo, H. and Pedersen, B. K. (1998)

Somatostatin attenuates the hyperthermia induced increase in neutrophil concentration. *European Journal of Applied Physiology and Occupational Physiology* 77: 149–56.

Kargarfard, M., Poursafa, P., Rezanejad, S. and Mousavinasab, F. (2011) Effects of exercise in polluted air on the aerobic power, serum lactate level and cell blood count of active individuals. *International Journal of Preventive Medicine* 2: 145–50.

Kasapis, C. and Thompson, P. D. (2005) The effects of physical activity on serum C-reactive protein and inflammatory markers: a systematic review. *Journal of the American College of Cardiology* 45: 1563–9.

Kastello, G. M., Sothmann, M. S. and Murthy, V. S. (1993) Young and old subjects matched for aerobic capacity have similar noradrenergic responses to exercise. *Journal of Applied Physiology* 74: 49–54.

Katelaris, C. H., Carrozzi, F. M., Burke, T. V. and Byth, K. (2000) A springtime Olympics demands special consideration for allergic athletes. *Journal of Allergy and Clinical Immunology* 106: 260–6.

Katelaris, C. H., Carrozzi, F. M. and Burke, T. V. (2003) Allergic rhinoconjunctivitis in elite athletes: optimal management for quality of life and performance. *Sports Medicine* 33: 401–6.

Katschinski, D. M., Benndorf, R., Wiedemann, G. J., Mulkerin, D. L., Touhidi, R. and Robins, H. I. (1999) Heat shock protein antibodies in sarcoma patients undergoing 41.8 degrees C whole body hyperthermia. *Journal of Immunotherapy* 22: 67–70.

Kaur, I., Simons, E. R., Castro, V. A., Mark, O. C. and Pierson, D. L. (2004) Changes in neutrophil functions in astronauts. *Brain, Behavior and Immunity* 18: 443–50.

Kaur, I., Simons, E. R., Castro, V. A., Ott, C. M. and Pierson, D. L. (2005) Changes in monocyte functions of astronauts. *Brain, Behavior and Immunity* 19: 547–54.

Kawanishi, N., Yano, H., Yokogawa, Y. and Suzuki, K. (2010) Exercise training inhibits inflammation in adipose tissue via both suppression of macrophage infiltration and acceleration of phenotypic switching from M1 to M2 macrophages in high-fat-diet-induced obese mice. *Exercise Immunology Review* 16: 105–18.

Keast, D., Arstein, D., Harper, W., Fry, R. W. and Morton, A. R. (1995) Depression of plasma glutamine concentration after exercise stress and its possible influence on the immune system. *Medical Journal* 162: 15–18.

Keatinge, W. R., Khartchenko, M., Lando, N. and Lioutov, V. (2001) Hypothermia during sports swimming in water below 11 degrees C. *British Journal of Sports Medicine* 35: 352–3.

Keen, P., McCarthy, D. A., Passfield, L., Shaker, H. A. A. and Wade, A. J. (1995) Leucocyte and erythrocyte counts during a multi-stage cycling race ('The Milk Race'). *British Journal of Sports Medicine* 29: 61–5.

Kehl-Fie, T. E. and Skaar, E. P. (2010) Nutritional immunity beyond iron: a role for manganese and zinc. *Current Opinion in Chemical Biology* 14: 218–24.

Kekkonen, R. A., Vasankari, T. J., Vuorimaa, T., Haahtela, T., Julkunen, I. and Korpela, R. (2007) The effect of probiotics on respiratory infections and gastrointestinal symptoms during training in marathon runners. *International Journal of Sport Nutrition and Exercise Metabolism* 17: 352–63.

Keller, C., Keller, P., Marshal, S. and Pedersen, B. K. (2003) IL-6 gene expression in human adipose tissue in response to exercise: effect of carbohydrate ingestion. *Journal of Physiology* 550: 927–31.

Keller, C., Steensberg, A., Hansen, A. K., Fischer, C. P., Plomgaard, P. and Pedersen, B. K. (2005) Effect of exercise, training, and glycogen availability on IL-6 receptor expression in human skeletal muscle. *Journal of Applied Physiology* 99: 2075–9.

Kendall, A., Hoffman-Goetz, L., Houston, M., MacNeil, B. and Arumugam, Y. (1990) Exercise and blood lymphocyte subset responses: intensity, duration, and subject fitness effects. *Journal of Applied Physiology* 69: 251–60.

Khansari, D. N., Murgo, A. J. and Faith, R. E. (1990) Effects of stress on the immune system. *Immunology Today* 11: 170–5.

Kimura, F., Aizawa, K., Tanabe, K., Shimizu, K., Kon, M., Lee, H., Akimoto, T., Akama, T. and Kono, I. (2008) A rat model of saliva secretory immunoglobulin: a suppression caused by intense exercise. *Scandinavian Journal of Medicine and Science in Sports* 18: 367–72.

Kingsbury, K. J., Kay, L. and Hjelm, M. (1998) Contrasting plasma amino acid patterns in elite athletes: association with fatigue and infection. *British Journal of Sports Medicine* 32: 25–33.

Kizaki, T., Takemasa, T., Sakurai, T., Izawa, T., Hanawa, T., Kamiya, S., Haga, S., Imaizumi, K. and Ohno, H. (2008) Adaptation of macrophages to exercise training improves innate immunity. *Biochemical and Biophysical Research Communications* 372: 152–6.

Kleessen, B., Schroedl, W., Stueck, M., Richter, A., Rieck, O. and Krueger, M. (2005) Microbial and immunological responses relative to high-altitude exposure in mountaineers. *Medicine and Science in Sports and Exercise* 37: 1313–18.

Klentrou, P., Cieslak, T., MacNeil, M., Vintinner, A. and Plyley, M. (2002) Effect of moderate exercise on salivary immunoglobulin A and infection risk in humans. *European Journal of Applied Physiology* 87: 153–8.

Kliesch, W. F., Cruse, J. M., Lewis, R. E., Bishop, G. R., Brackin, B. and Lampton, J. A. (1996) Restoration of depressed immune function in spinal cord injury patients receiving rehabilitation therapy. *Paraplegia* 34: 82–90.

Klokker, M., Kjaer, M., Secher, N. H., Hanel, B., Worm, L., Kappel, M. and Pedersen, B. K. (1995) Natural killer cell response to exercise in humans: effect of hypoxia and epidural anesthesia. *Journal of Applied Physiology* 78: 709–16.

Knighton, D. R., Halliday, B. and Hunt, T. K. (1984) Oxygen as an antibiotic. The effect of inspired oxygen on infection. *Archives of Surgery* 119: 199–204.

Koch, A. (2010) Immune response to resistance exercise. *American Journal of Lifestyle Medicine* 4: 244–52.

Kohut, M. L., Davis, J. M., Jackson, D. A., Colbert, L., Strasner, A., Essig, D. A., Pate, R. R., Ghaffar, A. and Mayer, E. P. (1998) The role of stress hormones in exercise-induced suppression of alveolar macrophage antiviral function. *Journal of Neuroimmunology* 81: 193–200.

Kohut, M. L., Davis, J. M., Jackson, D. A., Jani, P., Ghaffar, A., Mayer, E. P. and Essig, D. A. (1998) Exercise effects on IFN-beta expression and viral replication in lung macrophages after HSV-1 infection. *American Journal of Physiology* 275: L1089–94.

Kohut, M. L., Cooper, M. M., Nickolaus, M. D., Russell, D. R. and Cunnick, J. E. (2002) Exercise and psychosocial factors modulate immunity to influenza vaccine in elderly individuals. *Journals of Gerontology A Biological Sciences and Medical Sciences* 57: M557–62.

Kohut, M. L., Arntson, B. A., Lee, W., Rozeboom, K., Yoon, K.-J., Cunnick, J. E. and McElhaney, J. (2004) Moderate exercise improves antibody response to influenza immunisation in older adults. *Vaccine* 22: 2298–306.

Konig, D., Berg, A., Weinstock, C., Keul, J. and Northoff, H. (1997) Essential fatty acids, immune function, and exercise. *Exercise Immunology Review* 3, 1–31.

Konstantinova, I. V., Rykova, M. P., Lesnyak, A. T. and Antropova, E. A. (1993) Immune changes during long-duration missions. *Journal of Leukocyte Biology* 54: 189–201.

Kopp-Hoolihan, L. (2001) Prophylactic and therapeutic uses of probiotics: a review. *Journal of the American Dietetic Association* 101: 229–38.

Kraus, W. E., Houmard, J. A., Duscha, B. D., Knetzger, K. J., Wharton, M. B., McCartney, J. S., Bales, C. W., Henes, S., Samsa, G. P., Otvos, J. D., Kulkarni, K. R. and Slentz, C. A. (2002) Effects of the amount and intensity of exercise on plasma lipoproteins. *New England Journal of Medicine* 347: 1483–92.

Kregel, K. C. (2002) Heat shock proteins: modifying factors in physiological stress responses and acquired thermotolerance. *Journal of Applied Physiology* 92: 2177–86.

Kruger, K., Lechtermann, A., Fobker, M., Volker, K. and Mooren, F. C. (2008) Exercise-induced redistribution of T lymphocytes is regulated by adrenergic mechanisms. *Brain, Behavior and Immunity* 22: 324–38.

Kruger, K., Frost, S., Most, E., Volker, K., Pallauf, J. and Mooren, F. C. (2009) Exercise affects tissue lymphocyte apoptosis via redox-sensitive and Fas-dependent signaling pathways. *American Journal of Physiology – Regulatory, Integrative and Comparative Physiology* 296: R1518–27.

Kuennen, M., Gillum, T., Dokladny, K., Bedrick, E., Schneider, S. and Moseley, P. (2011) Thermotolerance and heat acclimation may share a common mechanism in humans. *American Journal of Physiology – Regulatory, Integrative and Comparative Physiology* 301: R524–33.

Kurz, A., Sessler, D. I. and Lenhardt, R. (1996) Perioperative normothermia to reduce the incidence of surgical-wound infection and shorten hospitalization. Study of Wound Infection and Temperature Group. *New England Journal of Medicine* 334: 1209–15.

Kvetnansky, R., Davydova, N. A., Noskov, V. B., Vigas, M., Popova, I. A., Usakov, A. C., Macho, L. and Grigoriev, A. I. (1988) Plasma and urine catecholamine levels in cosmonauts during long-term stay on Space Station Salyut-7. *Acta Astronautica* 17: 181–6.

La Cava, A. and Matarese, G. (2004) The weight of leptin in immunity. *Nature Reviews Immunology* 4: 371–9.

Laaksi, I. (2012) Vitamin D and respiratory infection in adults. *Proceedings of the Nutrition Society* 71: 90–7.

Laaksi, I., Ruohola, J. P., Tuohimaa, P., Auvinen, A., Haataja, R., Pihlajamaki, H. and Ylikomi, T. (2007) An association of serum vitamin D concentrations < 40 nmol/L with acute respiratory tract infection in young Finnish men. *American Journal of Clinical Nutrition* 86: 714–17.

Laaksi, I., Ruohola, J. P., Mattila, V., Auvinen, A., Ylikomi, T. and Pihlajamaki, H. (2010) Vitamin D supplementation for the prevention of acute respiratory tract infection: a randomized, double-blinded trial among young Finnish men. *Journal of Infectious Disease* 202: 809–14.

Laing, S. J., Oliver, S. J., Wilson, S., Walters, R., Bilzon, J. L. and Walsh, N. P. (2008) Neutrophil-degranulation and lymphocyte-subset response after 48 hr of fluid and/or energy restriction. *International Journal of Sport Nutrition and Exercise Metabolism* 18: 443–56.

Lakier, S. L. (2003) Overtraining, excessive exercise, and altered immunity: is this a T helper-1 versus T helper-2 lymphocyte response? *Sports Medicine* 33: 347–64.

Lamm, M. E. (1998) Current concepts in mucosal immunity IV. How epithelial transport of IgA antibodies related to host defense. *American Journal of Physiology* 274: G614–17.

Lancaster, G. I., Halson, S. L., Khan, Q., Drysdale, P., Jeukendrup, A. E., Drayson, M. T. and Gleeson, M. (2003) Effect of acute exhaustive exercise and a 6-day period of intensified training on immune function in cyclists. *Journal of Physiology* 548.P: O96.

Lancaster, G. I., Halson, S. L., Khan, Q., Drysdale, P., Wallace, F., Jeukendrup, A. E., Drayson, M. T. and Gleeson, M. (2004) Effects of acute exhaustive exercise and chronic exercise training on type 1 and type 2 T lymphocytes. *Exercise Immunology Review* 10: 91–106.

Lancaster, G. I., Khan, Q., Drysdale, P., Wallace, F., Jeukendrup, A. E., Drayson, M. T. and Gleeson, M. (2005a) Effect of prolonged strenuous exercise and carbohydrate ingestion on type 1 and type 2 T lymphocyte intracellular cytokine production in humans. *Journal of Applied Physiology* 98: 565–71.

Lancaster, G. I., Khan, Q., Drysdale, P., Wallace, F., Jeukendrup, A. E., Drayson, M. T. and Gleeson, M. (2005b) The physiological regulation of toll–like receptor expression and function in humans. *Journal of Physiology* 563: 945–55.

LaPerriere, A., Antoni, M. H., Schneiderman, N., Ironson, G., Klimas, N., Caralis, P. and Fletcher, M. A. (1990) Exercise intervention attenuates emotional distress and natural killer cell decrements following notification of positive serologic status for HIV-1. *Biofeedback and Self-Regulation* 15: 229–42.

LaPerriere, A., Fletcher, M. A., Antoni, M. H., Klimas, N. G., Ironson, G. and Schneiderman, N. (1991) Aerobic exercise training in an AIDS risk group. *International Journal of Sports Medicine* 12(Suppl 1): S53–7.

Larrabee, R. C. (1902) Leucocytosis after violent exercise. *Journal of Medical Research* 7: 76–82.

Larson-Meyer, D. E. and Willis, K. S. (2010) Vitamin D and athletes. *Current Sports Medicine Reports* 9: 220–6.

Leeder, J., Glaister, M., Pizzoferro, K., Dawson, J. and Pedlar, C. (2012) Sleep duration and quality in elite athletes measured using wristwatch actigraphy. *Journal of Sports Sciences* 30: 541–5.

Lehmann, M., Foster, C., Dickuth, H. H. and Gastmann, U. (1998) Autonomic imbalance hypothesis and overtraining syndrome. *Medicine and Science in Sports and Exercise* 30: 1140–5.

Lehtonen, O. P., Tenovuo, J., Aaltonen, A. S. and Vilja, P. (1987) Immunoglobulins and innate factors of immunity in saliva of children prone to respiratory infections. *Acta Pathologica, Microbiologica et Immunologica Scandinavica* 95: 35–40.

Leicht, C. A., Bishop, N. C. and Goosey-Tolfrey, V. L. (2011) Mucosal immune responses to treadmill exercise in elite wheelchair athletes. *Medicine and Science in Sports and Exercise* 43:1414–21.

Leicht, C.A., Bishop, N. C. and Goosey-Tolfrey, V. L. (2012a) Mucosal immune responses during court training in elite tetraplegic athletes. *Spinal Cord* 50: 760–5.

Leicht, C. A., Bishop, N. C., Paulson, T. A. W., Griggs, K. E. and Goosey-Tolfrey, V. L. (2012b) Salivary immunoglobulin A and upper respiratory symptoms during five months of training in elite tetraplegic athletes. *International Journal of Sports Physiology and Performance* 7: 210–13.

Leon, L. R. and Helwig, B. G. (2010) Heat stroke: role of the systemic inflammatory response. *Journal of Applied Physiology* 109: 1980–8.

Leon, L. R., Blaha, M. D. and DuBose, D. A. (2006) Time course of cytokine, corticosterone, and tissue injury responses in mice during heat strain recovery. *Journal of Applied Physiology* 100: 1400–9.

Lesourd, B., Raynaud-Simon, A. and Mazari, L. (2002) Nutrition and ageing of the immune system. In: P. C. Calder, C. J. Field and H. S. Gill (Editors), *Nutrition and Immune Function.* Oxford: CABI Publishing, pp. 357–74.

Levy, S. M., Herberman, R. B., Lee, J., Whiteside, T., Beadle, M., Heiden, L. and Simons, A. (1991) Persistently low natural killer cell activity, age, and environmental stress as predictors of infectious morbidity. *Nature Immunology and Cell Growth Regulation* 10: 289–307.

Lewicki, R., Tchorzewski, H., Denys, A., Kowalska, M. and Golinska, A. (1987) Effect of physical exercise on some parameters of immunity in conditioned sportsmen. *International Journal of Sports Medicine* 8: 309–14.

Li, P., Yin, Y. L., Li, D., Kim, S. W. and Wu, G. (2007) Amino acids and immune function. *British Journal of Nutrition* 98: 237–52.

Li, T. L. and Gleeson, M. (2004) The effect of single and repeated bouts of prolonged cycling and circadian variation on saliva flow rate, immunoglobulin A and alpha-amylase responses. *Journal of Sports Sciences* 22: 1015–24.

Liao, H. F., Chiang, L. M., Yen, C. C., Chen, Y. Y., Zhuang, R. R., Lai, L. Y., Chiang, J. and Chen, Y. J. (2006) Effect of a periodized exercise training and active recovery program on antitumor activity and development of dendritic cells. *Journal of Sports Medicine and Physical Fitness* 46: 307–14.

Libicz, S., Mercier, B., Bigou, N., Le Gallais, D. and Castex, F. (2006) Salivary IgA response of triathletes participating in the French Iron Tour. *International Journal of Sports Medicine* 27: 389–94.

Liew, F. Y. (2002) T(H)1 and T(H)2 cells: a historical perspective. *Nature Reviews Immunology* 2: 55–60.

Lim, C. L. and Mackinnon, L. T. (2006) The roles of exercise-induced immune system disturbances in the pathology of heat stroke : the dual pathway model of heat stroke. *Sports Medicine* 36: 39–64.

Lim, C. L., Wilson, G., Brown, L., Coombes, J. S. and Mackinnon, L. T. (2007) Pre-existing inflammatory state compromises heat tolerance in rats exposed to heat stress. *American Journal of Physiology – Regulatory, Integrative and Comparative Physiology* 292: R186–94.

Lin, M. T. (1997) Heatstroke-induced cerebral ischemia and neuronal damage. Involvement of cytokines and monoamines. *Annals of the New York Academy of Sciences* 813: 572–80.

Linde, K., Barrett, B., Wolkart, K., Bauer, R. and Melchart, D. (2006) Echinacea for preventing and treating the common cold. *Cochrane Database of Systematic Reviews* CD000530.

Lumme, A., Haahtela, T., Ounap, J., Rytila, P., Obase, Y., Helenius, M., Remes, V. and Helenius, I. (2003) Airway inflammation, bronchial hyperresponsiveness and asthma in elite ice hockey players. *European Respiratory Journal* 22: 113–17.

Lundby, C., Calbet, J. A., Sander, M., van Hall, G., Mazzeo, R. S., Stray-Gundersen, J., Stager, J. M., Chapman, R. F., Saltin, B. and Levine, B. D. (2007) Exercise economy does not change after acclimatization to moderate to very high altitude. *Scandinavian Journal of Medicine and Science in Sports* 17: 281–91.

Lykkesfeldt, J., Rose, A. J., Fischer, C. P. and Pedersen, B. K. (2010) Antioxidant supplementation does not alter endurance training adaptation. *Medicine and Science in Sports Exercise* 42: 1388–95.

McAnulty, S.R., Nieman, D.C., Fox-Rabinovich, M., Duran, V., McAnulty, L.S., Henson, D.A., Jin, F. and Landram, M.J. (2010) Effect of n-3 fatty acids and antioxidants on oxidative stress after exercise. *Medicine and Science in Sports Exercise* 42: 1704–1711.

McAuley, E., Hu, L., Chapman-Novakofski, K. and Woods, J. A. (2008) Cardiovascular exercise intervention improves the primary antibody response to keyhole limpet hemocyanin (KLH) in previously sedentary older adults. *Brain, Behavior and Immunity* 22: 923–32.

McCarthy, D. A. and Dale, M. M. (1988) The leukocytosis of exercise. *Journal of Sports Medicine* 6: 333–63.

McCarthy, D. A., Macdonald, I., Grant, M., Marbut, M., Watling, M., Nicholson, S., Deeks, J. J., Wade, A. J. and Perry, J. D. (1992a) Studies on the immediate and delayed leukocytosis elicited by brief (30-min) strenuous exercise. *European Journal of Applied Physiology* 64: 513–17.

McCarthy, D. A., Macdonald, I. A., Shaker, H. A., Hart, P., Georgiannos, S., Deeks, J. and Wade, A. J. (1992b) Changes in the leukocyte count during and after brief intense exercise. *European Journal of Applied Physiology* 64: 518–22.

McClung, J. P., Hasday, J. D., He, J. R., Montain, S. J., Cheuvront, S. N., Sawka, M. N. and Singh, I. S. (2008) Exercise-heat acclimation in humans alters baseline levels and ex vivo heat inducibility of HSP72 and HSP90 in peripheral blood mononuclear cells. *American Journal of Physiology – Regulatory, Integrative and Comparative Physiology* 294: R185–91.

McElroy, B. H. and Miller, S. P. (2002) Effectiveness of zinc gluconate glycine lozenges (Cold–Eeze) against the common cold in school-aged subjects: a retrospective chart review. *American Journal of Therapy* 9: 472–5.

McFadden, E. R., Pichurko, B. M., Bowman, H. F., Ingenito, E., Burns, S., Dowling, N. and Solway, J. (1985) Thermal mapping of the airways in humans. *Journal of Applied Physiology* 58: 564–70.

McFarlin, B. K., Flynn, M. G., Campbell, W. W., Stewart, L. K. and Timmerman, K. L. (2004) TLR4 is lower in resistance-trained older women and related to inflammatory cytokines. *Medicine and Science in Sports Exercise* 36: 1876–83.

McFarlin, B. K., Flynn, M. G., Phillips, M. D., Stewart, L. K. and Timmerman, K. L. (2005) Chronic resistance exercise training improves natural killer cell activity in older women. *Journals of Gerontology Series A: Biological Sciences and Medical Sciences* 60: 1315–18.

McFarlin, B. K., Flynn, M. G., Stewart, L. K. and Timmerman, K. L. (2004) Carbohydrate intake during endurance exercise increases natural killer cell responsiveness to IL-2. *Journal of Applied Physiology* 96: 271–5.

McGuirk, P. and Mills, K. H. (2002) Pathogen-specific regulatory T cells provoke a shift in the Th1/Th2 paradigm in immunity to infectious diseases. *Trends in Immunology* 23: 450–5.

Macha, M., Shlafer, M. and Kluger, M. J. (1990) Human neutrophil hydrogen peroxide generation following physical exercise. *Journal of Sports Medicine and Physical Fitness* 30: 412–19.

Mackinnon, L. T. (1996) Exercise, immunoglobulin and antibody. *Exercise Immunology Review* 2: 1–35.

Mackinnon, L. T. (1998) Effects of overreaching and overtraining on immune function. In: R. B. Kreider, A. C. Fry and M. L. O'Toole (Editors). *Overtraining In Sport.* Champaign IL: Human Kinetics. pp. 219–41.

Mackinnon, L. T. (2000) Overtraining effects on immunity and performance in athletes. *Immunology and Cell Biology* 78: 502–9.

Mackinnon, L. T. and Hooper, S. (1994) Mucosal (secretory) immune system responses to exercise of varying intensity and during overtraining. *International Journal of Sports Medicine* 15: S179–83.

Mackinnon, L. T. and Hooper, S. L. (1996) Plasma glutamine and upper respiratory tract infection during intensified training in swimmers. *Medicine and Science in Sports Exercise* 28: 285–90.

Mackinnon, L. T., Chick, T. W., van As, A. and Tomasi, T. B. (1989) Decreased secretory immunoglobulins following intense endurance exercise. *Sports Medicine, Training and Rehabilitation* 1: 209–18.

Mackinnon, L. T., Ginn, E. and Seymour, G. J. (1991) Temporal relationship between exercise-induced decreases in salivary IgA concentration and subsequent appearance of upper respiratory illness in elite athletes. *Medicine and Science in Sports Exercise* 23: S45.

Macknin, M. L. (1999) Zinc lozenges for the common cold. *Cleveland Clinic Journal of Medicine* 66: 27–32.

MacNeil, B. and Hoffman-Goetz, L. (1993) Chronic exercise enhances in vivo and in vitro cytotoxic mechanisms of natural immunity in mice. *Journal of Applied Physiology* 74: 388–95.

Maffei, M., Funicello, M., Vottari, T., Gamucci, O., Costa, M., Lisi, S., Viegi, A., Ciampi, O., Bardi, G., Vitti, P., Pinchera, A. and Santini, F. (2009) The obesity and inflammatory marker haptoglobin attracts monocytes via interaction with chemokine (C-C motif) receptor 2 (CCR2). *BMC Biology* 17: 87.

Main, L. C., Dawson, B., Heel, J.K., Grove, R., Landers G. J. and Goodman, C. (2010) Relationship between inflammatory cytokines and self-report measures of training overload. *Research in Sports Medicine* 2: 127–39.

Makinen, T. M., Juvonen, R., Jokelainen, J., Harju, T. H., Peitso, A., Bloigu, A., Silven-noinen-Kassinen, S., Leinonen, M. and Hassi, J. (2009) Cold temperature and low humidity are associated with increased occurrence of respiratory tract infections. *Respiratory Medicine* 103: 456–62.

Malm, C. (2006) Susceptibility to infections in elite athletes: the S curve. *Scandinavian Journal of Medicine and Science in Sports* 16: 4–6.

Maloy, K. J. and Powrie, F. (2001) Regulatory T cells in the control of immune pathology. *Nature Immunology* 2: 816–22.

Maloy, K. J., Salaun, L., Cahill, R., Dougan, G., Saunders, N. J. and Powrie, F. (2003) CD4+CD25+ T(R) cells suppress innate immune pathology through cytokine-dependent mechanisms. *Journal of Experimental Medicine* 197: 111–19.

Maron, M. B., Wagner, J. A. and Horvath, S. M. (1977) Thermoregulatory responses during competitive marathon running. *Journal of Applied Physiology* 42: 909–14.

Mars, M., Govender, S., Weston, A., Naicker, V. and Chuturgoon, A. (1998) High intensity exercise: a cause of lymphocyte apoptosis? *Biochemical and Biophysical Research Communications* 249: 366–70.

Marshall, I. (2000) Zinc for the common cold. *Cochrane Database of Systematic Reviews* CD001364.

Martinez, F. O., Sica, A., Mantovani, A. and Locati, M. (2008) Macrophage activation and polarization. *Frontiers in Bioscience* 13: 453–61.

Mathis, D. and Shoelson, S. (2011) Immunometabolism: an emerging frontier. *Nature Reviews Immunology* 11: 81.

Mathur, N. and Pedersen, B. K. (2008) Exercise as a mean to control low-grade inflammation. *Mediators of Inflammation* 2008:109502.

Matsui, M., Araya, S., Wang, H. Y., Onai, N., Matsushima, K. and Saida, T. (2003) Circulating lymphocyte subsets linked to intracellular cytokine profiles in normal humans. *Clinical Experimental Immunology* 134: 225–31.

Matsui, T., Ishikawa, T., Ito, H., Okamoto, M., Inoue, K., Lee, M.C., Fujikawa, T., Ichitani, Y., Kawanaka, K. and Soya, H. (2012) Brain glycogen supercompensation following exhaustive exercise. *Journal of Physiology* 590: 607–16.

Matsuzaki, T. (1998) Immunomodulation by treatment with Lactobacillus casei strain Shirota. *International Journal of Food Microbiology* 41: 133–40.

Matthews, C. E., Ockene, I. S., Freedson, P. S., Rosal, M. C., Merriam, P. A. and Hebert, J. R. (2002) Moderate to vigorous physical activity and the risk of upper-respiratory tract infection. *Medicine and Science in Sports Exercise* 34: 1242–8.

Mattusch, F., Dufaux, B., Heine, O., Mertens, I. and Rost, R. (2000) Reduction of the plasma concentration of C-reactive protein following nine months of endurance training. *International Journal of Sports Medicine* 21: 21–4.

Maynard, C. L. and Weaver, C. T. (2008) Diversity in the contribution of IL-10 to cell-mediated immune regulation. *Immunology Review* 226: 219–33.

Mazzeo, R. S. (2005) Altitude, exercise and immune function. *Exercise Immunology Review* 11: 6–16.

Mazzeo, R. S. and Reeves, J. T. (2003) Adrenergic contribution during acclimatization to high altitude: perspectives from Pikes Peak. *Exercise and Sport Sciences Reviews* 31: 13–18.

Mazzeo, R. S., Rajkumar, C., Rolland, J., Blaher, B., Jennings, G. and Esler, M. (1998) Immune response to a single bout of exercise in young and elderly subjects. *Mechanisms of Ageing and Development* 100: 121–32.

Meckel, Y., Eliakim, A., Seraev, M., Zaldivar, F., Cooper, D. M., Sagiv, M. and Nemet, D. (2009) The effect of a brief sprint interval exercise on growth factors and inflammatory mediators. *Journal of Strength and Conditioning Research* 23: 225–30.

Medzhitov, R. (2001) Toll-like receptors and innate immunity. *Nature Reviews Immunology* 1: 135–45.

Meehan, R., Duncan, U., Neale, L., Taylor, G., Muchmore, H., Scott, N., Ramsey, K., Smith, E., Rock, P. and Goldblum, R. (1988) Operation Everest II: alterations in the immune system at high altitudes. *Journal of Clinical Immunology* 8: 397–406.

Meeusen, R., Duclos, M., Foster, C., Fry, A., Gleeson, M., Nieman, D., Raglin, J., Rietjens, G., Steinacker, J. and Urhausen, A. (2013) Prevention, diagnosis and treatment of the Overtraining Syndrome. Joint consensus statement of the European College of Sport Science (ECSS) and the American College of Sports Medicine (ACSM). *European Journal of Sport Science* 13: 1–24.

Mehta, S. K., Stowe, R. P., Feiveson, A. H., Tyring, S. K. and Pierson, D. L. (2000) Reactivation and shedding of cytomegalovirus in astronauts during spaceflight. *Journal of Infectious Disease* 182: 1761–4.

Melhus, A. (2005) Fluoroquinolones and tendon disorders. *Expert opinion on drug safety* 4: 299–309.

Mengheri, E. (2008) Health, probiotics, and inflammation. *Journal of Clinical Gastroenterology* 42: S177–8.

Meyer, T. M., Gabriel, H., Ratz, M., Muller, H. J. and Kindermann, W. (2001) Anaerobic exercise induces moderate acute phase response. *Medicine and Science in Sports Exercise* 33: 549–55.

Michishita, R., Shono, N., Inoue, T., Tsuruta, T. and Node, K. (2008) Associations of monocytes, neutrophil count, and C-reactive protein with maximal oxygen uptake in overweight women. *Journal of Cardiology* 52: 247–53.

Michishita, R., Shono, N., Inoue, T., Tsuruta, T. and Node, K. (2010) Effect of exercise therapy on monocyte and neutrophil counts in overweight women. *American Journal of Medical Science* 339: 152–6.

Miles, M.P., Mackinnon, L.T., Grove, D.S., Williams, N.I., Bush, J.A., Marx, J.O., Kraemer, W.J. and Mastro, A.M. (2002) The relationship of natural killer cell counts, perforin mRNA and CD2 expression to post–exercise natural killer cell activity in humans. *Acta Physiologica Scandinavica* 174: 317–325.

Miles, M. P., Kraemer, W. J., Nindl, B. C., Grove, D. S., Leach, S. K., Dohi, K., Marx, J. O., Volek, J. S. and Mastro, A. M. (2003) Strength, workload, anaerobic intensity and the immune response to resistance exercise in women. *Acta Physiologica Scandinavica* 178: 155–63.

Miller, G. E. and Cohen, S. (2001) Psychological interventions and the immune system: a meta-analytic review and critique. *Health Psychology* 20: 47–63.

Mills, P. J., Hong, S., Redwine, L., Carter, S.M., Chiu, A., Ziegler, M. G., Dimsdale, J. E. and Maisel, A. S. (2006) Physical fitness attenuates leukocyte-endothelial adhesion in response to acute exercise. *Journal of Applied Physiology* 101: 785–8.

Minocha, A. (2009) Probiotics for preventive health. *Nutrition in Clinical Practice* 24: 227–41.

Mitchell, J. B., Pizza, F. X., Paquet, A., Davis, B. J., Forrest, M. B. and Braun, W. A. (1998) Influence of carbohydrate status on immune responses before and after endurance exercise. *Journal of Applied Physiology* 84: 1917–25.

Miyagi, M., Aoyama, H., Morishits, M., Iwamoto, Y. (1992) Effects of sex hormones on chemotaxis of human peripheral polymorphonuclear leukocytes and monocytes. *Journal of Periodontology* 63: 28–32.

Miyashita, M., Burns, S. F. and Stensel, D. J. (2008) Accumulating short bouts of brisk walking reduces postprandial plasma triacylglycerol concentrations and resting blood pressure in healthy young men. *American Journal of Clinical Nutrition* 88: 1225–31.

Moll, H. (2003) Dendritic cells and host resistance to infection. *Cellular Microbiology* 5: 493–500.

Moore, G. E., Holbein, M. E. and Knochel, J. P. (1995) Exercise-associated collapse in cyclists is unrelated to endotoxemia. *Medicine and Science in Sports and Exercise* 27: 1238–42.

Moore, K. W., de Waal Malefyt, R., Coffman, R. L. and O'Garra, A. (2001) Interleukin-10 and the interleukin-10 receptor. *Annual Review of Immunology* 19: 683–765.

Mooren, F. C., Bloming, D., Lechtermann, A., Lerch, M. M. and Volker, K. (2002) Lymphocyte apoptosis after exhaustive and moderate exercise. *Journal of Applied Physiology* 93: 147–53.

Mooren, F. C., Lechtermann, A. and Volker, K. (2004) Exercise-induced apoptosis of lymphocytes depends on training status. *Medicine and Science in Sports Exercise* 36: 1476–83.

Moraska, A., Deak, T., Spencer, R. L., Roth, D. and Fleshner, M. (2000) Treadmill running produces both positive and negative physiological adaptations in Sprague-Dawley rats. *American Journal of Physiology – Regulatory, Integrative and Comparative Physiology* 279: R1321–9.

Morgado, J. M., Rama, L., Matos, A., Silva I., Inacio M. J., Henriques A., Laranjeira, P., Rosado, F., Alves, F., Gleeson, M., Pais, M. L., Paiva, A. and Teixeira, A. M. (2012) Cytokine production by monocytes, neutrophils and dendritic cells is hampered by long term intensive training in elite swimmers. *European Journal of Applied Physiology* 112: 471–82.

Morgan, W. P., Brown, D. R. and Raglin, J. S. (1987) Mood disturbance following increased training in swimmers. *British Journal of Sports Medicine* 21: 107–14.

Morimoto, A., Murakami, N., Ono, T. and Watanabe, T. (1986) Dehydration enhances endotoxin fever by increased production of endogenous pyrogen. *American Journal of Physiology* 251: R41–7.

Mosmann, T. R. and Sad, S. (1996) The expanding universe of T-cell subsets: Th1, Th2 and more. *Immunology Today* 17: 138–46.

Moyna, N. M., Acker, G. R., Fulton, J. R., Weber, K., Goss, F. L., Robertson, R. J., Tollerud, D. J. and Rabin, B. S. (1996a) Lymphocyte function and cytokine production during incremental exercise in active and sedentary males and females. *International Journal of Sports Medicine* 17: 585–91.

Moyna, N. M., Acker, G. R., Weber, K. M., Fulton, J. R., Goss, F. L., Robertson, R. J. and Rabin, B. S. (1996b) The effects of incremental submaximal exercise on circulating leukocytes in physically active and sedentary males and females. *European Journal of Applied Physiology Occupational Physiology* 74: 211–18.

Moynihan, J. A., Callahan, T. A., Kelley, S. P. and Campbell, L. M. (1998) Adrenal hormone modulation of type 1 and type 2 cytokine production by spleen cells: dexamethasone and dehydroepiandrosterone suppress interleukin-2, interleukin-4, and interferon-gamma production in vitro. *Cellular Immunology* 184: 58–64.

Muldoon, S., Deuster, P., Brandom, B. and Bunger, R. (2004) Is there a link between malignant hyperthermia and exertional heat illness? *Exercise and Sport Sciences Reviews* 32: 174–9.

Munegowda, M. A., Xu, S., Freywald, A. and Xiang, J. (2012) CD4+ Th2 cells function alike effector Tr1 and Th1 cells through the deletion of a single cytokine IL-6 and IL-10 gene. *Molecular Immunology* 51: 143–9.

Munoz, C., Rios, E., Olivos, J., Brunser, O. and Olivares, M. (2007) Iron, copper and immunocompetence. *British Journal of Nutrition* 98(Suppl1): S24–8.

Murdoch, D. R. (1995) Symptoms of infection and altitude illness among hikers in the Mount Everest region of Nepal. *Aviation, Space, and Environmental Medicine* 66: 148–51.

Murphy, E. A., Davis, J. M., Brown, A. S., Carmichael, M. D., Van Rooijen, N., Ghaffar, A. and Mayer, E. P. (2004) Role of lung macrophages on susceptibility to respiratory infection following short-term moderate exercise training. *American Journal of Physiology* 287: R1354–8.

Mustafa, A., Ward, A., Treasure, J. and Peakman, M. (1997) T lymphocyte subpopulations in anorexia nervosa and refeeding. *Clinical Immunology and Immunopathology* 82: 282–9.

Mustafa, T., Sy, F. S., Macera, C. A., Thompson, S. J., Jackson, K. L., Selassie, A. and Dean, L. L. (1999) Association between exercise and HIV disease progression in a cohort of homosexual men. *Annals of Epidemiology* 9: 127–31.

Mylona, E., Fahlman, M. M., Morgan, A. L., Boardley, D. and Tsivitse, S. K. (2002) s-IgA response in females following a single bout of moderate intensity exercise in cold and thermoneutral environments. *International Journal of Sports Medicine* 23: 453–6.

Nagao, F., Suzuki, M., Takeda, K., Yagita, H. and Okumura, K. (2000) Mobilization of NK cells by exercise: downmodulation of adhesion molecules on NK cells by catecholamines. *American Journal of Physiology* 279: R1251–6.

Nagler-Anderson, C. (2001) Man the barrier! Strategic defences in the intestinal mucosa. *Nature Reviews Immunology* 1: 59–67.

Nahas, G. G., Tannieres, M. L. and Lennon, J. F. (1971) Direct measurement of leukocyte motility: effects of pH and temperature. *Proceedings of the Society for Experimental Biology and Medicine* 138: 350–2.

Nairz, M., Schroll, A., Sonnweber, T. and Weiss, G. (2010) The struggle for iron – a metal at the host–pathogen interface. *Cellular Microbiology* 12: 1691–702.

Nance, D. M. and Sanders, V. M. (2007) Autonomic innervation and regulation of the immune system (1987–2007). *Brain, Behavior and Immunity* 21: 736–45.

Nash, M. S. (2000) Immune dysfunction and illness susceptibility after spinal cord injury: an overview of probable causes, likely consequences, and potential treatments. *Journal of Spinal Cord Medicine* 23: 109–10.

Nehlsen-Cannarella, S. L., Fagoaga, O. R., Nieman, D. C., Henson, D. A., Butterworth, D. E., Schmitt, R. L., Bailey, E. M., Warren, B. J., Utter, A. and Davis, J. M. (1997) Carbohydrate and the cytokine response to 2.5 h of running. *Journal of Applied Physiology* 82: 1662–7.

Nehlsen-Cannarella, S. L., Nieman, D. C., Jesson, J., Chang, G., Gusewitch, G. G., Blix, G. G. and Ashley, E. (1991) The effects of acute moderate exercise on lymphocyte function and serum immunoglobulin levels. *International Journal of Sports Medicine* 12: 391–8.

Neville, V., Gleeson, M. and Folland, J. P. (2008) Salivary IgA as a risk factor for upper respiratory infections in elite professional athletes. *Medicine and Science in Sports and Exercise* 40: 1228–36.

Newsholme, E. A. (1994) Biochemical mechanisms to explain immunosuppression in well-trained and overtrained athletes. *International Journal of Sports Medicine* 15: S142–7.

Newsholme, E. A and Leech, A. R. (1983) *Biochemistry for the Medical Sciences.* New York: John Wiley and Sons.

Newsholme, E. A. and Leech, A. R. (1983) *Functional Biochemistry in Health and Disease.* New York: Wiley-Blackwell.

Newsholme, E. A. and Start, C. (1973) *Regulation in Metabolism.* New York: John Wiley and Sons.

Nicholson, J. P. and Case, D. B. (1983) Carboxyhemoglobin levels in New York city runners. *Physician Sportsmedicine* 11: 134–8.

Nickel, T., Emslander, I., Sisic, Z., David, R., Schmaderer, C., Marx, N., Schmidt-Trucksass, A., Hoster, E., Halle, M., Weis, M. and Hanssen, H. (2011) Modulation of dendritic cells and toll–like receptors by marathon running. *European Journal of Applied Physiology* 112: 1699–708.

Nickerson, C. A., Ott, C. M., Mister, S. J., Morrow, B. J., Burns-Keliher, L. and Pierson, D. L. (2000) Microgravity as a novel environmental signal affecting Salmonella enterica serovar Typhimurium virulence. *Infectious Immunity* 68: 3147–52.

Nielsen, H. B., Secher, N. H., Christensen, N. J. and Pedersen, B. K. (1996) Lymphocytes and NK cell activity during repeated bouts of maximal exercise. *American Journal of Physiology* 271: R222–7.

Nielsen, H. B., Secher, N. H., Kristensen, J. H., Christensen, N. J., Espersen, K. and Pedersen, B. K. (1997) Splenectomy impairs lymphocytosis during maximal exercise. *American Journal of Physiology* 272: R1847–52.

Nielsen, H. B., Secher, N. H., Kappel, M. and Pedersen, B. K. (1998) N-acetylcysteine does not affect the lymphocyte proliferation and natural killer cell activity responses to exercise. *American Journal of Physiology* 275: R1227–31.

Nielsen, H. G. and Lyberg, T. (2004) Long-distance running modulates the expression of leucocyte and endothelial adhesion molecules. *Scandinavian Journal of Immunology* 60: 356–62.

Nieman, D. C. (1994a) Exercise, infection and immunity. *International Journal of Sports Medicine* 15: S131–41.

Nieman, D. C. (1994b) Exercise, upper respiratory tract infection, and the immune system. *Medicine and Science in Sports and Exercise* 26: 128–39.

Nieman, D. C. (1998) Influence of carbohydrate on the immune response to intensive, prolonged exercise. *Exercise Immunology Review* 4: 64–76.

Nieman, D. C. (2000) Is infection risk linked to exercise workload? *Medicine and Science in Sports and Exercise* 32: S406–11.

Nieman, D. C. and Nehlsen-Cannarella, S. L. (1992) Exercise and Infection. In: R. R. Watson and M. Eisinger (Editors), *Exercise and Disease*. Boca Raton, LA: CRC Publishers, pp. 121–48.

Nieman, D. C., Johansen, L. M. and Lee, J. W. (1989a) Infectious episodes in runners before and after a road race. *Journal of Sports Medicine and Physical Fitness* 29: 289–96.

Nieman, D. C., Berk, L. S., Simpson-Westerberg, M., Arabatzis, K., Youngberg, S., Tan, S. A., Lee, J. W. and Eby, W. C. (1989b) Effects of long-endurance running on immune system parameters and lymphocyte function in experienced marathoners. *International Journal of Sports Medicine* 10: 317–23.

Nieman, D. C., Buckley, K. S., Henson, D. A., Warren, B. J., Suttles, J., Ahle, J. C., Simandle, S., Fagoaga, O. R. and Nehlsen-Cannarella, S. L. (1995) Immune function in marathon runners versus sedentary controls. *Medicine and Science in Sports and Exercise* 27: 986–92.

Nieman, D. C., Tan, S. A., Lee, J. W. and Berk, L. S. (1989c) Complement and immunoglobulin levels in athletes and sedentary controls. *International Journal of Sports Medicine* 10: 124–8.

Nieman, D. C., Johansen, L. M., Lee, J. W. and Arabatzis, K. (1990a) Infectious episodes in runners before and after the Los Angeles Marathon. *Journal of Sports Medicine and Physical Fitness* 30: 316–28.

Nieman, D. C., Nehlsen-Cannarella, S. L., Markoff, P. A., Balk-Lamberton, A. J., Yang, H., Chritton, D. B., Lee, J. W. and Arabatzis, K. (1990b) The effects of moderate exercise training on natural killer cells and acute upper respiratory tract infections. *International Journal of Sports Medicine* 11: 467–73.

Nieman, D. C., Henson, D. A., Gusewitch, G., Warren, B. J., Dotson, R. C., Butterworth, D. E. and Nehlsen-Cannarella, S. L. (1993a) Physical activity and immune function in elderly women. *Medicine and Science in Sports and Exercise* 25: 823–31.

Nieman, D. C., Miller, A. R., Henson, D. A., Warren, B. J., Gusewitch, G., Johnson, R. L., Davis, J. M., Butterworth, D. E. and Nehlsen-Cannarella, S. L. (1993b) Effect of high- versus moderate-intensity exercise on natural killer activity. *Medicine and Science in Sports and Exercise* 25: 1126–34.

Nieman, D. C., Miller, A. R., Henson, D. A., Warren, B. J., Gusewitch, G., Johnson, R. L., Davis, J. M., Butterworth, D. E., Herring, J. L. and Nehlsen-Cannarella, S. L. (1994) Effect of high- versus moderate-intensity exercise on lymphocyte subpopulations and proliferative response. *International Journal of Sports Medicine* 15: 199–206.

Nieman, D. C., Buckley, K. S., Henson, D. A., Warren, B. J., Suttles, J., Ahle, J. C., Simandle, S., Fagoaga, O. R. and Nehlsen-Cannarella, S. L. (1995) Immune function in marathon runners versus sedentary controls. *Medicine and Science in Sports and Exercise* 27: 986–92.

Nieman, D. C., Henson, D. A., Garner, E. B., Butterworth, D. E., Warren, B. J., Utter, A., Davis, J. M., Fagoaga, O. R. and Nehlsen-Cannarella, S. L. (1997) Carbohydrate affects natural killer cell redistribution but not activity after running. *Medicine and Science in Sports and Exercise* 29: 1318–24.

Nieman, D. C., Nehlsen-Cannarella, S. L., Fagoaga, O. R., Henson, D. A., Utter, A., Davis, J. M., Williams, F. and Butterworth, D. E. (1998a) Effects of mode and carbohydrate on the granulocyte and monocyte response to intensive, prolonged exercise. *Journal of Applied Physiology* 84: 1252–9.

Nieman, D. C., Nehlsen-Cannarella, S. L., Fagoaga, O. R., Henson, D. R. U. A., Utter, A., Davis, J., Williams, F. and Butterworth, D. E. (1998b) Influence of mode and carbohydrate on the cytokine response to heavy exertion. *Medicine and Science in Sports and Exercise* 30: 671–8.

Nieman, D. C., Henson, D. A., Smith, L. L., Utter, A. C., Vinci, D. M., Davis, M. J., Kaminsky, D. E. and Shute, M. (2001) Cytokine changes after a marathon race. *Journal of Applied Physiology* 91:109–14.

Nieman, D. C., Henson, D. A., Nehlsen-Cannarella, S. L., Ekkens, M., Utter, A. C., Butterworth, D. E. and Fagoaga, O. R. (1999) Influence of obesity on immune function. *Journal of the American Dietetic Association* 99: 294–9.

Nieman, D. C., Henson, D. A., Fagoaga, O. R., Utter, A. C., Vinci, D. M., Davis, J. M. and Nehlsen-Cannarella, S. L. (2002a) Change in salivary IgA following a competitive marathon race. *International Journal of Sports Medicine* 23: 69–75.

Nieman, D. C., Henson, D. A., McAnulty, S. R., McAnulty, L., Swick, N. S., Utter, A. C., Vinci, D. M., Opiela, S. J. and Morrow, J. D. (2002b) Influence of vitamin C supplementation on oxidative and immune changes after an ultramarathon. *Journal of Applied Physiology* 92: 1970–7.

Nieman, D. C., Davis, J. M., Henson, D. A., Walberg-Rankin, J., Shute, M., Dumke, C. L., Utter, A. C., Vinci, D. M., Carson, J. A., Brown, A., Lee, W. J., McAnulty, S. R. and McAnulty, L. S. (2003a) Carbohydrate ingestion influences skeletal muscle cytokine mRNA and plasma cytokine levels after a 3-h run. *Journal of Applied Physiology* 94: 1917–25.

Nieman, D. C., Dumke, C. I., Henson, D. A., McAnulty, S. R., McAnulty, L. S., Lind, R. H. and Morrow, J. D. (2003b) Immune and oxidative changes during and following the Western States Endurance Run. *International Journal of Sports Medicine* 24: 541–7.

Nieman, D.C., Davis, J.M., Brown, V.A., Henson, D.A., Dumke, C.L., Utter, A.C., Vinci, D.M., Downs, M.F., Smith, J.C., Carson, J., Brown, A., McAnulty, S.R. and McAnulty, L.S. (2004) Influence of carbohydrate ingestion on immune changes after 2 h of intensive resistance training. *Journal of Applied Physiology* 96: 1292–8.

Nieman, D. C., Dumke, C. L., Henson, D. A., McAnulty, S. R., Gross, S. J. and Lind, R. H. (2005a) Muscle damage is linked to cytokine changes following a 160-km race. *Brain, Behavior and Immunity* 19: 398–403.

Nieman, D. C., Henson, D. A., Austin, M. D. and Brown, V. A. (2005b) Immune response to a 30-minute walk. *Medicine and Science in Sports and Exercise* 37: 57–62.

Nieman, D. C., Henson, D. A., Dumke, C. L., Lind, R. H., Shooter, L. R. and Gross, S. J. (2006) Relationship between salivary IgA secretion and upper respiratory tract infection following a 160-km race. *Journal of Sports Medicine and Physical Fitness* 46: 158–62.

Nieman, D. C., Henson, D. A., Gross, S. J., Jenkins, D. P., Davis, J. M., Murphy, E. A., Carmichael, M. D., Dumke, C. L., Utter, A. C., McAnulty, S. R., McAnulty, L. S. and Mayer, E. P. (2007) Quercetin reduces illness but not immune perturbations after intensive exercise. *Medicine and Science in Sports and Exercise* 39: 1561–9.

Nieman, D. C., Henson, D. A., McMahon, M., Wrieden, J. L., Davis, J. M., Murphy, E. A.,

Gross, S. J., McAnulty, L. S. and Dumke, C. L. (2008) Beta-glucan, immune function, and upper respiratory tract infections in athletes. *Medicine and Science in Sports and Exercise* 40: 1463–71.

Nieman, D. C., Henson, D. A., Maxwell, K. R., Williams, A. S., McAnulty, S. R., Jin, F., Shanely, R. A. and Lines, T. C. (2009a) Effects of quercetin and EGCG on mitochondrial biogenesis and immunity. *Medicine and Science in Sports and Exercise* 41: 1467–1475.

Nieman, D. C., Henson, D. A., McAnulty, S. R., Jin, F. and Maxwell, K. R. (2009b) n-3 polyunsaturated fatty acids do not alter immune and inflammation measures in endurance athletes. *International Journal of Sport Nutrition and Exercise Metabolism* 19: 536–46.

Nieman, D. C., Henson, D. A., Austin, M. D. and Sha, W. (2011a) Upper respiratory tract infection is reduced in physically fit and active adults. *British Journal of Sports Medicine* 45: 987–92.

Nieman, D. C., Konrad, M., Henson, D. A., Kennerly, K., Shanely, R. A. and Wallner-Liebmann, S. J. (2011b) Variance in the acute inflammatory response to prolonged cycling is linked to exercise intensity. *Journal of Interferon and Cytokine Research* 32: 12–17.

Niess, A. M., Fehrenbach, E., Strobel, G., Roecker, K., Schneider, E. M., Buergler, J., Fuss, S., Lehmann, R., Northoff, H. and Dickhuth, H. H. (2003) Evaluation of stress responses to interval training at low and moderate altitudes. *Medicine and Science in Sports and Exercise* 35: 263–9.

Noakes, T. D. (1992) *Lore of Running* (2nd ed.). Cape Town: Oxford University Press.

Northoff, H. and Berg, A. (1991) Immunologic mediators as parameters of the reaction to strenuous exercise. *International Journal of Sports Medicine* 12(Suppl 1): S9–15.

Northoff, H., Weinstock, C. and Berg, A. (1994) The cytokine response to strenuous exercise. *International Journal of Sports Medicine* 15(Suppl 3): S167–71.

Northoff, H., Berg, A. and Weinstock, C. (1998) Similarities and differences of the immune response to exercise and trauma: the IFN-gamma concept. *Canadian Journal of Physiology and Pharmacology* 76: 497–504.

Northoff, H., Synon, S., Zieker, D., Schaible, E., Schaefer, K., Thoma, S., Loeffler, M., Abbasi, A., Simon, P., Niess, A. M. and Fehrenbach, E. (2008) Gender- and menstrual-phase dependent regulation of inflammatory gene expression in response to aerobic exercise. *Exercise Immunology Review* 14: 86–103.

Novas, A. M., Rowbottom, D. G. and Jenkins, D. G. (2003) Tennis, incidence of URTI and salivary IgA. *International Journal of Sports Medicine* 24: 223–9.

Nuckton, T. J., Claman, D. M., Goldreich, D., Wendt, F. C. and Nuckton, J. G. (2000) Hypothermia and afterdrop following open water swimming: the Alcatraz/San Francisco Swim Study. *American Journal of Emergency Medicine* 18: 703–7.

Nybo, L., Nielsen, B., Pedersen, B. K., Møller, K. and Secher, N. H. (2002) Interleukin-6 release from the human brain during prolonged exercise. *Journal of Physiology* 542: 991–5.

O'Brien, K., Nixon, S., Tynan, A. M. and Glazier, R. (2010) Aerobic exercise interventions for adults living with HIV/AIDS. *Cochrane Database of Systematic Reviews* 4: CD001796.

O'Connell, E. J. (2004) The burden of atopy and asthma in children. *Allergy* 59 (Suppl 78): 7–11.

Oertelt-Prigione, S. (2012) The influence of sex and gender on the immune response. *Autoimmunity Reviews* 11: A479–85.

Ogata, K., An, E., Shioi, Y., Nakamura, K., Luo, S., Yokose, N., Minami, S. and Dan, K. (2001) Association between natural killer cell activity and infection in immunologically normal elderly people. *Clinical Experimental Immunology* 124: 392–7.

Okutsu, M., Ishii, K., Niu, K. J. and Nagatomi, R. (2005) Cortisol-induced CXCR4 augmentation mobilizes T lymphocytes after acute physical stress. *American Journal of Physiology – Regulatory, Integrative and Comparative Physiology* 288: R591–9.

Okutsu, M., Suzuki, K., Ishijima, T., Peake, J. and Higuchi, M. (2008) The effects of acute exercise-induced cortisol on CCR2 expression on human monocytes. *Brain, Behavior and Immunity* 22: 1066–71.

Oliveira, M. and Gleeson, M. (2010) The influence of prolonged cycling on monocyte Toll-like receptor 2 and 4 expression in healthy men. *European Journal of Applied Physiology* 109: 251–7.

Oliver, S. J., Laing, S. J., Wilson, S., Bilzon, J. L., Walters, R. and Walsh, N. P. (2007) Salivary immunoglobulin A response at rest and after exercise following a 48 h period of fluid and/or energy restriction. *British Journal of Nutrition* 97: 1109–16.

Oliver, S. J., Gallagher, C. A., Di Felice, U., Harper Smith, A. D., Macdonald, J. H. and Walsh, N. P. (2011) High-altitude impairs the induction phase of an in vivo T-cell-mediated immune response in humans. In: ISEI, *Proceedings of the 10th International Society of Exercise Immunology Symposium, Exercise and Immunity in Athletic Performance and a Healthy Life, St Catherine's College, University of Oxford, July 11th–13th, 2011.* Abstract p. 54, p. 79. Available online at www.isei.dk/index.php?pageid=21

Oliver, S. J., Sanders, S. J., Williams, C. J., Smith, Z. A., Lloyd-Davies, E., Roberts, R., Arthur, C., Hardy, L. and Macdonald, J. H. (2012) Physiological and psychological illness symptoms at high altitude and their relationship with acute mountain sickness: a prospective cohort study. *Journal of Travel Medicine* 19: 210–19.

Ortega, E. (2003) Neuroendocrine mediators in the modulation of phagocytosis by exercise: physiological implications. *Exercise Immunology Review* 9: 70–93.

Ortega, E., Barriga, C. and de la Fuente, M. (1993a) Study of the phagocytic process in neutrophils from elite sportswomen. *European Journal of Applied Physiology* 66: 37–42.

Ortega, E., Collazos, M. E., Maynar, M., Barriga, C. and de la Fuente, M. (1993b) Stimulation of the phagocytic function of neutrophils in sedentary men after acute moderate exercise. *European Journal of Applied Physiology* 66: 60–4.

Ortega, E., Rodriguez, M. J., Barriga, C. and Forner, M. A. (1996) Corticosterone, prolactin and thyroid hormones as hormonal mediators of the stimulated phagocytic capacity of peritoneal macrophages after high-intensity exercise. *International Journal of Sports Medicine* 17: 149–55.

Ortega, E., Forner, M. A. and Barriga, C. (1997) Exercise-induced stimulation of murine macrophage chemotaxis: role of corticosterone and prolactin as mediators. *Journal of Physiology* 498: 729–34.

Ostrowski, K., Hermann, C., Bangash, A., Schjerling, P., Nielsen, J. N. and Pedersen, B. K. (1998a) A trauma-like elevation of plasma cytokines in humans in response to treadmill running. *Journal of Physiology* 513: 889–94.

Ostrowski, K., Rohde, T., Zacho, M., Asp, S. and Pedersen, B. K. (1998b) Evidence that interleukin-6 is produced in human skeletal muscle during prolonged running. *Journal of Physiology* 508: 949–53.

Ostrowski, K., Rohde, T., Asp, S., Schjerling, P. and Pedersen, B. K. (1999) Pro- and anti-inflammatory cytokine balance in strenuous exercise in humans. *Journal of Physiology* 515: 287–91.

Ostrowski, K., Rohde, T., Asp, S., Schjerling, P. and Pedersen, B. K. (2001) Chemokines are elevated in plasma after strenuous exercise in humans. *European Journal of Applied Physiology* 84: 244–5.

Ouchi, N., Parker, J. L., Lugus, J. J. and Walsk, K. (2011) Adipokines in inflammation and metabolic disease. *Nature Reviews Immunology* 11: 85–97.

Overbeck, S., Rink, L. and Haase, H. (2008) Modulating the immune response by oral zinc supplementation: a single approach for multiple diseases. *Archivum Immunologiae et Therapia Experimentalis (Warszaw)* 56: 15–30.

Park, M. M., Hornback, N. B., Endres, S. and Dinarello, C. A. (1990) The effect of whole body hyperthermia on the immune cell activity of cancer patients. *Lymphokine Research* 9: 213–23.

Parker, A. J., Hamlin, G. P., Coleman, C. J. and Fitzpatrick, L. A. (2003) Dehydration in stressed ruminants may be the result of a cortisol-induced diuresis. *Journal of Animal Science* 81: 512–19.

Parry-Billings, M., Blomstrand, E., McAndrew, N. and Newsholme, E. A. (1990) A communicational link between skeletal muscle, brain, and cells of the immune system. *International Journal of Sports Medicine* 11: S122–8.

Parry-Billings, M., Budgett, R., Koutedakis, Y., Blomstrand, E., Brooks, S., Williams, C., Calder, P. C., Pilling, S., Baigrie, R. and Newsholme, E. A. (1992) Plasma amino acid concentrations in the overtraining syndrome: possible effects on the immune system. *Medicine and Science in Sports and Exercise* 24: 1353–8.

Paulson, T., Goosey-Tolfrey, V., Lenton, J., Leicht, C. and Bishop, N. C. (2013) Spinal cord injury level and the circulating cytokine response to strenuous exercise. *Medicine and Science in Sports and Exercise* published online 11 March. DOI: 10.1249/MSS.06013e31828f9666

Peake, J., Wilson, G., Hordern, M., Suzuki, K., Yamaya, K., Nosaka, K., Mackinnon, L. and Coombes, J. S. (2004) Changes in neutrophil surface receptor expression, degranulation, and respiratory burst activity after moderate- and high-intensity exercise. *Journal of Applied Physiology* 97: 612–18.

Peake, J. M. (2002) Exercise-induced alterations in neutrophil degranulation and respiratory burst activity: possible mechanisms of action. *Exercise Immunology Review* 8: 49–100.

Pedersen, B. K. (1991) Influence of physical activity on the cellular immune system: mechanisms of action. *International Journal of Sports Medicine* 12: S23–9.

Pedersen, B. K. (2009) Edward F. Adolph distinguished lecture: muscle as an endocrine organ: IL-6 and other myokines. *Journal of Applied Physiology* 107: 1006–14.

Pedersen, B. K. and Bruunsgaard, H. (1995) How physical exercise influences the establishment of infections. *Sports Medicine* 19: 393–400.

Pedersen, B. . and Febbraio, M. A. (2008) Muscle as an endocrine organ: focus on muscle-derived interleukin-6. *Physiological Review* 88: 1379–406.

Pedersen, B. K. and Fischer, C. P. (2007) Beneficial health effects of exercise: the role of IL-6 as a myokine. *Trends in Pharmacological Science* 28: 152–6.

Pedersen, B. K. and Hoffman-Goetz, L. (2000) Exercise and the immune system: regulation, integration, and adaptation. *Physiological Review* 80: 1055–81.

Pedersen, B. K. and Saltin, B. (2006) Evidence for prescribing exercise as therapy in chronic disease. *Scandinavian Journal of Medicine and Science in Sports* 16(Suppl 1): 5–65.

Pedersen, B. K. and Ullum, H. (1994) NK cell response to physical activity; possible mechanisms of action. *Medicine and Science in Sports and Exercise* 26: 104–46.

Pedersen, B. K., Tvede, N., Hansen, F. R., Andersen, V., Bendix, T., Bendixen, G., Bendtzen,

K., Galbo, H., Haahr, P. M., Klarlund, K., Sylvest, J., Thomsen, B. and Halkjaer-Kristensen, J. (1988) Modulation of natural killer cell activity in peripheral blood by physical exercise. *Scandinavian Journal of Immunology* 26: 673–8.

Pedersen, B. K., Tvede, N., Christensen, L. D., Klarlund, K., Kragbak, S. and Halkjaer-Kristensen, J. (1989) Natural killer cell activity in peripheral blood of highly trained and untrained persons. *International Journal of Sports Medicine* 10: 129–31.

Pedersen, B. K., Tvede, N., Klarlund, K., Christensen, L. D., Hansen, F. R., Galbo, H., Kharazmi, A. and Halkjaer-Kristensen, J. (1990) Indomethacin in vitro and in vivo abolishes post-exercise suppression of natural killer cell activity in peripheral blood. *International Journal of Sports Medicine* 11: 127–31.

Pedersen, B. K., Ostrowski, K., Rohde, T. and Bruunsgaard, H. (1998) The cytokine response to strenuous exercise. *Canadian Journal of Physiology and Pharmacology* 76: 505–11.

Pedersen, B. K., Helge, J. W., Richter, E. A., Rohde, T. and Kiens, B. (2000) Training and natural immunity: effects of diets rich in fat or carbohydrate. *European Journal of Applied Physiology* 82: 98–102.

Pedersen, B. K., Steensberg, A., Fischer, C., Keller, C., Ostrowski, K. and Schjerling, P. (2001) Exercise and cytokines with particular focus on muscle-derived IL-6. *Exercise Immunology Review* 7: 18–31.

Pedersen, B. K., Steensberg, A., Keller, P., Keller, C., Fischer, C., Hiscock, N., van Hall, G., Plomgaard, P. and Febbraio, M. A. (2003) Muscle-derived interleukin-6: lipolytic, anti-inflammatory and immune regulatory effects. *Pflugers Archives* 446: 9–16.

Pennell, L. M., Galligan, C. L. and Fish, E. N. (2012) Sex affects immunity. *Journal of Autoimmunity* 38: J282–91.

Peralbo, E., Alonso, C. and Solana, R. (2007) Invariant NKT and NKT-like lymphocytes: two different T cell subsets that are differentially affected by ageing. *Experimental Gerontology* 42: 703–8.

Perna, F. M., LaPerriere, A., Klimas, N., Ironson, G., Perry, A., Pavone, J., Goldstein, A., Majors, P., Makemson, D., Talutto, C., Schneiderman, N., Fletcher, M. A., Meijer, O. G. and Koppes, L. (1999) Cardiopulmonary and CD4 cell changes in response to exercise training in early symptomatic HIV infection. *Medicine and Science in Sports and Exercise* 31: 973–9.

Peters, C., Lotzerich, H., Niemeier, B., Schule, K. and Uhlenbruck, G. (1994) Influence of a moderate exercise training on natural killer cytotoxicity and personality traits in cancer patients. *Anticancer Research* 14: 1033–6.

Peters, E. M. and Bateman, E. D. (1983) Ultramarathon running and upper respiratory tract infections. An epidemiological survey. *South African Medical Journal* 64: 582–4.

Peters, E. M., Goetzsche, J. M., Grobbelaar, B. and Noakes, T. D. (1993) Vitamin C supplementation reduces the incidence of postrace symptoms of upper-respiratory-tract infection in ultramarathon runners. *American Journal of Clinical Nutrition* 57: 170–4.

Peters, E. M., Goetzsche, J. M., Joseph, L. E. and Noakes, T. D. (1996) Vitamin C as effective as combinations of anti-oxidant nutrients in reducing symptoms of upper respiratory tract infections in ultramarathon runners. *South African Journal of Sports Medicine* 11: 23–7.

Petersen, A. M. and Pedersen, B. K. (2005) The anti-inflammatory effect of exercise. *Journal of Applied Physiology* 98: 1154–62.

Phillips, T., Childs, A. C., Dreon, D. M., Phinney, S. and Leeuwenburgh, C. (2003) A dietary supplement attenuates IL-6 and CRP after eccentric exercise in untrained males. *Medicine and Science in Sports and Exercise* 35: 2032–7.

Pierson, D. L., Stowe, R. P., Phillips, T. M., Lugg, D. J. and Mehta, S. K. (2005) Epstein-Barr virus shedding by astronauts during space flight. *Brain, Behavior and Immunity* 19: 235–42.

Pischon, T., Boeing, H., Hoffmann, K., Bergmann, M., Schulze, M. B., Overvad, K., van der Schouw, Y. T., Spencer, E., Moons, K. G., Tjønneland, A., Halkjaer, J., Jensen, M. K., Stegger, J., Clavel-Chapelon, F., Boutron-Ruault, M. C., Chajes, V., Linseisen, J., Kaaks, R., Trichopoulou, A., Trichopoulos, D., Bamia, C., Sieri, S., Palli, D., Tumino, R., Vineis, P., Panico, S., Peeters, P. H., May, A. M., Bueno-de-Mesquita, H. B., van Duijnhoven, F. J., Hallmans, G., Weinehall, L., Manjer, J., Hedblad, B., Lund, E., Agudo, A., Arriola, L., Barricarte, A., Navarro, C., Martinez, C., Quirós, J. R., Key, T., Bingham, S., Khaw, K. T., Boffetta, P., Jenab, M., Ferrari, P. and Riboli, E. (2008) General and abdominal adiposity and risk of death in Europe. *New England Journal of Medicine* 359: 2105–20.

Poli, A., Michel, T., Theresine, M., Andres, E., Hentges, F. and Zimmer, J. (2009) CD56bright natural killer (NK) cells: an important NK cell subset. *Immunology* 126: 458–65.

Poole, J. G., Lawrenson, L., Kim, J., Brown, C. and Richardson, R. S. (2003) Vascular and metabolic response to cycle exercise in sedentary humans: effect of age. *American Journal of Physiology – Heart and Circulatory Physiology* 284: H1251–9.

Potteiger, J. A., Chan, M. A., Haff, G. G., Mathew, S., Schroeder, C. A., Haub, M. D., Chirathaworn, C., Tibbetts, S. A., McDonald, J., Omoike, O. and Benedict, S. H. (2001) Training status influences T-cell responses in women following acute resistance exercise. *Journal of Strength and Conditioning Research* 15: 185–91.

Powers, S., Nelson, W. B. and Larson-Meyer, E. (2011) Antioxidant and vitamin D supplements for athletes: sense or nonsense? *Journal of Sports Sciences* 29: S47–S55.

Powers, S. K., DeRuisseau, K. C., Quindry, J. and Hamilton, K. L. (2004) Dietary antioxidants and exercise. *Journal of Sports Sciences* 22: 81–94.

Pradhan, A. D., Manson, J. E., Rifai, N., Buring, J. E. and Ridker, P. M. (2001) C-reactive protein, interleukin 6, and risk of developing type 2 diabetes mellitus. *Journal of the American Medical Association* 286: 327–34.

Prasad, A. S. (2009) Zinc: role in immunity, oxidative stress and chronic inflammation. *Current Opinion in Clinical Nutrition and Metabolic Care* 12: 646–52.

Prieto, A., Knight, A., Compton, C., Gleeson, M. and Travers, P. J. (2013) Premature immune senescence in elite athletes. *Journal of Immunology* (in press).

Proctor, G. B. and Carpenter, G. H. (2007) Regulation of salivary gland function by autonomic nerves. *Autonomic Neuroscience* 133: 3–18.

Proctor, G. B., Garrett, J. R., Carpenter, G. H. and Ebersole, L. E. (2003) Salivary secretion of immunoglobulin A by submandibular glands in response to autonomimetic infusions in anaesthetised rats. *Journal of Neuroimmunology* 136: 17–24.

Provinciali, M., Moresi, R., Donnini, A. and Lisa, R. M. (2009) Reference values for CD4+ and CD8+ T lymphocytes with naive or memory phenotype and their association with mortality in the elderly. *Gerontology* 55: 314–21.

Pugh, L. G. (1967) Cold stress and muscular exercise, with special reference to accidental hypothermia. *British Medical Journal* 2: 333–7.

Pugh, L. G., Corbett, J. L. and Johnson, R. H. (1967) Rectal temperatures, weight losses, and sweat rates in marathon running. *Journal of Applied Physiology* 23: 347–52.

Pyne, D., McDonald, W. A., Morton, D. S., Swigget, J. P., Foster, M., Sonnenfeld, G. and Smith, J. A. (2000) Inhibition of interferon, cytokine, and lymphocyte proliferative responses in elite swimmers with altitude exposure. *Journal of Interferon and Cytokine Research* 20: 411–18.

Pyne, D. B. (1994) Regulation of neutrophil function during exercise. *Sports Medicine* 17: 245–58.

Pyne, D. B. and Gleeson, M. (1998) Effects of intensive exercise training on immunity in athletes. *International Journal of Sports Medicine.* 19(Suppl 3): S183–91.

Pyne, D. B., Baker, M. S., Fricker, P. A., McDonald, W. A., Telford, R. D. and Weidemann, M. J. (1995) Effects of an intensive 12-wk training program by elite swimmers on neutrophil oxidative activity. *Medicine and Science in Sports and Exercise* 27: 536–42.

Pyne, D. B., Baker, M. S., Smith, J. A. and Telford, R. D. (1996) Exercise and the neutrophil oxidative burst: biological and experimental variability. *European Journal of Applied Physiology* 74: 564–71.

Pyne, D. B., McDonald, W. A., Gleeson, M., Flanagan, A., Clancy, R. L. and Fricker, P. A. (2000) Mucosal immunity, respiratory illness and competitive performance in elite swimmers. *Medicine and Science in Sports and Exercise* 33: 348–53.

Quadrilatero, J. and Hoffman-Goetz, L. (2004) N-Acetyl-L-cysteine prevents exercise–induced intestinal lymphocyte apoptosis by maintaining intracellular glutathione levels and reducing mitochondrial membrane depolarization. *Biochemical and Biophysical Research Communications* 319: 894–901.

Radogna, F., Diederich, M. and Ghibelli, L. (2010) Melatonin: a pleiotropic molecule regulating inflammation. *Biochemical Pharmacology* 80: 1844–52.

Radom-Aizik, S., Zaldivar, F. Jr, Leu, S. Y., Adams, G. R., Oliver, S. and Cooper, D. M. (2012) Effects of exercise on microRNA expression in young males peripheral blood mononuclear cells. *Clinical and Translational Science* 5: 32–8.

Rae, D. E., Knobel, G. J., Mann, T., Swart, J., Tucker, R. and Noakes, T. D. (2008) Heatstroke during endurance exercise: is there evidence for excessive endothermy? *Medicine and Science in Sports and Exercise* 40: 1193–204.

Raison, C. L., Capuron, L. and Miller, A. H. (2006) Cytokines sing the blues: inflammation and the pathogenesis of depression. *Trends in Immunology* 27: 24–31.

Rajan, K. B., Wetmore, C. M., Potter, J. D. and Ulrich, C. M. (2006) Moderate-intensity exercise reduces the incidence of colds among postmenopausal women. *American Journal of Medicine* 119: 937–42.

Rama, L., Teixeira, A. M., Matos, A., Borges, G., Henriques, A., Gleeson, M., Pedreiro, S., Filaire, E., Alves, F. and Paiva, A. (2013) Changes in natural killer cell subpopulations over a winter training season in elite swimmers. *European Journal of Applied Physiology* 113: 859–68.

Raso, V., Benard, G., Da Silva Duarte, A. J. and Natale, V. M. (2007) Effect of resistance training on immunological parameters of healthy elderly women. *Medicine and Science in Sports and Exercise* 39: 2152–9.

Rav-Acha, M., Hadad, E., Epstein, Y., Heled, Y. and Moran, D. S. (2004) Fatal exertional heat stroke: a case series. *American Journal of Medical Sciences* 328: 84–7.

Raven, P. B., Drinkwater, B. L., Ruhling, R. O., Bolduan, N., Taguchi, S., Gliner, J. and Horvath, S. M. (1974) Effect of carbon monoxide and peroxyacetyl nitrate on man's maximal aerobic capacity. *Journal of Applied Physiology* 36: 288–93.

Rebelo, A. N., Candeias, J. R., Fraga, M. M., Duarte, J. A., Soares, J. M., Magalhaes, C. and Torrinha, J. A. (1998) The impact of soccer training on the immune system. *Journal of Sports Medicine and Physical Fitness* 38: 258–61.

Reid, V. L., Gleeson, M., Williams, N. and Clancy, R. L. (2004) Clinical investigation of athletes with persistent fatigue and/or recurrent infections. *British Journal of Sports Medicine* 38: 42–5.

Rennie, M. J., Edwards, R. H., Krywawych, S., Davies, C. T., Halliday, D., Waterlow, J. C. and Millward, D. J. (1981) Effect of exercise on protein turnover in man. *Clinical Science (London)* 61: 627–39.

Rhind, S. G., Gannon, G. A., Shek, P. N., Brenner, I. K., Severs, Y., Zamecnik, J., Buguet, A., Natale, V. M., Shephard, R. J. and Radomski, M. W. (1999) Contribution of exertional hyperthermia to sympathoadrenal-mediated lymphocyte subset redistribution. *Journal of Applied Physiology* 87: 1178–85.

Rhind, S. G., Gannon, G. A., Shephard, R. J., Buguet, A., Shek, P. N. and Radomski, M. W. (2004) Cytokine induction during exertional hyperthermia is abolished by core temperature clamping: neuroendocrine regulatory mechanisms. *International Journal of Hyperthermia* 20: 503–16.

Rigsby, L. W., Dishman, R. K., Jackson, A. W., Maclean, G. S., Raven, P. B. (1992) Effects of training on men seropositive for the human immunodeficiency virus-1. *Medicine and Science in Sports and Exercise* 24: 6–12.

Ristow, M., Zarse, K., Oberbach, A., Kloting, N., Birringer, M., Kiehntopf, M., Stumvoll, M., Kahn, C. R. and Bluher, M. (2009) Antioxidants prevent health-promoting effects of physical exercise in humans. *Proceedings of the National Academy of Sciences* 106: 8665–70.

Rivier, A., Pene, J., Chanez, P., Anselme, F., Caillaud, C., Prefaut, C., Godard, P. and Bousquet, J. (1994) Release of cytokines by blood monocytes during strenuous exercise. *International Journal of Sports Medicine* 15: 192–8.

Roberts, C., Pyne, D. B. and Horn, P. L. (2004) CD94 expression and natural killer cell activity after acute exercise. *Journal of Science and Medicine in Sport* 7: 237–47.

Roberts, N. J. and Sandberg, K. (1979) Hyperthermia and human leukocyte function. II. Enhanced production of and response to leukocyte migration inhibition factor (LIF). *Journal of Immunology* 122: 1990–3.

Roberts, W. O. (1989) Exercise-associated collapse in endurance events: A classification system. *Physician Sportsmedicine* 17: 49–55.

Robson, P. J. (2003) Elucidating the unexplained underperformance syndrome: the cytokine hypothesis revisited. *Sports Medicine* 33: 771–81.

Robson, P. J., Blannin, A. K., Walsh, N. P., Bishop, N. C. and Gleeson, M. (1999a) The effect of an acute period of intense interval training on human neutrophil function and plasma glutamine in endurance-trained male runners. *Journal of Physiology* 515P: 84–5.

Robson, P. J., Blannin, A. K., Walsh, N. P., Castell, L. M. and Gleeson, M. (1999b) Effects of exercise intensity, duration and recovery on in vitro neutrophil function in male athletes. *International Journal of Sports Medicine* 20: 128–35.

Robson-Ansley, P. and Toit, G. D. (2010) Pathophysiology, diagnosis and management of exercise-induced anaphylaxis. *Current Opinion in Allergy and Clinical Immunology* 10: 312–17.

Robson-Ansley, P., Barwood, M., Canavan, J., Hack, S., Eglin, C., Davey, S., Hewitt, J., Hull, J. and Ansley, L. (2009) The effect of repeated endurance exercise on IL-6 and sIL-6R and their relationship with sensations of fatigue at rest. *Cytokine* 45: 111–16.

Robson-Ansley, P., Howatson, G., Tallent, J., Mitcheson, K., Walshe, I., Toms, C., Du Toit, G., Smith, M. and Ansley, L. (2012) Prevalence of allergy and upper respiratory tract symptoms in runners of the London Marathon. *Medicine and Science in Sports and Exercise* 44: 999–1004.

Robson-Ansley, P. J., de Milander, L., Collins, M. and Noakes, T. D. (2004) Acute interleukin-6 administration impairs athletic performance in healthy, trained male runners. *Canadian Journal of Applied Physiology* 29: 411–18.

Robson-Ansley, P. J., Blannin, A. and Gleeson, M. (2007) Elevated plasma interleukin-6 levels in trained male triathletes following and acute period of intense interval training. *European Journal of Applied Physiology* 99:353–60.

Rodriguez, A. B., Barriga, C. and De la Fuente, M. (1991) Phagocytic function of blood neutrophils in sedentary young people after physical exercise. *International Journal of Sports Medicine* 12: 276–80.

Rodriguez, N. R., Di Marco, N. M. and Langley, S. (2009) American College of Sports Medicine position stand. Nutrition and athletic performance. *Medicine and Science in Sports and Exercise* 41: 709–31.

Rohde, T., Ullum, H., Rasmussen, J. P., Kristensen, J. H., Newsholme, E. and Pedersen, B. K. (1995) Effects of glutamine on the immune system: influence of muscular exercise and HIV infection. *Journal of Applied Physiology* 79: 146–50.

Rohde, T., MacLean, D. A. and Pedersen, B. K. (1998) Effect of glutamine supplementation on changes in the immune system induced by repeated exercise. *Medicine and Science in Sports and Exercise* 30: 856–62.

Ronsen, O. (2005) Prevention and management of respiratory tract infections in athletes. *New Studies in Athletics* 20: 49–56.

Ronsen, O., Haug, E., Pedersen, B. K. and Bahr, R. (2001a) Increased neuroendocrine response to a repeated bout of endurance exercise. *Medicine and Science in Sports and Exercise* 33: 568–75.

Ronsen, O., Pedersen, B. K., Oritsland, T. R., Bahr, R. and Kjeldsen-Kragh, J. (2001b) Leukocyte counts and lymphocyte responsiveness associated with repeated bouts of strenuous endurance exercise. *Journal of Applied Physiology* 91: 425–34.

Rose-John, S., Scheller, J., Elson, G. and Jones, S. A. (2006) IL-6 biology is co-ordinated by membrane bound and soluble receptors: role in inflammation and cancer. *Journal of Leukocyte Biology* 80: 27–36.

Rosenthal, L. A., Taub, D. D., Moors, M. A. and Blank, K. J. (1992) Methylxanthine-induced inhibition of the antigen- and superantigen-specific activation of T and B lymphocytes. *Immunopharmacology and Immunology* 24: 203–17.

Ross, A. C., Manson, J. E., Abrams, S. A., Aloia, J. F., Brannon, P. M., Clinton, S. K., Durazo-Arvizu, R. A., Gallagher, J. C., Gallo, R. L., Jones, G., Kovacs, C. S., Mayne, S. T., Rosen, C. J. and Shapses, S. A. (2011) The 2011 report on dietary reference intakes for calcium and vitamin D from the Institute of Medicine: what clinicians need to know. *Journal of Clinical Endocrinology Metabolism* 96: 53–8.

Ross, R. and Bradshaw, A. J. (2009) The future of obesity reduction: beyond weight loss. *Nature Reviews Endocrinology* 5: 319–25.

Rossen, R. D., Butler, W. T., Waldman, R. H., Alford, R. H., Hornick, R. B., Togo, Y. and Kasel, J. A. (1970) The proteins in nasal secretion. II. A longitudinal study of IgA and neutralizing antibody levels in nasal washings from men infected with influenza virus. *Journal of the American Medical Association* 211: 1157–61.

Rowbottom, D. G., Keast, D., Goodman, C. and Morton, A. R. (1995) The haematological, biochemical and immunological profile of athletes suffering from the Overtraining

Syndrome. *European Journal of Applied Physiology* 70: 502–9.

Roxas, M. and Jurenka, J. (2007) Colds and influenza: a review of diagnosis and conventional, botanical, and nutritional considerations. *Alternative Medicine Review* 12: 25–48.

Rueda, R. (2007) The role of dietary gangliosides on immunity and the prevention of infection. *British Journal of Nutrition* 98: S68–S73.

Rushall, B. S. (1990) A tool for measuring stress tolerance in elite athletes. *Journal of Applied Sports Psychology* 2: 51–66.

Sacheck, J. M., Milbury, P. E., Cannon, J. G., Roubenoff, R. and Blumberg, J. B. (2003) Effect of vitamin E and eccentric exercise on selected biomarkers of oxidative stress in young and elderly men. *Free Radical Biology & Medicine* 34: 1575–88.

Sackstein, R. (2005) The lymphocyte homing receptors: gatekeepers of the multistep paradigm. *Current Opinion in Hematology* 12: 444–50.

Sakaguchi, S. (2005) Naturally arising Foxp3-expressing CD25+CD4+ regulatory T cells in immunological tolerance to self and non-self. *Nature Immunology* 6: 345–52.

Sallusto, F., Lenig, D., Forster, R., Lipp, M. and Lanzavecchia, A. (1999) Two subsets of memory T lymphocytes with distinct homing potentials and effector functions. *Nature* 401: 708–12.

Sallusto, F., Geginat, J. and Lanzavecchia, A. (2004) Central memory and effector memory T cell subsets: function, generation, and maintenance. *Annual Review Immunology* 22: 745–63.

Sarnquist, F. H. (1983) Physicians on Mount Everest. A clinical account of the 1981 American medical research expedition to Everest. *Western Journal of Medicine* 139: 480–5.

Savendahl, L. and Underwood, L. E. (1997) Decreased interleukin-2 production from cultured peripheral blood mononuclear cells in human acute starvation. *Journal of Clinical Endocrinology and Metabolism* 82: 1177–80.

Schedlowski, M., Jacobs, R., Stratmann, G., Richter, S., Hadicke, A., Tewes, U., Wagner, T. O. and Schmidt, R. E. (1993) Changes of natural killer cells during acute psychological stress. *Journal of Clinical Immunology* 13: 119–26.

Schedlowski, M., Hosch, W., Oberbeck, R., Benschop, R. J., Jacobs, R., Raab, H. R. and Schmidt, R. E. (1996) Catecholamines modulate human NK cell circulation and function via spleen-independent beta 2-adrenergic mechanisms. *Journal of Immunology* 156: 93–9.

Schelegle, E. S. and Adams, W. C. (1986) Reduced exercise time in competitive simulations consequent to low level ozone exposure. *Medicine and Science in Sports and Exercise* 18: 408–14.

Schlitt, A., Heine, G. H., Blankenberg, S., Espinola-Klein, C., Dopheide, J. F., Bickel, C., Lackner, K. J., Iz, M., Meyer, J., Darius, H. and Rupprecht, H. J. (2004) CD14+CD16+ monocytes in coronary artery disease and their relationship to serum TNF-alpha levels. *Journal of Thrombosis and Haemostasis* 92: 419–24.

Schouten, W. J., Verschuur, R. and Kemper H. C. G. (1988) Physical activity and upper respiratory tract infections in a normal population of young men and women: the Amsterdam Growth and Health Study. *International Journal of Sports Medicine* 9: 451–5.

Schwellnus, M., Kiessig, M., Dermam, W. and Noakes, T. D. (1997) Fusafungine reduced symptoms of upper respiratory tract infections (URTI) in runners after a 56 km race. *Medicine and Science in Sports and Exercise* 29: S296.

Scrimshaw, N. S. and SanGiovanni, J. P. (1997) Synergism of nutrition, infection and immunity: an overview. *American Journal of Clinical Nutrition* 66: 464S–77S.

Segerstrom, S. C. and Miller, G. E. (2004) Psychological stress and the human immune system: a meta-analytic study of 30 years of inquiry. *Psychological Bulletin* 130: 601–30.

Selkirk, G. A., McLellan, T. M., Wright, H. E. and Rhind, S. G. (2008) Mild endotoxemia, NF-kappaB translocation, and cytokine increase during exertional heat stress in trained and untrained individuals. *American Journal of Physiology – Regulatory, Integrative and Comparative Physiology* 295: R611–23.

Seltzer, J., Bigby, B. G., Stulbarg, M., Holtzman, M. J., Nadel, J. A., Ueki, I. F., Leikauf, G. D., Goetzl, E. J. and Boushey, H. A. (1986) O3-induced change in bronchial reactivity to methacholine and airway inflammation in humans. *Journal of Applied Physiology* 60: 1321–6.

Semple, S. J., Smith, L. L. and McKune, A. J. (2004) Alterations in acute phase reactants (CRP, rheumatoid factor, complement, Factor B, and immune complexes) following an ultramarathon. *South African Journal of Sports Medicine* 16: 17–21.

Semple, S. J., Smith, L. L., McKune, A. J., Hoyos, J., Mokgethwa, B., San Juan, A. F., Lucia, A. and Wadee, A. A. (2006) Serum concentrations of C reactive protein, alpha1 antitrypsin, and complement (C3, C4, C1 esterase inhibitor) before and during the Vuelta a Espana? *British Journal of Sports Medicine* 40: 124–7.

Severs, Y., Brenner, I., Shek, P. N. and Shephard, R. J. (1996) Effects of heat and intermittent exercise on leukocyte and sub-population cell counts. *European Journal of Applied Physiology and Occupational Physiology* 74: 234–45.

Shaw, A. C., Joshi, S., Greenwood, H., Panda, A. and Lord, J. M. (2010) Aging of the innate immune system. *Current Opinion in Immunology* 22: 507–13.

Shaw, A. C., Panda, A., Joshi, S. R., Qian, F., Allore, H. G. and Montgomery, R. R. (2011) Dysregulation of human Toll-like receptor function in aging. *Ageing Research Review* 10: 346–53.

Shek, P. N., Sabiston, B. H., Buguet, A. and Radomski, M. W. (1995) Strenuous exercise and immunological changes: a multiple-time-point analysis of leukocyte subsets CD4/CD8 ratio, immunoglobulin production and NK cell response. *International Journal of Sports Medicine* 16: 466–74.

Shephard, R. J. (1997) *Physical Activity, Training and the Immune Response*. Carmel, IN: Cooper.

Shephard, R. J. (1998) Immune changes induced by exercise in an adverse environment. *Canadian Journal of Physiology and Pharmacology* 76: 539–46.

Shephard, R. J. (2001) Sepsis and mechanisms of inflammatory response: is exercise a good model? *British Journal of Sports Medicine* 35: 223–30.

Shephard, R. J. (2003) Adhesion molecules, catecholamines and leucocyte redistribution during and following exercise. *Sports Medicine* 33: 261–84.

Shephard, R. J. and Shek, P. N. (1999a) Effects of exercise and training on natural killer cell counts and cytolytic activity: a meta-analysis. *Sports Medicine* 28: 177–95.

Shephard, R. J. and Shek, P. N. (1999b) Immune dysfunction as a factor in heat illness. *Critical Review Immunology* 19: 285–302.

Shephard, R. J., Rhind, S. and Shek, P. N. (1994) Exercise and the immune system. Natural killer cells, interleukins and related responses. *Sports Medicine* 18: 340–69.

Shimizu, K., Kimura, F., Akimoto, T., Akama, T., Tanabe, K., Nishijima, T., Kuno, S. and Kono, I. (2008) Effect of moderate exercise training on T-helper cell subpopulations in elderly people. *Exercise Immunology Review* 14: 24–37.

Shimizu, K., Suzuki, N., Imai, T., Aizawa, K., Nanba, H., Hanaoka, Y., Kuno, S., Mesaki, N., Kono, I. and Akama, T. (2011) Monocyte and T-cell responses to exercise training in elderly subjects. *Journal of Strength and Conditioning Research* 25: 2565–72.

Shinkai, S., Kohno, H., Kimura, K., Komura, T., Asai, H., Inai, R., Oka, K., Kurokawa, Y. and Shephard, R. (1995) Physical activity and immune senescence in men. *Medicine and Science in Sports and Exercise* 27: 1516–26.

Simonson, S. R. and Jackson, C. G. (2004) Leukocytosis occurs in response to resistance exercise in men. *Journal of Strength and Conditioning Research* 18: 266–71.

Simpson, A. and Custovic, A. (2005) Pets and the development of allergic sensitization. *Current Allergy and Asthma Reports* 5: 212–20.

Simpson, R. J. (2011) Aging, persistent viral infections, and immunosenescence: can exercise 'make space'? *Exercise and Sport Sciences Reviews* 39: 23–33.

Simpson, R. J. and Guy, K. (2010) Coupling aging immunity with a sedentary lifestyle: has the damage already been done? A mini-review. *Gerontology* 56: 449–58.

Simpson, R. J., Florida-James, G. D., Whyte, G. P. and Guy, K. (2006a) The effects of intensive, moderate and downhill treadmill running on human blood lymphocytes expressing the adhesion/activation molecules CD54 (ICAM–1), CD18 (beta2 integrin) and CD53. *European Journal of Applied Physiology* 97: 109–21.

Simpson, R. J., Guy, K., Whyte, G. P., Middleton, N., Black, J. R., Ross, J. A., Shave, R. and Florida-James, G. D. (2006b) Lymphocyte phenotype alterations, pro-inflammatory cytokines and acute phase proteins following repeated bouts of mountainous hill-running. *Medicine and Science in Sports and Exercise* 38: S412–13.

Simpson, R. J., Florida-James, G. D., Cosgrove, C., Whyte, G. P., Macrae, S., Pircher, H. and Guy, K. (2007a) High-intensity exercise elicits the mobilization of senescent T lymphocytes into the peripheral blood compartment in human subjects. *Journal of Applied Physiology* 103: 396–401.

Simpson, R. J., Florida-James, G. D., Whyte, G. P., Black, J. R., Ross, J. A. and Guy, K. (2007b) Apoptosis does not contribute to the blood lymphocytopenia observed after intensive and downhill treadmill running in humans. *Research in Sports Medicine* 15: 157–74.

Simpson, R. J., Cosgrove, C., Ingram, L. A., Florida-James, G. D., Whyte, G. P., Pircher, H. and Guy, K. (2008) Senescent T-lymphocytes are mobilised into the peripheral blood compartment in young and older humans after exhaustive exercise. *Brain, Behavior and Immunity* 22: 544–51.

Simpson, R. J., McFarlin, B. K., McSporran, C., Spielmann, G., ó Hartaigh, B. and Guy, K. (2009) Toll-like receptor expression on classic and pro-inflammatory blood monocytes after acute exercise in humans. *Brain, Behavior and Immunity* 23: 232–9.

Simpson, R. J., Cosgrove, C., Chee, M. M., McFarlin, B. K., Bartlett, D. B., Spielmann, G., O'Connor, D. P., Pircher, H. and Shiels, P. G. (2010) Senescent phenotypes and telomere lengths of peripheral blood T-cells mobilized by acute exercise in humans. *Exercise Immunology Review* 16: 36–51.

Simpson, R. J., Lowder, T. W., Spielmann, G., Bigley, A. B., Lavoy, E. C. and Kunz, H. (2012) Exercise and the aging immune system. *Ageing Research Review* 11: 404–20.

Singh, A., Failla, M. L. and Deuster, P. A. (1994) Exercise-induced changes in immune function: effects of zinc supplementation. *Journal of Applied Physiology* 76: 2298–303.

Singh, I., Chohan, I. S., Lal, M., Khanna, P. K., Srivastava, M. C., Nanda, R. B., Lamba, J. S. and Malhotra, M. S. (1977) Effects of high altitude stay on the incidence of common diseases in man. *International Journal of Biometeorology* 21: 93–122.

Sivertsen, B. (2006) Global ambient air pollution concentrations and trends, In: *World Health Organization Air Quality Guidelines: Global Update 2005*, (edited by M. Chan and M. Danzon). Germany: Druckpartner Moser.

Skinner, N. A., MacIsaac, C. M., Hamilton, J. A. and Visvanathan, K. (2005) Regulation of Toll-like receptor (TLR)2 and TLR4 on CD14dimCD16+ monocytes in response to sepsis-related antigens. *Clinical Experimental Immunology* 141: 270–8.

Skrzeczynska-Moncznik, J., Bzowska, M., Loseke, S., Grage-Griebenow, E., Zembala, M. and Pryjma, J. (2008) Peripheral blood CD14high CD16+ monocytes are main producers of IL-10. *Scandinavian Journal of Immunology* 67: 152–9.

Sloan, R. P., Shapiro, P. A., Demeersman, R. E., McKinley, P. S., Tracey, K. J., Slavov, I., Fang, Y. and Flood, P. D. (2007) Aerobic exercise attenuates inducible TNF production in humans. *Journal of Applied Physiology* 103: 1007–11.

Smith, D. J. and Norris, S. R. (2000) Changes in glutamine and glutamate concentrations for tracking training tolerance. *Medicine and Science in Sports and Exercise* 32: 684–9.

Smith, J. A., Telford, R. D., Mason, I. B. and Weidemann, M. J. (1990) Exercise, training and neutrophil microbicidal activity. *International Journal of Sports Medicine* 11: 179–87.

Smith, L. L. (2000) Cytokine hypothesis of overtraining: a physiological adaptation to excessive stress? *Medicine and Science in Sports and Exercise* 32: 317–31.

Smith, L. L. (2003) Overtraining, excessive exercise, and altered immunity. Is this a T Helper-1 versus T Helper-2 lymphocyte response? *Sports Medicine* 33: 347–64.

Smith, L. L. (2004) Tissue trauma: the underlying cause of overtraining syndrome? *Journal of Strength and Conditioning Research* 18: 185–93.

Smith, R. (2005) Investigating the previous studies of a fraudulent author. *British Medical Journal* 331: 288–91.

Soppi, E., Varjo, P., Eskola, J. and Laitinen, L. A. (1982) Effect of strenuous physical stress on circulating lymphocyte number and function before and after training. *Journal of Clinical Laboratory Immunology* 8: 43–6.

Souza, P. M., Jacob-Filho, W., Santarém, J. M., Silva, A. R., Li, H. Y. and Burattini, M. N. (2008) Progressive resistance training in elderly HIV-positive patients: does it work? *Clinics* 63: 619–24.

Spence, L., Brown, W. J., Pyne, D. B., Nissen, M. D., Sloots, T. P., McCormack, J. G., Locke, A. S. and Fricker, P. A. (2007) Incidence, etiology, and symptomatology of upper respiratory illness in elite athletes. *Medicine and Science in Sports and Exercise* 39: 577–86.

Spielmann, G., McFarlin, B. K., O'Connor, D. P., Smith, P. J., Pircher, H. and Simpson, R. J. (2011) Aerobic fitness is associated with lower proportions of senescent blood T-cells in man. *Brain, Behavior and Immunity* 25: 1521–9.

Starkie, R., Ostrowski, S. R., Jauffred, S., Febbraio, M. and Pedersen, B. K. (2003) Exercise and IL-6 infusion inhibit endotoxin-induced TNF-alpha production in humans. *FASEB Journal* 17: 884–6.

Starkie, R. L., Angus, D. J., Rolland, J., Hargreaves, M. and Febbraio, M. A. (2000) Effect of prolonged, submaximal exercise and carbohydrate ingestion on monocyte intracellular cytokine production in humans. *Journal of Physiology* 528: 647–55.

Starkie, R. L., Rolland, J., Angus, D. J., Anderson, M. J. and Febbraio, M. A. (2001a) Circulating monocytes are not the source of elevations in plasma IL-6 and TNF-alpha levels after prolonged running. *American Journal of Physiology – Cell Physiology* 280: C769–74.

Starkie, R. L., Arkinstall, M. J., Koukoulas, I., Hawley, J. A. and Febbraio, M. A. (2001b) Carbohydrate ingestion attenuates the increase in plasma interleukin-6, but not skeletal muscle interleukin-6 mRNA, during exercise in humans. *Journal of Physiology* 533: 585–91.

Starkie, R. L., Rolland, J. and Febbraio, M. A. (2001c) Effect of adrenergic blockade on lymphocyte cytokine production at rest and during exercise. *American Journal of Physiology – Cell Physiology* 281: C1233–40.

Steensberg, A. (2003) The role of IL-6 in exercise-induced immune changes and metabolism. *Exercise Immunology Review* 9: 40–7.

Steensberg, A., van Hall, G., Osada, T., Sacchetti, M., Saltin, B. and Pedersen, B. K. (2000) Production of interleukin-6 in contracting human skeletal muscles can account for the exercise-induced increase in plasma interleukin-6. *Journal of Physiology* 529: 237–42.

Steensberg, A., Febbraio, M. A., Osada, T., Schjerling, P., van Hall, G., Saltin, B. and Pedersen, B. K. (2001a) Interleukin-6 production in contracting human skeletal muscle is influenced by pre-exercise muscle glycogen content. *Journal of Physiology* 537: 633–9.

Steensberg, A., Toft, A. D., Bruunsgaard, H., Sandmand, M., Halkjaer-Kristensen, J. and Pedersen, B. K. (2001b) Strenuous exercise decreases the percentage of type 1 T cells in the circulation. *Journal of Applied Physiology* 91: 1708–12.

Steensberg, A., Morrow, J., Toft, A. D., Bruunsgaard, H. and Pedersen, B. K. (2002) Prolonged exercise, lymphocyte apoptosis and F2-isoprostanes. *European Journal of Applied Physiology* 87: 38–42.

Steensberg, A., Fischer, C. P., Keller, C., Moller, K. and Pedersen, B. K. (2003) IL-6 enhances plasma IL-1ra, IL-10, and cortisol in humans. *American Journal of Physiology – Endocrinology and Metabolism* 285: E433–7.

Stenvinkel, P., Ketteler, M., Johnson, R. J., Lindholm, B., Pecoits-Filho, R., Riella, M., Heimbürger, O., Cederholm, T. and Girndt, M. (2005) IL-10, IL-6, and TNF-alpha: central factors in the altered cytokine network of uremia: the good, the bad, and the ugly. *Kidney International* 67: 1216–33.

Steppich, B., Dayyani, F., Gruber, R., Lorenz, R., Mack, M. and Ziegler-Heitbrock, H.W. (2000) Selective mobilization of CD14(+)CD16(+) monocytes by exercise. *American Journal of Physiology – Cell Physiology* 279: C578–86.

Steptoe, A., Hamer, M. and Chida, Y. (2007) The effects of acute psychological stress on circulating inflammatory factors in humans: a review and meta-analysis. *Brain Behavior and Immunity* 21: 901–12.

Stewart, L. K., Flynn, M. G., Campbell, W. W., Craig, B. A., Robinson, J. P., McFarlin, B. K., Timmerman, K. L., Coen, P. M., Felker, J. and Talbert, E. (2005) Influence of exercise training and age on CD14+ cell surface expression of toll-like receptor 2 and 4. *Brain, Behavior and Immunity* 19: 389–97.

Stowe, R. P., Pierson, D. L., Feeback, D. L. and Barrett, A. D. (2000) Stress-induced reactivation of Epstein-Barr virus in astronauts. *Neuroimmunomodulation* 8: 51–8.

Stowe, R. P., Mehta, S. K., Ferrando, A. A., Feeback, D. L. and Pierson, D. L. (2001) Immune responses and latent herpesvirus reactivation in spaceflight. *Aviation, Space, and Environmental Medicine* 72: 884–91.

Stowe, R. P., Sams, C. F. and Pierson, D. L. (2011) Adrenocortical and immune responses following short- and long-duration spaceflight. *Aviation, Space, and Environmental Medicine* 82: 627–34.

Stowe, R. P., Sams, C. F. and Pierson, D. L. (2003) Effects of mission duration on neuroimmune responses in astronauts. *Aviation, Space, and Environmental Medicine* 74: 1281–4.

Strachan, D. P. (2000) Family size, infection and atopy: the first decade of the 'hygiene hypothesis'. *Thorax* 55(Suppl 1): S2–S10.

Stray-Gundersen, J. and Levine, B. D. (2008) Live high, train low at natural altitude. *Scandinavian Journal of Medicine and Science in Sports* 18: 21–8.

Strazdins, L., Meyerkort, S., Brent, V., D'Souza, R. M., Broom, D. H. and Kyd, J. M. (2005) Impact of saliva collection methods on SIgA and cortisol assays and acceptability to participants. *Journal of Immunology Methods* 307: 167–71.

Stringer, W. W., Berezovskaya, M., O'Brien, W. A., Beck, C. K. and Casaburi, R. (1998) The effect of exercise training on aerobic fitness, immune indices, and quality of life in HIV+ patients. *Medicine and Science in Sports and Exercise* 30: 11–16.

Suchanek, O., Podrazil, M., Fischerova, B., Bocinska, H., Budinsky, V., Stejskal, D., Spisek, R., Bartunkova, J. and Kolar, P. (2010) Intensive physical activity increases peripheral blood dendritic cells. *Cellular Immunology* 266: 40–5.

Sugiura, H., Nishida, H., Sugiura, H. and Mirbod, S. M. (2002) Immunomodulatory action of chronic exercise on macrophage and lymphocyte cytokine production in mice. *Acta Physiologica Scandinavica* 174: 247–56.

Sulowska, Z. and Lewicki, R. (1994) Immunological status of competitive cyclists before and after the training season. *International Journal of Sports Medicine* 15: 319–24.

Sun, J. C. and Lanier, L. L. (2011) NK cell development, homeostasis and function: parallels with CD8(+) T cells. *Nature Reviews Immunology* 11: 645–57.

Sunyer, J., Jarvis, D., Pekkanen, J., Chinn, S., Janson, C., Leynaert, B., Luczynska, C., Garcia-Esteban, R., Burney, P. and Anto, J. M. (2004) Geographic variations in the effect of atopy on asthma in the European Community Respiratory Health Study. *Journal of Allergy and Clinical Immunology* 114: 1033–9.

Suzui, M., Kawai, T., Kimura, H., Takeda, K., Yagita, H., Okumura, K., Shek, P. N. and Shephard, R. J. (2004) Natural killer cell lytic activity and CD56(dim) and CD56(bright) cell distributions during and after intensive training. *Journal of Applied Physiology* 96: 2167–73.

Suzuki, K., Naganuma, S., Totsuka, M., Suzuki, K. J., Mochizuki, M., Shiraishi, M., Nakaji, S. and Sugawara, K. (1996) Effects of exhaustive endurance exercise and its one-week daily repetition on neutrophil count and functional status in untrained men. *International Journal of Sports Medicine* 17: 205–12.

Suzuki, K., Totsuka, M., Nakaji, S., Yamada, M., Kudoh, S., Liu, Q., Sugawara, K., Yamaya, K. and Sato, K. (1999) Endurance exercise causes interaction among stress hormones, cytokines, neutrophil dynamics, and muscle damage. *Journal of Applied Physiology* 87: 1360–7.

Suzuki, K., Nakaji, S., Yamada, M., Totsuka, M., Sato, K. and Sugawara, K. (2002) Systemic inflammatory response to exhaustive exercise. Cytokine kinetics. *Exercise Immunology Review* 8: 6–48.

Suzuki, K., Nakaji, S., Yamada, M., Liu, Q., Kurakake, S., Okamura, N., Kumae, T., Umeda, T. and Sugawara, K. (2003) Impact of a competitive marathon race on systemic cytokine and neutrophil responses. *Medicine and Science in Sports and Exercise* 35: 348–55.

Takashi, I., Umeda, T. Mashiko, T., Chinda, D., Oyama, T., Sugawara, K., Nakaji, S. (2007) Effects of rugby sevens matches on human neutrophil-related non-specific immunity. *British Journal of Sports Medicine* 41: 13–18.

Takeda, K., Kaisho, T. and Akira, S. S. (2003) Toll-like receptors. *Annual Review of Immunology* 21: 335–76.

Tam, M., Gomez, S., Gonzalez-Gross, M. and Marcos, A. (2003) Possible roles of magnesium on the immune system. *European Journal of Clinical Nutrition* 57: 1193–7.

Tanasescu, M., Leitzmann, M. F., Rimm, E. B., Willett, W. C., Stampfer, M. J. and Hu, F. B. (2002) Exercise type and intensity in relation to coronary heart disease in men. *Journal of the American Medical Association* 288: 1994–2000.

Taylor, G. R. (1974) Space microbiology. *Annual Review Microbiology* 28: 121–37.

Taylor, G. R. (1993) Immune changes during short-duration missions. *Journal of Leukocyte Biology* 54: 202–8.

Taylor, G. R. and Dardano, J. R. (1983) Human cellular immune responsiveness following space flight. *Aviation, Space, and Environmental Medicine* 54: S55–9.

Taylor, G. R. and Janney, R. P. (1992) In vivo testing confirms a blunting of the human cell-mediated immune mechanism during space flight. *Journal of Leukocyte Biology* 51: 129–32.

Taylor, G. R., Neale, L. S. and Dardano, J. R. (1986) Immunological analyses of U.S. Space Shuttle crewmembers. *Aviation, Space, and Environmental Medicine* 57: 213–17.

Thalacker-Mercer, A. E., Dell'Italia, L. J., Cui, X., Cross, J. M., Bamman, M. M. (2010) Differential genomic responses in old vs. young humans despite similar levels of modest muscle damage after resistance loading. *Physiological Genomics* 40: 141–9.

Thies, F., Nebe-von-Caron, G., Powell, J. R., Yaqoob, P., Newsholme, E. A. and Calder, P. C. (2001) Dietary supplementation with eicosapentaenoic acid, but not with other long-chain n-3 or n-6 polyunsaturated fatty acids, decreases natural killer cell activity in healthy subjects aged >55 y. *American Journal of Clinical Nutrition* 73: 539–48.

Tidball, J. G. (2002) Interactions between muscle and the immune system during modified musculoskeletal loading. *Clinical Orthopaedics and Related Research* 403(Suppl): S100–9.

Timmerman, K. L., Flynn, M. G., Coen, P. M., Markofski, M. M. and Pence, B. D. (2008) Exercise training-induced lowering of inflammatory (CD14+CD16+) monocytes: a role in the anti-inflammatory influence of exercise? *Journal of Leukocyte Biology* 84: 1271–8.

Timmons, B. W. and Cieslak, T. (2008) Human natural killer cell subsets and acute exercise: a brief review. *Exercise Immunology Review* 14: 8–23.

Timmons, B. W., Hamadeh, M. J., Devries, M. C. and Tarnopolsky, M. A. (2005) Influence of gender, menstrual phase and oral contraceptive use on immunological responses to prolonged cycling. *Journal of Applied Physiology* 99: 979–85.

Timmons, B. W., Tarnopolsky, M. A. and Bar-Or, O. (2006) Sex-based effects on the distribution of NK cell subsets in response to exercise and carbohydrate intake in adolescents. *Journal of Applied Physiology* 100: 1513–19.

Tintinger, G. R., Theron, A. J., Anderson, R. and Ker, J. A. (2001) The anti-inflammatory interactions of epinephrine with human neutrophils in vitro are achieved by cyclic AMP-mediated accelerated resequestration of cytosolic calcium. *Biochemical Pharmacology* 61: 1319–28.

Tiollier, E., Gomez-Merino, D., Burnat, P., Jouanin, J. C., Bourrilhon, C., Filaire, E., Guezennec, C. Y. and Chennaoui, M. (2005a) Intense training: mucosal immunity and incidence of respiratory infections. *European Journal of Applied Physiology* 93: 421–8.

Tiollier, E., Schmitt, L., Burnat, P., Fouillot, J. P., Robach, P., Filaire, E., Guezennec, C. and Richalet, J. P. (2005b) Living high-training low altitude training: effects on mucosal immunity. *European Journal of Applied Physiology* 94: 298–304.

Tiollier, E., Chennaoui, M., Gomez-Merino, D., Drogou, C., Filaire, E. and Guezennec, C. Y. (2007) Effect of a probiotics supplementation on respiratory infections and immune and hormonal parameters during intense military training. *Military Medicine* 172: 1006–11.

Tomasi, T. B., Trudeau, F. B., Czerwinski, D. and Erredge, S. (1982) Immune parameters in athletes before and after strenuous exercise. *Journal of Clinical Immunology* 2: 173–8.

Tonnesen, E., Christensen, N. J. and Brinklov, M. M. (1987) Natural killer cell activity during cortisol and adrenaline infusion in healthy volunteers. *European Journal of Clinical Investigation* 17: 497–503.

Tuomilehto, J., Lindstrom, J., Eriksson, J. G., Valle, T. T., Hamalainen, H., Ilanne-Parikka, P., Keinanen-Kiukaanniemi, S., Laakso, M., Louheranta, A., Rastas, M., Salminen, V. and Uusitupa, M. (2001) Prevention of type 2 diabetes mellitus by changes in lifestyle among subjects with impaired glucose tolerance. *New England Journal of Medicine* 344: 1343–50.

Turner, J. E., Aldred, S., Witard, O. C., Drayson, M. T., Moss, P. M. and Bosch, J. A. (2010) Latent cytomegalovirus infection amplifies CD8 T-lymphocyte mobilisation and egress in response to exercise. *Brain, Behavior and Immunity* 24: 1362–70.

Turner, J. E., Bosch, J. A. and Aldred, S. (2011) Measurement of exercise-induced oxidative stress in lymphocytes. *Biochemical Society Transactions* 39: 1299–304.

Tvede, N., Heilmann, C., Halkjaer-Kristensen, J. and Pedersen, B. K. (1989) Mechanisms of B-lymphocyte suppression induced by acute physical exercise. *Journal of Clinical Laboratory Immunology* 30: 169–73.

Tvede, N., Kappel, M., Halkjaer-Kristensen, J., Galbo, H. and Pedersen, B. K. (1993) The effect of light, moderate and severe bicycle exercise on lymphocyte subsets, natural and lymphokine activated killer cells, lymphocyte proliferative response and interleukin 2 production. *International Journal of Sports Medicine* 14: 275–82.

Tvede, N., Kappel, M., Klarlund, K., Duhn, S., Halkjaer-Kristensen, J., Kjaer, M., Galbo, H. and Pedersen, B. K. (1994) Evidence that the effect of bicycle exercise on blood mononuclear cell proliferative responses and subsets is mediated by epinephrine. *International Journal of Sports Medicine* 15: 100–4.

Ueta, M., Furusawa, K., Takahashi, M., Akatsu, Y., Nakamura, T. and Tajima, F. (2008) Attenuation of natural killer cell activity during 2-h exercise in individuals with spinal cord injuries. *Spinal Cord* 46: 26–32.

Ullum, H., Haahr, P. M., Diamant, M., Palmø, J., Halkjaer-Kristensen, J. and Pedersen, B. K. (1994a) Bicycle exercise enhances plasma IL-6 but does not change IL-1 alpha, IL-1 beta, IL-6, or TNF-alpha pre-mRNA in BMNC. *Journal of Applied Physiology* 77: 93–7.

Ullum, H., Palmø, J., Halkjaer-Kristensen, J., Diamant, M., Klokker, M., Kruuse, A., LaPerriere, A., Pedersen, B. K. (1994b) The effect of acute exercise on lymphocyte subsets, natural killer cells, proliferative responses and cytokines in HIV-seropositive persons. *Journal of Acquired Immune Deficiency Syndromes* 7: 1122–33.

van Eeden, S. F., Granton, J., Hards, J. M., Moore, B. and Hogg, J. C. (1999) Expression of the cell adhesion molecules on leukocytes that demarginate during acute maximal exercise. *Journal of Applied Physiology* 86: 970–6.

van Hall, G., Steensberg, A., Sacchetti, M., Fischer, C., Keller, C., Schjerling, P., Hiscock, N., Møller, K., Saltin, B., Febbraio, M. A. and Pedersen, B. K. (2003) Interleukin-6 stimulates lipolysis and fat oxidation in humans. *Journal of Clinical Endocrinology and Metabolism* 88: 3005–10.

Verde, T., Thomas, S. and Shephard, R. J. (1992) Potential markers of heavy training in highly trained endurance runners. *British Journal of Sports Medicine* 26: 167–75.

Veverka, D. V., Wilson, C., Martinez, M. A., Wenger, R. and Tamosuinas, A. (2009) Use of zinc supplements to reduce upper respiratory infections in United States Air Force Academy cadets. *Complementary Therapies in Clinical Practice* 15: 91–5.

Viana, J. L., Smith, A. C., Kosmadakis, G., Bevington, A., Clapp, E. L., Feehally, J. and

Bishop, N. C. (2011) Antigen-stimulated monocyte and T-lymphocyte activation and systemic inflammatory cytokine concentration in chronic kidney disease: effect of regular moderate intensity aerobic exercise. In: International Society of Exercise Immunology, *Proceedings of the 10th ISEI Symposium, St Catherine's College, University of Oxford, July 11th–13th, 2011*. Abstract O.9, p.23.

Vider, J., Lehtmaa, J., Kullisaar, T., Vihalemm, T., Zilmer, K., Kairane, C., Landor, A., Karu, T. and Zilmer, M. (2001) Acute immune response in respect to exercise-induced oxidative stress. *Pathophysiology* 7: 263–70.

Vieira, R. D., Toledo, A. C., Silva, L. B., Almeida, F. M., Damaceno-Rodrigues, N. R., Caldini, E. G., Santos, A. B., Rivero, D. H., Hizume, D. C., Lopes, F. D., Olivo, C. R., Castro-Faria-Neto, H. C., Martins, M. A., Saldiva, P. H. and Dolhnikoff, M. (2012) Anti-inflammatory effects of aerobic exercise in mice exposed to air pollution. *Medicine and Science in Sports and Exercise* 44: 1227–34.

Vieira, V. J., Valentine, R. J., Wilund, K. R., Antao, N., Baynard, T. and Woods, J. A. (2009a) Effects of exercise and low-fat diet on adipose tissue inflammation and metabolic complications in obese mice. *American Journal of Physiology – Endocrinology and Metabolism* 296: E1164–71.

Vieira, V. J., Valentine, R. J., Wilund, K. R. and Woods, J. A. (2009b) Effects of diet and exercise on metabolic disturbances in high-fat diet-fed mice. *Cytokine* 46: 339–45.

Volman, J. J., Ramakers, J. D. and Plat, J. (2008) Dietary modulation of immune function by beta-glucans. *Physiology and Behavior* 94: 276–84.

Voss, E. W. (1984) Prolonged weightlessness and humoral immunity. *Science* 225: 214–15.

WADA (2013) List of Prohibited Substances and Methods. Montreal: World Anti Doping Agency. Available online at http://list.wada-ama.org

Wahle, M., Stachetzki, U., Krause, A., Pierer, M., Hantzschel, H. and Baerwald, C. G. (2001) Regulation of beta2-adrenergic receptors on CD4 and CD8 positive lymphocytes by cytokines in vitro. *Cytokine* 16: 205–9.

Walburn, J., Vedhara, K., Hankins, M., Rixon, L. and Weinman, J. (2009) Psychological stress and wound healing in humans: a systematic review and meta-analysis. *Journal of Psychosomatic Research* 67: 253–71.

Walker, G. J., Caudwell, P., Dixon, N. and Bishop, N. C. (2006) The effect of caffeine ingestion on neutrophil oxidative burst responses following prolonged cycling. *International Journal of Sport Nutrition and Exercise Metabolism* 16: 24–35.

Wallenius, V., Wallenius, K., Ahren, B., Rudling, M., Carlsten, H., Dickson, S. L., Ohlsson, C. and Jansson, J. O. (2002) Interleukin-6-deficient mice develop mature-onset obesity. *Nature Medicine* 8: 75–9.

Walrand, S., Moreau, K., Caldefie, F., Tridon, A., Chassagne, J., Portefaix, G., Cynober, L., Beaufrere, B., Vasson, M. P. and Boirie, Y. (2001) Specific and nonspecific immune responses to fasting and refeeding differ in healthy young adult and elderly persons. *American Journal of Clinical Nutrition* 74: 670–8.

Walsh, N. P. and Whitham, M. (2006) Exercising in environmental extremes: a greater threat to immune function? *Sports Medicine* 36: 941–976.

Walsh, N. P., Blannin, A. K., Clark, A. M., Cook, L., Robson, P. J. and Gleeson, M. (1998a) The effects of high intensity intermittent exercise on the plasma concentration of glutamine and organic acids. *European Journal of Applied Physiology* 77: 434–8.

Walsh, N. P., Blannin, A. K., Robson, P. J. and Gleeson, M. (1998b) Glutamine, exercise and immune function: links and possible mechanisms. *Sports Medicine* 26: 177–91.

Walsh, N. P., Blannin, A. K., Clark, A. M., Cook, L., Robson, P. J. and Gleeson, M. (1999) The effects of high-intensity intermittent exercise on saliva IgA, total protein and alpha-amylase. *Journal of Sports Sciences* 17: 129–34.

Walsh, N. P., Blannin, A. K., Bishop, N. C., Robson, P. J. and Gleeson, M. (2000) Effect of oral glutamine supplementation on human neutrophil lipopolysaccharide-stimulated degranulation following prolonged exercise. *International Journal of Sport Nutrition and Exercise Metabolism* 10: 39–50.

Walsh, N. P., Bishop, N. C., Blackwell, J., Wierzbicki, S. G. and Montague, J. C. (2002) Salivary IgA response to prolonged exercise in a cold environment in trained cyclists. *Medicine and Science in Sports and Exercise* 34: 1632–7.

Walsh, N. P., Laing, S. J., Oliver, S. O., Montague, J. C., Walters, R. and Bilzon, J. L. (2004) Saliva parameters as potential indices of hydration status during acute dehydration. *Medicine and Science in Sports and Exercise* 36: 1535–42.

Walsh, N. P., Gleeson, M., Shephard, R. J., Gleeson, M., Woods, J. A., Bishop, N. C., Fleshner, M., Green, C., Pedersen, B. K., Hoffman-Goetz, L., Rogers, C. J., Northoff, H., Abbasi, A. and Simon, P. (2011a) Position Statement Part one: Immune function and exercise. *Exercise Immunology Review* 17: 6–63.

Walsh, N. P., Gleeson, M., Pyne, D. B., Nieman, D. C., Dhabhar, F. S., Shephard, R. J., Oliver, S. J., Bermon, S. and Kajeniene, A. (2011b) Position Statement Part two: Maintaining immune health. *Exercise Immunology Review* 17: 64–103.

Walshe, I., Robson-Ansley, P., St Clair Gibson, A., Lawrence, C., Thompson, K. G. and Ansley, L. (2010) The reliability of the IL-6, sIL-6R and sgp130 response to a preloaded time trial. *European Journal of Applied Physiology* 110: 619–25.

Wang, J., Song, H., Tang, X., Yang, Y., Niu, Y. and Ma, Y. (2012) Effect of exercise training intensity on murine T-regulatory cells and vaccination response. *Scandinavian Journal of Medicine and Science in Sports* 22: 643–52.

Wang, J. S. and Chiu, Y. T. (2009) Systemic hypoxia enhances exercise-mediated bactericidal and subsequent apoptotic responses in human neutrophils. *Journal of Applied Physiology* 107: 1213–22.

Wang, J. S. and Lin, C. T. (2010) Systemic hypoxia promotes lymphocyte apoptosis induced by oxidative stress during moderate exercise. *European Journal of Applied Physiology* 108: 371–82.

Wang, J. S. and Wu, C. K. (2009) Systemic hypoxia affects exercise-mediated antitumor cytotoxicity of natural killer cells. *Journal of Applied Physiology* 107: 1817–24.

Wang, J. S., Chung, Y. and Chow, S. E. (2009) Exercise affects platelet-impeded antitumor cytotoxicity of natural killer cell. *Medicine and Science in Sports and Exercise* 41: 115–22.

Wang, T. D., Wang, Y. H., Huang, T. S., Su, T. C., Pan, S. L. and Chen, S. Y. (2007) Circulating levels of markers of inflammation and endothelial activation are increased in men with chronic spinal cord injury. *Journal of the Formosan Medical Association* 106: 919–28.

Warren, T. Y., Barry, V., Hooker, S. P., Sui, X., Church, T. S. and Blair, S. N. (2010) Sedentary behaviors increase risk of cardiovascular disease mortality in men. *Medicine and Science in Sports and Exercise* 42: 879–85.

Webb, P. (1992) Temperatures of skin, subcutaneous tissue, muscle and core in resting men in cold, comfortable and hot conditions. *European Journal of Applied Physiology and Occupational Physiology* 64: 471–6.

Weidner, T. G., Cranston, T., Schurr, T. and Kaminsky, L. A. (1998) The effect of exercise training on the severity and duration of a viral upper respiratory illness. *Medicine and Science in Sports and Exercise* 30: 1578–83.

Weight, L. M., Alexander, D. and Jacobs, P. (1991) Strenuous exercise: analogous to the acute-phase response? *Clinical Science (London)* 81: 677–83.

Wenisch, C., Narzt, E., Sessler, D. I., Parschalk, B., Lenhardt, R., Kurz, A. and Graninger, W. (1996) Mild intraoperative hypothermia reduces production of reactive oxygen intermediates by polymorphonuclear leukocytes. *Anesthesia and Analgesia* 82: 810–16.

West, N. P., Pyne, D. B, Renshaw, G. and Cripps, A. W. (2006) Antimicrobial peptides and proteins, exercise and innate mucosal immunity. *FEMS Immunology and Medical Microbiology* 48: 293–304.

West, N. P., Pyne, D. B., Peake, J. M. and Cripps, A. W. (2009) Probiotics, immunity and exercise: a review. *Exercise Immunology Review* 15: 107–26.

West, N. P., Pyne, D. B., Kyd, J. M., Renshaw, G. M., Fricker, P. A. and Cripps, A. W. (2010) The effect of exercise on innate mucosal immunity. *British Journal of Sports Medicine* 44: 227–31.

White, R. J. and Averner, M. (2001) Humans in space. *Nature* 409: 1115–18.

Whitham, M., Laing, S. J., Dorrington, M., Walters, R., Dunklin, S., Bland, D., Bilzon, J. L. and Walsh, N. P. (2006) The influence of an arduous military training program on immune function and upper respiratory tract infection incidence. *Military Medicine* 171: 703–9.

Whitmer, R. A., Gustafson, D. R., Barrett-Connor, E., Haan, M. N., Gunderson, E. P., and Yaffe, K. (2008) Central obesity and increased risk of dementia more than three decades later. *Neurology* 71: 1057–64.

Wilder, R. L. (1998) Hormones, pregnancy, and autoimmune diseases. *Annals of the New York Academy of Sciences* 840: 45–50.

William, J. L., Radu, S., Aziz, S. A., Rahim, R. A., Cheah, Y. K., Liwan, A. and Lihan, S. (2004) Prevalence of Staphylococcus aureus carriage by young Malaysian footballers during indoor training. *British Journal of Sports Medicine* 38: 12–14.

Williams, L. A., Ulrich, C. M., Larson, T., Wener, M. H., Wood, B., Campbell, P. T., Potter, J. D., McTiernan, A. and De Roos, A. J. (2009) Proximity to traffic, inflammation, and immune function among women in the Seattle, Washington, area. *Environmental Health Perspectives* 117: 373–8.

Wilson, J. W., Ott, C. M., zu Honer, B. K., Ramamurthy, R., Quick, L., Porwollik, S., Cheng, P., McClelland, M., Tsaprailis, G., Radabaugh, T., Hunt, A., Fernandez, D., Richter, E., Shah, M., Kilcoyne, M., Joshi, L., Nelman-Gonzalez, M., Hing, S., Parra, M., Dumars, P., Norwood, K., Bober, R., Devich, J., Ruggles, A., Goulart, C., Rupert, M., Stodieck, L., Stafford, P., Catella, L., Schurr, M.J., Buchanan, K., Morici, L., McCracken, J., Allen, P., Baker-Coleman, C., Hammond, T., Vogel, J., Nelson, R., Pierson, D. L., Stefanyshyn-Piper, H. M. and Nickerson, C. A. (2007) Space flight alters bacterial gene expression and virulence and reveals a role for global regulator Hfq. *Proceedings of the National Academy of Sciences* U.S.A 104: 16299–304.

Wintergerst, E. S., Maggini, S. and Hornig, D. H. (2007) Contribution of selected vitamins and trace elements to immune function. *Annals of Nutrition and Metabolism* 51: 301–23.

Wolin, K. Y., Yan, Y. and Colditz, G. A. (2011) Physical activity and risk of colon adenoma: a meta-analysis. *British Journal of Cancer* 104: 882–5.

Woods, J. A., Davis, J. M., Mayer, E. P., Ghaffar, A. and Pate, R. R. (1993) Exercise increases inflammatory macrophage antitumor cytotoxicity. *Journal of Applied Physiology* 75: 879–86.

Woods, J. A., Davis, J. M., Mayer, E. P., Ghaffar, A. and Pate, R. R. (1994) Effects of exercise on macrophage activation for antitumor cytotoxicity. *Journal of Applied Physiology* 76: 2177–85.

Woods, J. A., Ceddia, M. A., Kozak, C. and Wolters, B. W. (1997) Effects of exercise on the macrophage MHC II response to inflammation. *International Journal of Sports Medicine* 18: 483–8.

Woods, J. A., Evans, J. K., Wolters, B. W., Ceddia, M. A. and McAuley, E. (1998) Effects of maximal exercise on natural killer (NK) cell cytotoxicity and responsiveness to interferon-alpha in the young and old. *Journals of Gerontology Series A: Biological Sciences and Medical Sciences* 53: B430–7.

Woods, J. A., Ceddia, M. A., Wolters, B. W., Evans, J. K., Lu, Q. and McAuley, E. (1999) Effects of 6 months of moderate aerobic exercise training on immune function in the elderly. *Mechanisms of Ageing and Development* 109: 1–19.

Woods, J. A., Lowder, T. W. and Keylock, K. T. (2002) Can exercise training improve immune function in the aged? *Annals of the New York Academy of Sciences* 959: 117–27.

Woods, J. A., Keylock, K. T., Lowder, T., Vieira, V. J., Zelkovich, W., Dumich, S., Colantuano, K., Lyons, K., Leifheit, K., Cook, M., Chapman-Novakofski, K. and McAuley, E. (2009) Cardiovascular exercise training extends influenza vaccine seroprotection in sedentary older adults: the immune function intervention trial. *Journal of the American Geriatric Society* 57: 2183–91.

Xue, F. and Michels, K. B. (2007) Diabetes, metabolic syndrome, and breast cancer: a review of the current evidence. *American Journal of Clinical Nutrition* 86: 823–35.

Yamanaka, M., Furusawa, K., Sugiyama, H., Goto, M., Kinoshita, T., Kanno, N., Takaoka, K. and Tajima, F. (2010) Impaired immune response to voluntary arm-crank ergometer exercise in patients with cervical spinal cord injury. *Spinal Cord* 48: 734–9.

Yan, H., Kuroiwa, A., Tanaka, H., Shindo, M., Kiyonaga, A., Nagayama, A. (2001) Effect of moderate exercise on immune senescence in men. *European Journal of Applied Physiology* 86: 105–11.

Yeh, S. H., Chuang, H., Lin, L. W., Hsiao, C. Y. and Eng, H. L. (2006) Regular tai chi chuan exercise enhances functional mobility and CD4CD25 regulatory T cells. *British Journal of Sports Medicine* 40: 239–43.

Yeh, S. H., Chuang, H., Lin, L. W., Hsiao, C. Y., Wang, P. W., Liu, R. T. and Yang, K. D. (2009) Regular Tai Chi Chuan exercise improves T cell helper function of patients with type 2 diabetes mellitus with an increase in T-bet transcription factor and IL-12 production. *British Journal of Sports Medicine* 43: 845–50.

Yfanti, C., Akerström, T., Nielsen, S., Nielsen, A. R., Mounier, R., Mortensen, O. H., Lykkesfeldt, J., Rose, A. J., Fischer, C. P. and Pedersen, B. K. (2010) Antioxidant supplementation does not alter endurance training adaptation. *Medicine and Science in Sports and Exercise* 42: 1388–95.

Yoshino, Y., Yamane, A., Suzuki, M. and Nakagawa, Y. (2009) Availability of saliva for the assessment of alterations in the autonomic nervous system caused by physical exercise training. *Archives of Oral Biology* 54: 977–85.

Young, T., Finn, L. and Kim, H. (1997) Nasal obstruction as a risk factor for sleep-disordered breathing. The University of Wisconsin Sleep and Respiratory Research Group. *Journal of Allergy and Clinical Immunology* 99: S757–62.

Yudkin, J. S. (2007) Inflammation, obesity, and the metabolic syndrome. *Hormone and Metabolic Research* 39: 707–9.

Zaldivar, F., Wang-Rodriguez, J., Nemet, D., Schwindt, C., Galassetti, P., Mills, P. J., Wilson, L. D. and Cooper, D. M. (2006) Constitutive pro- and anti-inflammatory cytokine and growth factor response to exercise in leukocytes. *Journal of Applied Physiology* 100: 1124–33.

Zeyda, M., Huber, J., Prager, G. and Stulnig, T. M. (2011) Inflammation correlates with markers of T-cell subsets including regulatory T cells in adipose tissue from obese patients. *Obesity* 19: 743–8.

Zhang, Y., Hu, Y. and Wang, F. (2007) Effects of a 28-day 'living high – training low' on T-lymphocyte subsets in soccer players. *International Journal of Sports Medicine* 28: 354–8.

Zielinski, M. R., Muenchow, M., Wallig, M. A., Horn, P. L. and Woods, J. A. (2004) Exercise delays allogeneic tumor growth and reduces intratumoral inflammation and vascularization. *Journal of Applied Physiology* 96: 2249–56.

Zoppini, G., Targher, G., Zamboni, C., Venturi, C., Cacciatori, V., Moghetti, P. and Muggeo, M. (2006) Effects of moderate–intensity exercise training on plasma biomarkers of inflammation and endothelial dysfunction in older patients with type 2 diabetes. *Nutrition, Metabolism and Cardiovascular Diseases* 16: 543–9.

Index

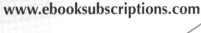
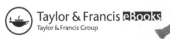